Atlas of X-Ray Diagnosis of Early Gastric Cancer

Atlas of X-Ray Diagnosis of Early Gastric Cancer

Second Edition

Hikoo Shirakabe, M.D.
Mamoru Nishizawa, M.D.
Masakazu Maruyama, M.D.
Shigeo Kobayashi, M.D.

IGAKU-SHOIN Ltd. Tokyo·New York

Published and distributed by
IGAKU-SHOIN Ltd.,
    5-24-3 Hongo, Bunkyo-ku, Tokyo
IGAKU-SHOIN Medical Publishers, Inc.,
    1140 Avenue of the Americas, New York, N.Y. 10036

Library of Congress Cataloging in Publication Data
Main entry under title:

Atlas of X-ray diagnosis of early gastric cancer.

    Includes index.
    1. Stomach — Cancer — Diagnosis. 2. Diagnosis,
Radioscopic. 3. Stomach — Radiography.
I. Shirakabe, Hikoo, 1921-   . [DNLM:
1. Stomach neoplasms — Radiography — Atlases.
WI 17 A881]
RC280.S8A86 1982   616.99′43307572   82-6255
ISBN 0-89640-075-1   AACR2

Printed and bound in Japan.

Preface to the Second Edition

The first edition of this Atlas was published 15 years ago. We believe that this Atlas played an important role in the diagnosis of early gastric cancer, in spite of the fact that the photographs and figures may not have been clear enough to explain our theory, especially in view of the high quality photographs of radiography and endoscopy available at the present time. This may explain why some controversial opinions arose in the book reviews of Western countries concerning the evidence for the diagnosis of early gastric cancer in the cases presented. We have therefore, since shortly after the first edition was published, devoted ourselves to performing our diagnostic methodology and obtaining excellent radiographic details in anticipations of this revision.

In February 1972, we first attempted to revise the first edition, by bringing together a collection of new cases. But this could not be accomplished for many reasons. In November 1977, the second attempt was made with a firm resolution to complete the work of revision. The cases prepared in the first meeting were critically reevaluated. Only those that deserved presentation at that time were selected. Many cases were replaced with newer cases having high quality radiographic details. After five years of preparation, we have accomplished publication of this book.

The diagnosis and the treatment of early gastric cancer have improved extensively in the last 15 years. In fact, we were obliged to rewrite the manuscript whenever new knowledge of each subject was reported. During this time, the composition of the editorial board changed considerably as several members were not able to participate in the publication of this book. Dr. Ichikawa and his colleagues at the National Cancer Center Hospital had taken a leading part in the first meeting held in February 1972, but their inevitable commitment to the tremendous volume of work at their hospital has prevented them from participating in the preparation of this book since the second attempt in 1977. Nevertheless, Dr. Ichikawa, who undertook the arduous task of Director of the National Cancer Center Hospital in 1976, has continually given us innumerable suggestions and encouragement along with a beautiful collection of cases. This book would have never been completed without his generosity and cooperation.

This new edition is characterized not only by the detailed descriptions and pictures of the radiographic diagnosis of early gastric cancer but also by a complete reference to other allied diseases of the stomach, namely malignant lymphoma, peptic ulcer and erosions and miscellaneous tumors, listing as many bibliographies as possible.

Chapter 1 deals with the definition and macroscopic classification of early gastric cancer. Herein are discussed some problems which were raised in Japan and abroad on the validity of the macroscopic classification of early gastric cancer.

Chapter 2 gives a full account of the methodology of double contrast radiography. Chapter 3 discusses the diagnosis of early gastric cancer by radiography, endoscopy and biopsy.

In order to make a positive diagnosis of early gastric cancer using radiographic findings, it is necessary to prove that the lesion is neither an advanced cancer nor another non-malignant lesion. This proof may not be as definitive as that shown by biopsy. However, in its own way, the analysis of the radiographic findings can authenticate the diagnosis of early cancer. In Chapters 4 and 6 basic principles composing the radiographic diagnosis of early cancer are described, followed by an explanation of how a positive diagnosis of early cancer is possible radiographically. In Chapter 5 the concept of atypical epithelium (ATP) or adenoma is discussed and differentiated from elevated early cancer (IIa) radiographically.

The main purpose of this book is to discuss the radiographic diagnosis of early gastric cancer as thoroughly as possible from every viewpoint. However, since most cases of early gastric cancer are macroscopically depressed or ulcerated lesions, and differentiation from benign peptic ulcer and erosions has always been a problem, merely giving a brief description of those benign lesions would be unsatisfactory. Therefore, Chapters 7 and 8 are devoted to the detailed description of peptic ulcers and erosions of the stomach. Not only is this for the purpose of discussing the differential diagnosis of early gastric cancer, but also it enables us to introduce the contributions of Japanese radiography in this field. These two chapters may be useful to readers in countries having a low incidence of gastric cancer.

In Chapter 9 malignant lymphoma and reactive lymphoreticular hyperplasia (pseudolymphoma) are discussed and differentiated from early depressed cancer. In addition, the concept of early malignant lymphoma is proposed with some case presentations.

Chapters 10 through 14 are concerned with selected features associated with the radiographic diagnosis of early gastric cancer. All relevant details are present for an up-to-date account of the radiography of early gastric cancer. In Chapter 15 radiographic details of miscellanous tumors are presented.

Radiologists, who are now being confronted with the high diagnostic yields of endoscopy, may be pessimistic with regard to their diagnostic ability. However, the diagnosis of gastric pathology cannot be done without radiography. The majority of radiologists and endoscopists in Japan have agreed that radiography and endoscopy are complimentary procedures in the diagnosis of gastric pathology, and cooperation between these two modalities is necessary.

This book's intentions are twofold. It serves a source of basic information about the radiographic diagnosis of early gastric cancer and its allied diseases for radiologists in countries having a high incidence of gastric cancer. It also emphasizes a certain uniformity of method and a certain philosophy which form the basis of our diagnostic approach to the radiography of the stomach. For these reasons, this book will provide a reliable guide to all radiologists who are interested in radiography of the stomach.

September, 1981

Hikoo Shirakabe, M.D.

Acknowledgements

I owe a special debt of gratitude to Prof. Kyoichi Nakamura, who has offered professional suggestions and instructions concerning gastric pathology as well as the technical support in preparing the histologic findings of cases presented. I am much indebted to the late Dr. Ryozo Sano, the former chief of the Pathology Department of the National Cancer Center, who kindly offered the microscopic preparations of the cases from the National Cancer Center Hospital and also to Dr. Teruyuki Hirota, the present chief of the Pathology Department of the National Cancer Center, who has kindly offered the microscopic preparations of the recent cases. My sincere gratitude is extended to Mr. Katsumi Takano, the chief of the Photolaboratory of the Cancer Institute Hospital for this technical assistance in reproducing the prints of the radiographic findings. Particular obligation is owed to Mrs. Junko Adachi, who has devoted herself to the completion of this new Atlas, not only as my secretary, but also as the excellent technician of the photolaboratory.

Finally, I should like to express my cordial appreciation for all doctors of my research group, who have been involved in the publication of this new Atlas. Most of them are originally from my research laboratory of the 1st Department of Internal Medicine, Chiba University and the Department of Gastroenterology, Juntendo University. There are also those from other universities, who have participated in my research group, and have shared my method of research in the diagnostic radiography and endoscopy of the stomach. Their names and present affiliations are listed on the following pages.

It is also our pleasant duty to express our cordial appreciation to Dr. William Kadner, Portland, Oregon, who patiently undertook the tremendous effort of copy-editing the manuscripts from our awkward English. If this book brings more than we have intended to express, it is exclusively due to his untiring efforts toward understanding our concepts on the radiographic diagnosis of the stomach and to his brilliant ability in the insight into gastroenterology in Japan.

Hikoo Shirakabe, M.D.

Preface of the First Edition

THE DIAGNOSTIC ROENTGENOLOGY of the stomach, especially for early detection of carcinoma, has been greatly developed by the efforts of R.A. Gutmann (1937 and 1956), R. Prévôt (1937 and 1957), J. Bücker (1941 and 1944), and R. Golden (1948), whose excellent achievements have been a good guide to us and to the roentgenologist. And the achievement done by W. Frik (1965) shown in the recent textbook of Schinz must be also highly appreciated. We have learned much from his descriptions.

In Japan, more than four hundred papers concerning early carcinoma of the stomach have been delivered at medical societies, while about two hundred papers have been issued in Japanese publications.

We have delivered many reports on the roentgenologic and endoscopic diagnosis of mucosal carcinoma, and this book is a compilation of our reports.

Our research group consists of the members of School of Medicine, Chiba University. Although some of them are now playing an active part in other hospitals or institutes, all are making efforts for the early detection of mucosal carcinoma, maintaining a certain uniformity in method and in philosophy of content and taking pride in their work.

We are tremendously indebted to Professor Tadashige Murakami of School of Medicine, Showa University, for his elucidation of the histological aspects of early gastric cancer. But for his great cooperation, our present work could not have been fulfilled. We also wish to express our thanks to the secretary, Miss J. Adachi for her photographic preparations.

1966, Fall

Hikoo Shirakabe, M.D.

Contributors and Collaborators

YASUMASA BABA, M.D.
Department of Internal Medicine, Cancer Institute Hospital, Japanese Foundation for Cancer Research, Tokyo

HIDETAKA DOI, M.D.
Professor and Chairman, Department of Radiology, Gifu University School of Medicine, Gifu

HISAO HAYAKAWA, M.D.
Associate Professor, Department of Gastroenterology, Juntendo University School of Medicine, Tokyo

Late **HIROSHI HORIKOSHI, M.D.**
Former Professor, Department of Radiology, Dokkyo University School of Medicine, Mibu

HEIZABURO ICHIKAWA, M.D.
Director, National Cancer Center Hospital, Tokyo

YUJI ITAI, M.D.
Department of Radiology, Tokyo University School of Medicine, Tokyo

ATUSHI KARIYA, M.D.
Chief, Department of Diagnostic Radiology, Chiba Prefectural Cancer Center, Chiba

SHIGEO KOBAYASHI, M.D.
Department of Gastroenterology, Juntendo University School of Medicine, Tokyo

KENJI KUMAKURA, M.D.
Professor, Department of Diagnostic Radiology, Keio University School of Medicine, Tokyo

MASAKAZU MARUYAMA, M.D.
Department of Internal Medicine, Cancer Institute Hospital, Japanese Foundation for Cancer Research, Tokyo

TOSHIHIDE MARUYAMA, M.D.
Department of Gastroenterology, Juntendo University School of Medicine, Tokyo

HIROTO MATSUE, M.D.
Department of Diagnostic Radiology, National Cancer Center Hospital, Tokyo

TETSUJI NAKAJIMA, M.D.
Chief, Department of Radiology, Toranomon Hospital, Tokyo

TAKESHI NINOMIYA, M.D.
Department of Internal Medicine, Cancer Institute Hospital, Japanese Foundation for Cancer Research, Tokyo

MAMORU NISHIZAWA, M.D.
Director, Tokyo Metropolitan Cancer Detection Center, Tokyo

KAZUO NOMOTO, M.D.
Chief, Department of Gastroenterology, Tokyo Metropolitan Cancer Detection Center, Tokyo

MICHIZO SASAGAWA, M.D.
Department of Diagnostic Radiology, National Cancer Center Hospital, Tokyo

HIKOO SHIRAKABE, M.D.
Professor and Chairman, Department of Gastroenterology, Juntendo University School of Medicine, Tokyo

NORIYOSHI SUGIYAMA, M.D.
Department of Internal Medicine, Cancer Institute Hospital, Japanese Foundation for Cancer Research, Tokyo

YOSHIYUKI TAKEDA, M.D.
Department of Radiology, Kyushu University School of Medicine, Fukuoka

TATSUYA YAMADA, M.D.
Chief, Department of Diagnostic Radiology, National Cancer Center Hospital, Tokyo

TADASHI YARITA, M.D.
Department of Gastroenterology, Juntendo University School of Medicine, Tokyo

Contents

The Origin of the Cases

Abbreviation in parentheses indicates the institution where photographs were prepared. It is followed by the age and sex of each case in this Atlas.

JU: Department of Gastroenterology, Juntendo University School of Medicine, Tokyo

NCCH: National Cancer Center Hospital, Tokyo

TMCDC: Tokyo Metropolitan Cancer Detection Center, Tokyo

CIH: Cancer Institute Hospital, Japanese Foundation for Cancer Research, Tokyo

TH: Toranomon Hospital, Tokyo

CU: First Department of Internal Medicine, Chiba University School of Medicine, Chiba

CPCC: Chiba Prefectural Cancer Center, Chiba

Chapter 1

Definition and Classification of Early Gastric Cancer

Definition

The definition and classification of early gastric cancer were first proposed at the annual meeting of Japan Gastroenterological Endoscopy Society in 1962. Early gastric cancer was defined as cancer in which invasion was limited to the mucosa and submucosa, regardless of the presence of lymph node or distant metastases. In 1963, at the annual meeting of Japanese Research Society for Gastric Cancer, this definition was temporarily modified as "cancer limited to the mucosa and submucosa without metastases". Due to advances in radiographic and endoscopic diagnosis and surgical techniques, both Societies later agreed on the original definition of 1962.

Macroscopic Classification

The macroscopic definition and classification of early gastric cancer (Fig. 1) were proposed on the grounds that, in most cases, the Borrmann's classification of gastric cancer (see page 10) was not applicable to early gastric cancer which is limited to the mucosa and submucosa. It should be stressed that this classification is not an endoscopic one but a macroscopic one. This classification is also applicable to radiographic and endoscopic diagnosis, based on the supposition that a one-to-one correspondence between macroscopic, radiographic and endoscopic findings is possible under ideal conditions.

The macroscopic classification of early gastric cancer consists of three basic types, namely Type I (Protruded Type), Type II (Superficial Type) and Type III (Excavated Type). The Type II cancer is further divided into three subtypes, i.e. Type IIa (Superficial, Depressed Type), Type IIb (Superficial, Flat Type) and Type IIc (Superficial, Depressed Type).

A polypoid early cancer is macroscopically diagnosed as type I if its protrusion into the gastric lumen is over 5 mm and it is diagnosed as type IIa if its protrusion is within 5 mm. Type IIb applies to a lesion with almost unrecognizable elevation or depression from the surrounding normal mucosa. This type was initially employed in the belief that an incipient phase of gastric cancer (Fig. 2) might have taken such a form, although this point had not been substantiated at the time of the classifica-

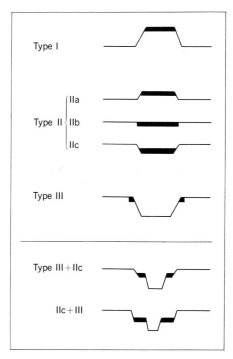

Fig. 1 Macroscopic classification of early gastric cancer proposed by Japan Gastroenterological Endoscopy Society (1962).

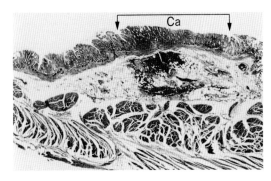

Fig. 2 Cross section of Type IIb microcarcinoma measuring 2 mm in the largest diameter, which was incidentally discovered on the histologic examination of the resected stomach (refer to Chapter 14).

tion's proposal. Recently, however, the type IIb has been understood in a wider sense than the original concept and it has been used in radiographic as well as endoscopic diagnosis as a term indicating a "visible and diagnosable" lesion with the slightest difference in elevation or depression from the neighboring mucosa (cf. chapter 11). This is called "type IIb-simulating" or "type IIb-like lesion". Type IIc applies to a lesion with a slightly depressed surface usually not penetrating the muscularis mucosae. Type III applies to a lesion with a prominent excavation which usually points to an ulceration. Occassionally a type III may not be ulcerated histologically.

When an early cancer reveals different morphologic patterns, two or more types are described together, with the predominant pattern preceding the others, e.g. type IIc + III or type I + IIa.

Some Problems Concerning the Macroscopic Classification of Early Gastric Cancer

More than ten years have passed since the macroscopic classification of early gastric cancer was proposed in Japan. During the first few years after the proposal was made, the classification of the three basic types was unquestionably effective in the overwhelming majority of cases. Consequently, cases in which the macroscopic classification did not apply were simply ignored. When such cases were present, it was sufficient merely to describe the macroscopic peculiarities found in those lesions.

Recently, however, after the years of routine

use, a movement towards redefining this macroscopic classification of early cancer was begun. One reason for this movement was that each hospital in Japan had been reporting extremely variable figures for the incidence of classifiable early gastric cancer. Well aware of the ability of each hospital shown to classify early gastric cancer cases macroscopically, Japanese reseachers had not considered those variable figures to be a target of critisism until Hermanek and Rösch pointed it out in 1973. The classification was brought up for rediscussion in 1976, the fourteenth year after it was instituted (*I to Cho*, vol. 11, No. 1). The second reason is that combined types gradually have been increasing relative to the basic types of early gastric cancer with the accumulation of many cases. Thirdly, macroscopic types of gastric cancer, including basic. types, have been changing their morphology with time. Thus, it is imperative to select the same year's figures reported from the various Japanese hospitals to discover the true incidence of classifiable early gastric cancer. Finally, there is a variable diagnostic ability among hospitals.

Table 1 Rate of agreement in macroscopic diagnosis of early gastric cancer by 14 authorities.

Rate of agreement	No. of cases
More than 91%	12
90 — 80%	15
79 — 70%	19
69 — 60%	11
59 — 50%	21
49 — 40%	13
Less than 39%	9
Total	100 Cases

(From Ichikawa, H. in discussion: *I to Cho*, 11:30-56, 1976)

Table 1 shows the result of macroscopic diagnosis of one hundred cases of early gastric cancer experienced in The National Cancer Center. The diagnosis was made by fourteen experts engaged in the research of early gastric cancer since the establishment of its macroscopic classification. 80 per cent of the experts agreed with classification in 27 cases (27%) demonstrating that about one-third of the cases are classified without any question. But the classification of two-thirds of the cases shows relative variability resulting from individual differences.

At the panel discussion, Ichikawa (1976) summerized the four problems of macroscopic classification of early gastric cancer, and proposed a modified classification (Figs. 3, 4).

Type IIa + IIc, type IIc + IIa (Fig. 3)

Type IIa + IIc is characterized by a central depression located in the type IIa superficial lesion. This original type of IIa + IIc was limited to such polypoid lesions as No. 1 and 2 in Figure 3. A central depression which has grown large enough to have a rectangular configuration like No. 6 of Figure 3 gave impetus to naming such a type IIc + IIa. This proposal has been accepted unanimously. A similar lesion with type IIc central depression causes a problem as in Case 7 (see Fig. 30 in Chapter 2). In this case the predominant lesion is the depression itself, surrounding type IIa elevation resulting from inflammation of the tip of the converging (mucosal) folds. There is one opinion that this type of lesion should originally be classified as type IIc, but another opinion states that it is better classified as type IIc + IIa, for the

depression rather than the elevation is noticeable. A majority opinion is that morphologically the initial state of the lesion is type IIa + IIc, and the apparent macroscopic presence of ulceration assists in adequately describing it as type IIa + IIc (UI). The location of the depression and elevation in the lesions such as Nos. 5, 7 and 8 in Figure 3 is different from the above types. But the same principle of macroscopic classification applies to them all, i.e. they are macroscopically classified as type IIc + IIa or type IIa + IIc with the more noticeable feature preceeding the other, as long as the transition from depression to elevation is smooth. Thus type IIa + IIc and type IIc + IIa are lesions with depression and surrounding elevation. They occur frequently.

Type IIc, type IIc + III, type III + IIc and type III

Figure 4 shows sketches of macroscopic types which have questionable classification. It is important to notice if ulceration is present or not

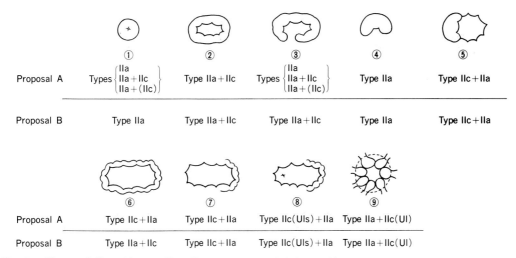

Fig. 3 Usage of IIa + IIc and IIc + IIa proposed by Ichikawa. Note: An emphasis is placed upon the "ring form" of the lesion in Proposal A (From Ichikawa, H. in discussion: *I to Cho*, 11: 30–56, 1976).

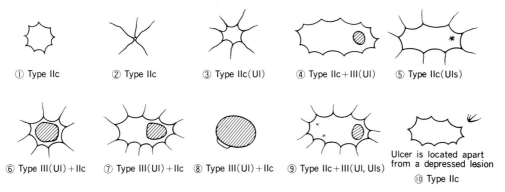

Fig. 4 Usage of IIc, IIc + III and III + IIc proposed by Ichikawa. (From Ichikawa, H. in discussion: *I to Cho*, 11: 30–56, 1976).

in a lesion and this finding should be written at the end of classification. (UI) is added if macroscopic findings reveal the presence of active ulceration in a depressed lesion, and (UIs) is added if ulcer scars are present. Nothing is added if the lesion is a simple depression without ulceration or if it is an erosion. According to this rule, only Nos. 1 and 2 in Figure 4 are the type IIc consisting of only erosion without (UI) nor (UIs) (cf. cases 30, 145, 148, 150). No. 2 is an exceptional case, however, as Sano (1967) noted, for the lesion was a scar-cancer i.e. a benign small ulcer scar surrounded by type IIc. The author considers it better to add (UIs) to it. It is possible to interpret No. 2 as a smaller version of No. 3. No. 10 in Figure 4 is written without (UIs) because there is no continuity between the lesions.

Whether a lesion is type IIc + III or type III + IIc is determined by which element is more prominent. Type III and type IIc + III differ in that type III applies exclusively to a lesion whose depression is deep and large, while type IIc + III applies to a lesion such as No. 4 in Figure 4, with a large area of type IIc containing a small area with a slightly deeper portion than type IIc.

Type III lesions have been regarded as peptic ulcers, but the principles of classification merely indicate a deep, large depression and nothing else. Therefore type III (UI) is the adequate classification in most cases. Type III indicates a deep depression, but it leaves open the question of how many of these lesions are macroscopically type III early cancer only. No hospital has any clear answer. According to Sano (1976), a type III lesion surrounded by type IIc with maximum width of 5 mm is indicated as type III. It is stated that peptic ulcer by macroscopic diagnosis may have a very small portion of cancer on its margin. In Japan a strict, objective standard has not been established to define type III as no agreement was ever reached in this regard. Johansen's assertion (1976) not to apply type III when classification is made macroscopically is a trial to solve the matter differently from the way the Japanese do. As shown in Figure 5, Johansen divides type III into type III + IIa, type III + IIb and type III + IIc, on the ground that cancer is located not in the depression indicated as type III but in the surrounding margin. This method is again a contradiction, if the principle presides that macroscopic classification should indicate the morphology of a cancerous lesion, because macroscopic morphology of the cancer-free portion of a lesion is indicated first by the preceding type III.

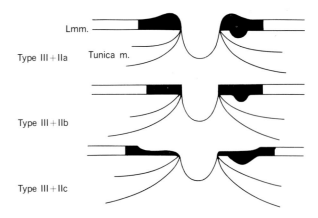

Fig. 5 Johansen's classification of early ulcer cancers. A chronic ulcer is surrounded by the three types of superficial cancers IIa, IIb and IIc. On the left intramucosal cancers are demonstrated and on the right, submucosal cancers (From Johansen, A. A. *in*: Pathology of the Gastro-intestinal Tract, ed. by B. C. Morson, Springer-Verlag, Berlin, 1976).

Differentiating between type I and type IIa (Table 2)

Type I is differentiated from type IIa by the lesion's height of elevation from the level of surrounding mucosa. If the height is 5 mm or above, it is classified as type I, and if less than 5 mm, as type IIa. In this classification, it is not the size or morphology, but only the height of a lesion that matters.

Table 2   Usage of types I and IIa.

Type I: Polypoid lesion more than 0.5cm in height
Type IIa: Superficial elevated lesion less than 5mm in height

(From Ichikawa, H. in discussion: *I to Cho*, 11: 30-56, 1976)

Usage of type IIb (Table 3)

Type IIb indicates a lesion which is neither higher nor lower than the surrounding mucosa; type IIb (IIa) is a lesion faintly elevated from its surrounding mucosa but not as much as to be indicated as type IIa; type IIb (IIc) is a lesion faintly depressed but not as much as type IIc. This classification was proposed a few years ago by Kumakura et al. (1972) who engaged in clinical diagnosis, not by pathologists, to indicate a type IIb-simulating lesion which was not a pure type IIb radiographically or endoscopically (cf. cases 129,

Table 3   Usage of type IIb.

Type IIb:	Lesion with surrounding mucosa neither higher nor lower than the lesion
Type IIb(IIa):	Lesion faintly elevated from its surrounding mucosa but not as much as type IIa
Type IIb(IIc):	Lesion faintly depressed but not as much as type IIc

(From Ichikawa, H. in discussion: *I to Cho*, 11: 30-56, 1976)

130, 131). The findings in this kind of lesion were not well defined enough to be indicated as either type IIa or type IIc. This will be discussed later. Another proposal was made at that time to call it a type IIb-simulating lesion, accompanying a type IIc part.

In any event, very few cases of pure type IIb lesions are recognizable as cancer since they are level with the surrounding mucosa and have similar colors and patterns therefore macroscopic diagnosis of cancer is almost impossible to discover. Type IIb is applied after histologic diagnosis is established.

Evaluation of the Macroscopic Classification

The Japanese classification of early gastric cancer seems to have been accepted internationally except for opposition offered by the Erlangen school in 1973 (Hermanek and Rösch). It seems there is an insufficient understanding of the description by the Japanese authors (Shirakabe et al. 1966, Nakamura et al. 1967, Ariga 1970, Hayashida and Kidokoro 1970, Ueno et al. 1970, Kasugai 1972, Kawai 1972, Murakami 1972, Okabe 1972, Okuda 1972, Sano 1972, Iwanaga and Taniguchi 1973, Okabe et al. 1973, Yamagata and Masuda 1973). They raise two major objections. One is the lack of reproducibility in the classification of each type because of a large discrepancy in the incidence of the macroscopic types reported from the various institutions in Japan. However, it would be unusual for the incidence of each classification in every hospital to exactly coincide. Take type IIa for instance. Its incidence varies because the compression method is not uniformly employed in each hospital, and because age distribution of patients is considerably different. In one hospital in Tokyo where patients are exclusively over 60 years of age, all the cases of detected early cancer were reported

to be polypoid form (Mochizuki 1976). The biggest discrepancy according to the Erlangen group is in the incidence of type IIc and type IIc + III. This discrepancy is due to whether or not an ulceration in a type IIc part is regarded as a component of type III. If one is aware of the presence of a minimum ulceration in a type IIc part, it may be classified as type IIc + III. If one ignores such a minimum ulceration, it is classified as type IIc. In addition, the characteristics of the lesion may change with time. This is the concept of malignant cycle of early gastric cancer which is discussed later (Murakami 1966). This discrepancy, therefore, cannot provide a basis for disputing the validity of the Japanese classification of early gastric cancer. The reported incidence of type IIc plus type IIc + III ranges from 56.9 per cent to 79.9 per cent (except for the reports by Takemoto et al. (1972) and Yamagata and Masuda (1973)). On the other hand, type IIc should not be eliminated from the diagnosis and classification of a small early cancer consisting of only pure cancerous erosion as shown in Figures 113 — 116 (Case 30 in Chapter 3).

Another objection is a question raised on the prognostic value of the Japanese classification of early gastric cancer. From a prognostic point of view, all cases of early gastric cancer are classified into two simple groups, i.e. polypoid and depressed (Hermanek and Rösch 1973). A report from the Cancer Institute Hospital (Takagi and Nakada 1976) favors their opinion because the reported five-year survival rates of polypoid intramucosal cancer without lymph node metastasis was 95 per cent and 78 per cent with submucosal involvement. This was due mainly to liver metastasis; for intramucosal cancer in the depressed form it was 94 per cent without and 89 per cent with submucosal involvement. Thus in cases of intramucosal cancer both forms reveal almost the same prognosis despite the presence of lymph node metastasis in the depressed form (Table 4, 5). On the other hand, in cases of early cancer with submucosal involvement, the prognosis is significantly worse with the polypoid form than with the depressed form. It is important to notice the risk of liver metastasis in the polypoid form which histologically always shows the differentiated type* of cancer (Nakamura et al. 1976). Thus it might be meaningless to make a simple comparison of the five-year survival rates according to the difference

---

* In the histological description about the presented cases "adenocarcinoma tubulare" means the differentiated type and "adenocarcinoma mucocellulare" and "adenocarcinoma scirrhosum" mean the undifferentiated type.

Table 4   Invasion depth, lymph nodes metastasis and prognosis of polypoid early cancer (1950 – 1968).

	Limited to mucosa		Involving submocosa		Total	
	5-year survival rate	Number of cases	5-year survival rate	Number of cases	5-year survival rate	Number of cases
n_0	95%	36/38	91%	42/46	93%	78/84
$n_1 (+)$			63%	12/19	63%	12/19
$n_2 (+)$			71%	5/7	71%	5/7
$n_3 (+)$			0%	0/3	0%	0/3
$n_4 (+)$						
Total	95%	36/38	78%	59/76	83%	95/114

(From Takagi, K and Nakada, K.: *Rinsho Geka*, 31: 19–27, 1976)

Table 5   Invasion depth, lymph node metastasis and prognosis of depressed early cancer (1950 – 1968).

	Limited to mucosa		Involving submocosa		Total	
	5-year survival rate	Number of cases	5-year survival rate	Number of cases	5-year survival rate	Number of cases
n_0	96%	113/118	94%	104/111	95%	217/229
n_1	86%	6/7	82%	13/16	83%	19/23
n_2	50%	2/4	64%	7/11	60%	9/15
n_3			100%	1/1	100%	1/1
n_4			0%	0/1	0%	0/1
Total	94%	121/129	89%	125/141	91%	246/270

(From Takagi, K. and Nakada, K.: *Risnho Geka*, 31: 19–27, 1976)

in histologic types of early gastric cancer. Depth of invasion obviously plays an important role in the evaluation of prognostic value in any type of the classification. Consequently, the radiologic investigation of early gastric cancer has recently been directed to the estimation of its depth of invasion (intramucosal cancer and submucosal involvement) and further, to distinguishing early gastric cancer from an advanced cancer simulating early cancer macroscopically. It is attributed to a merit of the Japanese classification that the transition phase of early gastric cancer into advanced cancer has been successfully revealed (Maruyama et al. 1976).

Pathologically, the Western concept of early gastric cancer has been described in detail by Johansen (1976) and Morson (1977). Johansen (1976) presented several cases of early gastric cancer and discussed its macroscopic and microscopic features. Morson (1977) stated that carcinoma of the stomach is still a common form of malignant disease in North America and Europe. He suggests the possibility that the Japanese experience in the radiologic diagnosis of early gastric cancer may make a contribution to Western radiologists.

Application of the Macroscopic Classification to the Radiographic Diagnosis

The classification of early gastric cancer is widely used in the actual practice of radiologic and endoscopic diagnosis. However, strictly speaking, the classification is a macroscopic one and moreover, it is exclusively used for that of early gastric cancer. The classification should be logically applied only to a lesion that has been proved to be early cancer by the histological examination (Llorens 1975). In other words, clinical usage of the classification might be incompatible with the basic principle of the classification, because a definite diagnosis of cancer cannot be established prior to surgery, and because there is no evidence that a lesion is early cancer even though it may appear so. There have been occasional cases of cancer which involves the subserosa or serosa despite certain macroscopic impressions of type IIc early cancer. For such cases, a concept of type IIc simulating advanced cancer has been applied (Maruyama et al. 1976), and is discussed in Chapter 10.

This classification, however, can be used for radiographic and endoscopic diagnosis. This is justifiable by the low error rate of diagnosing early gastric cancer macroscopically and by a one-to-one correspondence between the macroscopic and radiographic findings in an ideal state. Approximately 70 per cent of early gastric cancer have been correctly diagnosed radiographically (see page 72).

Prognosis of Early Gastric Cancer

Table 6 reveals the number of radical operations for all gastric cancers and the number of detected early gastric cancers in a period of 25 years from 1946 to 1970 at the Cancer Institute Hospital. In the first five years from 1946 to 1950, only one case of early gastric cancer was discovered, comprising 0.5 per cent of all the radical operations. In the fourth period from 1961 to 1965, 149 cases (19.2%) of early gastric cancers were discovered. This rapid increase in the detection rate of early gastric cancer during this period is closely correlated with the institution of double contrast radiography (Shirakabe et al. 1966), and the development of endoscopic examination with biopsy. In the final period from 1966 to 1970 the

detected number of early gastric cancers compromised 28.8 per cent of all radical operations. This remarkable increase corresponds with the increase in the 5-year survival rate folling radical operation (Table 7). The over-all 5-year survival of early gastric cancer was 90.4 per cent and that of advanced cancer alone was 41.8 per cent. In the latter two periods, it was 54.6 per cent and 59.0 per cent respectively. It is obvious that such an increase in the survival rate is related much more closely to the rapid increase in the number of detected early gastric cancer cases than the progress in the surgery for advanced gastric cancer.

The 10-year survival rate of all radical operation cases (Table 8) is 46 per cent for single

Table 6   Transitional number of detected early cancer.

Period	No. of radical operations	No. of early cancers	%
1946 − 1950	201	1	0.5
1951 − 1955	572	24	4.2
1956 − 1960	806	67	8.3
1961 − 1965	775	149	19.2
1966 − 1970	791	228	28.8
Total	3,145	469	14.9

(From Takagi, K. et al.: *Operation*, 32: 161−169, 1978)

Table 7   Transitional rate of radical operations for gastric cancer.

Period	5-year survival rate of early cancer	5-year survival rate of advanced cancer	5-year survival rate of total case
1946 − 1950	100.0% (1/ 1)	39.0% (78/200)	39.3% (79/201)
1951 − 1955	87.5% (21/ 24)	38.0% (208/548)	40.0% (229/572)
1956 − 1960	88.1% (59/ 67)	38.5% (284/739)	42.5% (343/806)
1961 − 1965	89.9% (134/149)	46.2% (289/626)	54.6% (423/775)
1966 − 1970	91.7% (209/228)	45.8% (258/563)	59.0% (467/791)
Total	90.4% (424/469)	41.8% (1,117/2,676)	49.0% (1,541/3,145)

(From Takagi, K. et al.: *Operation*, 32: 161−169, 1978)

Table 8   Final result of radical operations for gastric cancer.

Period	Survival Rate					
	Single cancer		Multiple cancer		Over-all	
	5-year	10-year	5-year	10-year	5-year	10-year
1946 − 1950	39% (79/201)	29% (59/201)	63% (5/ 8)	38% (3/ 8)	40% (84/209)	30% (62/209)
1951 − 1955	40% (229/572)	31% (178/572)	39% (12/ 27)	37% (10/ 27)	40% (241/599)	31% (188/599)
1956 − 1960	43% (343/806)	33% (266/806)	36% (28/ 78)	17% (13/ 78)	42% (371/884)	32% (279/884)
1961 − 1965	55% (423/775)	46% (359/775)	62% (38/ 61)	48% (29/ 61)	55% (461/836)	46% (388/836)
1966 − 1970	59% (467/791)		60% (71/118)		59% (538/909)	
Total	49% (1,541/3,145)	36% (862/2,390)	53% (154/292)	32% (55/174)	49% (1,695/3,437)	36% (917/2,564)

(From Takagi, K. et al.: *Operation*, 32: 161−169, 1978)

Table 9 Five-year survival rate and depth of invasion of cancer of the stomach (single lesion).
Cancer Institute Hospital, 1946–1969.

Invasion depth	Result of operation		Total
	Radical	Conservative	
Limited to mucosa (m)	94.1% (176/187)		94.1% (176/187)
Involving submucosa (sm)	87.1% (204/234)	0% (0/ 4)	85.7% (204/238)
Involving propria muscle layer (pm)	70.9% (239/337)	0% (0/ 18)	67.3% (239/355)
Involving subserosa (ss)	50.3% (490/973)	1.1% (2/167)	43.1% (492/1,140)
Involving serosa (s_1)	44.0% (196/445)	4.5% (5/110)	36.2% (201/555)
(s_2)	22.3% (114/510)	0% (0/319)	13.7% (114/829)
(s_3)	4.6% (13/280)	0% (0/159)	2.9% (13/439)
Total	48.2% (432/2,966)	0.9% (7/777)	38.4% (1,439/3,743)

(From Maruyama, M. et al.: *I to Cho*, 11: 855-868, 1976)

cancer and 48 per cent in multiple cancers. The total 10-year survival rate of radical operations is 46 per cent (Table 8).

As shown in Table 7, death occurs within five years in about 10 per cent of early cancer cases even though the detection is made at an early phase. Table 9 reveals the relation between 5-year survival rate and depth of invasion of gastric cancer in a period of 24 years from 1946 to 1969. In this table, the total 5-year survival rate is lower than that shown in Table 7, because Table 9 includes the cases of conservative operation (Maruyama et al. 1976). The 5-year survival rate of cancer involving the subserosa (ss) and deeper (s_0, s_1, s_2, s_3) is 27.7 per cent (820/2963). On the other hand, the 5-year survival rate of cancer limited to the propria muscle layer remains in between the former two rates. It is important to establish an accurate diagnosis of cancer involving propria muscle layer (pm), as well as the diagnosis of early cancer.

In this book the possibility of making radiographic diagnosis of early cancer and of cancer involving the propria muscle layer is discussed. There are two reasons why cancer involving this muscle layer should be diagnosed. One is because of its transitional place between early cancer and radiographically definite advanced cancer. Second is that from developmental point of view this cancer reveals a transitory morphology from an early to an advanced stage.

As mentioned above, early gastric cancer shows a good prognosis, although 10 per cent of the cases result in death within five postoperative years (Takagi and Nakada 1976). The causes of death in early gastric cancer are roughly divided into direct death, recurrence, and other diseases. The most important is recurrence with an incidence varying from 25.5 per cent to 53 per cent depending upon the series. Factors associated with recurrence include peritoneal dissemination (P-factor), liver

metastasis (H-factor) and lymph node metastasis (N-factor). Lymph node metastasis is most important. Table 10 is an analysis of the prognosis of early gastric cancer in relationship to depth of invasion and lymph node metastasis.

Polypoid early cancer (type I, type IIa, type IIa + IIc) is studied in terms of its depth of invasion, lymph node metastasis and prognosis. No lymph node metastasis is found in intramucosal cancer (n_0). Prognosis is also favourable, as the 5-year survival rate is 95 per cent. In contrast to this, lymph node metastasis is found in 29 of the 76 cases of cancers with submucosal involvement and the prognosis drops to 78 per cent. As to cases experienced at the Cancer Institute Hospital, the 5-year survival rate of lesions with metastasis to n_2 group (71%) is higher than that of the n_1 group (63%). Kitaoka and Miwa (1974) reported that the 5-year survival rate of polypoid early cancer with metastasis to n_1 group nodes was 62.5 per cent (10/16).

As to depressed early intramucosal cancer (Table 5) overall prognosis seems fairly good despite 8 cases (6.0%) of lymph node metastasis in 129 cases. But the prognosis worsens with increasing lymph nodes metastases. There are 21 cases (14.9%) of distant lymph node metastasis in 141 cases of submucosal cancer, with a 5-year survival rate of 89 per cent. Comparison of the 5-year survival rate of the cases with lymph node metastasis according to numbers of affected lymph nodes discloses that the rate is 83 per cent in the n_1 group, 60 per cent in the n_2 group with only one case in n_3 group living longer than five years.

In the studies made by Kitaoka and Miwa (1974) at National Cancer Center, 5 cases are reported to have lymph node metastasis in 100 cases of intramucosal cancer, showing 80 per cent 5-year survival rate (4/5), no difference in the 5-year survival rate was found between n_1 positive and n_2 positive group in the early cancer with submucosal involvement, excluding 3 cases of direct death and 12 cases of death due to other causes. Comparison of the 5-year survival rate between polypoid early cancer and depressed early cancer shows that the prognosis is essentially identical for intramucosal cancer, whereas in submucosal involvement the prognosis for polypoid early cancer is worse.

Further studies of the relationship between lymph node metastasis and prognosis of early gastric cancer suggest that liver metastasis is the factor most responsible for poorer prognosis (Takagi and Nakada 1976). As is shown in Table 10, in 17 cases of death by recurrence of early gastric cancer, 8 cases are due to liver metastasis, and 2 are without lymph node metastasis. It is noteworthy, however, that all the cases of liver metastasis belong to the polypoid early cancer with submucosal involvement group. In Takagi's analysis in differentiated types, 3 cases belong to type I, 1 case to type IIa, 1 case to type I + IIa, and 3 cases to type IIa + IIc.

Two cases in n_0 group lived longer than three years, but all cases in n_+ group died within a year. Sano et al. (1970) report that all 5 cases with liver metastasis were macroscopically polypoid cancer with submucosal involvement, and these patients died within three years. In Sano's experience the incidence of liver metastasis is 10 per cent (3/22) of polypoid submucosal cancer with lymph node metastasis. Takagi has a higher percentage of liver metastasis at 20.1 per cent (6/29).

Next to liver metastasis is local recurrence, with four cases. All are n_2 group. One case with peritoneal dissemination belongs to type IIc, positive in n_1 group. One case with lymph node metastasis is positive in n_4 group. One case with lung metastasis is type IIa with submucosal involvement and positive in n_1 group. A case of bone metastasis to the rib and vertebra is type IIc + III with submucosal involvement and positive in n_2 group. Sano (1976) reports two cases of peritoneal carcinomatosis in a depressed type submucosal cancer without lymph node metastasis among the cases of recurrence without liver metastases within five years. Takagi and Nakada (1976) thought it interesting that only 2 of 17 cases of death by recurrence within 5 years were free of lymph node metastasis compared to 11 of 19 cases dying of other causes. Only 2 of the 17 cases of death by recurrence within five years had no lymph node metastasis. Few deaths from local recurrence occur beyond 5 years. Two cases of stump recurrence and one case of local recurrence

Table 10 Relationship between lymph node and distance metastasis of early gastric cancer.

	n_0	n_1	n_2	n_3	n_4	Total
Liver	2	2	1	2		8*
Local			3			3
Peritoneal dissemination		1				1
Lymph node			1		1	2
Bone			1			1
Lung		1	1			2
Total	2/313 0.6%	4/42 9.5%	7/22 31.8%	2/4 50%	1/1	17/383 4.4%

* Includes 1 case without lymph node examination
(From Takagi, K. and Nakada, K.: *Rinsho Geka*, 31: 19–27, 1976)

are reported by Takagi and Nakada (1976), and two cases of stump recurrence are reported by Sano et al. (1970).

Advanced Cancer, Its Macroscopic Classification and Radiographic Diagnosis

An advanced cancer is defined as a lesion which involves at least the propria muscle layer or the deeper layer of the gastric wall (subserosa and serosa). The radiographic diagnosis of typical advanced cancers is not described in this book. An emphasis is mainly placed on the radiographic diagnosis of the advanced lesions which macroscopically simulate early lesions and the differentiation of a lesion involving the propria muscle layer from early cancer. Therefore, only a brief description of the macroscopic classification of so-called advanced cancer is given, with demonstrations of typical cases.

Although the classification of gastric cancer is said to be confusing in the Western literature (Palmer 1974), the Borrmann's (1926) (Fig. 6) classification, though very old, has been widely accepted and used in Japan. This classification is based upon pure macroscopic findings of the lesions and has proved to be significant in relation to the analysis of their biological behavior as well as prognosis after surgery. An old classification (Palmer 1974) has combined macroscopic and microscopic findings, thereby making it less meaningful. In the Japanese Research Society of Gastric Cancer general rules by another two types are

9

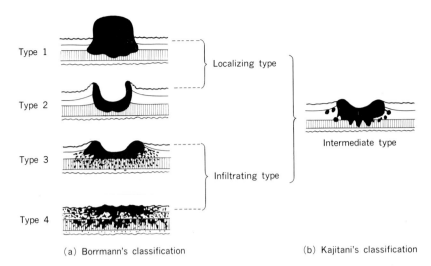

Type 1

Type 2

Localizing type

Type 3

Type 4

Infiltrating type

Intermediate type

(a) Borrmann's classification

(b) Kajitani's classification

Fig. 6 Schematization from Borrmann's concept (1926) on the classification of advanced gastric cancer and Kajitani's modified classification (1950). (From Japanese Society for Gastric Cancer: General Rules for the Gastric Cancer Study in Surgery and Pathology, 9th ed., Kanehara Shuppan, Tokyo, 1974).

added to the Borrmann's classification in order to include early cancer (Borrmann type 0) and lesions which are unclassifiable into Borrmann's variety (Borrmann type 5). Being a more simplified classification than Borrmann's, the Kajitani's classification is frequently used (Table 7) because it leads to an easy recognition of the infiltrating pattern of the advanced cancers.

Prognosis of Advanced Cancer in Relation to Borrmann's Classification

The prognosis of small Borrmann types 1 and 2 lesions are better than that of Borrmann types 3 and 4 lesions, but the opposite is true in the large advanced cancers (Fig. 7, Nishi et al. 1969). Concerning the relationship between the depth of invasion and the prognosis of the advanced cancers,

Fig. 7 Five-year survival rate of gastric cancer in relation to depth of invasion and Borrmann's classification (Modified from Nishi, M. et al.: *I to Cho*, 4: 1087–1100, 1969).

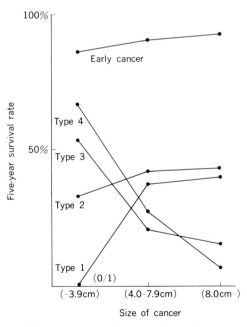

Fig. 8 Five-year survival rate of gastric cancer in relation to size and Borrmann's classification (Modified from Nishi, M. et al.: *I to Cho*, 4: 1087–1100, 1969).

10

the 5-year survival rate of Borrmann type 1 and 2 is worse than that of Borrmann types 3 and 4 with invasion limited to the propria muscle layer, but it is reversed when the muscle is penetrated (Fig. 8, Nishi et al. 1969).

As Nakamura (1972) stated, since Borrmann types 1 and 2 are histologically differentiated cancers in most cases, and Borrmann types 3 and 4 are undifferentiated, the prognosis of the two groups can be equated with advanced cancers having two different histological types. The 5-year survival rate of differentiated cancer is worse than that of undifferentiated cancer if their largest diameter is smaller than 39 mm. But, it is reversed for size over 40 mm in largest diameter. In terms of their depth of invasion, the 5-year survival rate of differentiated cancers is worse than that of undifferentiated cancers with invasion limited to the propria muscle layer, and it becomes reversed if invasion has reached the serosa. Such a clear difference in the 5-year survival rate between the two histological types is explained by the difference in their biological behavior types.

Venous permeation occurs frequently in differentiated cancer of small size, and consequently there is a high risk of liver metastasis. With large differentiated cancer, surgical resection is easier than in the undifferentiated cancer, the latter infiltrating diffusely into the neighboring tissues, resulting in peritoneal carcinomatosis.

Typical Radiographic Features of Advanced Cancer

Representative radiographic and macroscopic findings of the four types of Borrmann's variety are presented (Figs. 9–21). The Borrmann type 3 is most frequently encountered, followed by Borrmann type 2 and Borrmann type 4. Borrmann type 1 is extremely rare. A big polypoid lesion is often early cancer, as was suggested by Borrmann (1926).

Case 1   Typical Borrmann Type 1 Advanced Cancer.
A 76-year-old woman (CIH). (Figs. 9-12)

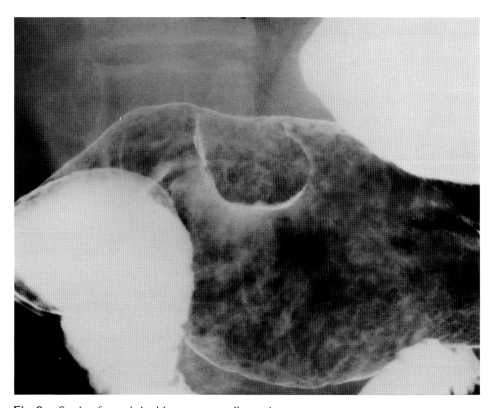

Fig. 9   Supine frontal double contrast radiograph.

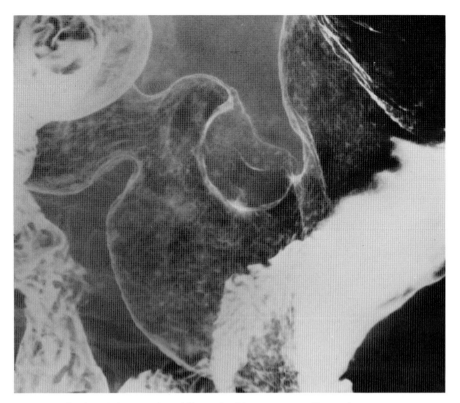

Fig. 10   Supine right anterior oblique double contrast radiograph.

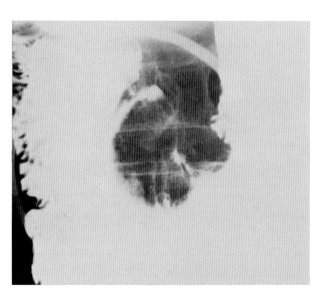

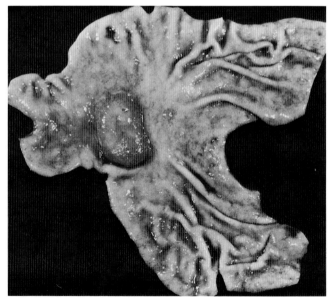

Fig. 11   Fig. 12

Fig. 11   Compression radiograph.

Fig. 12   Photograph of the resected specimen. The lesion measures 35 × 20 mm, with invasion into the propria muscle layer. Adenocarcinoma papillotubulare, with lymph node metastasis (1/18).

Case 2   Typical Borrmann Type 2 Advanced Cancer.
A 65-year-old man (CIH). (Figs. 13-16)

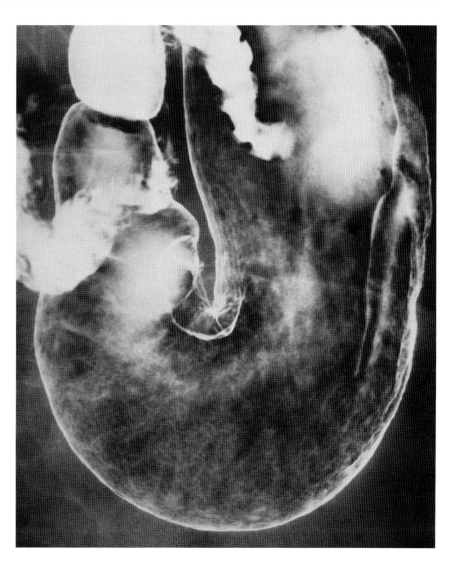

Fig. 13   Supine frontal double contrast radiograph.

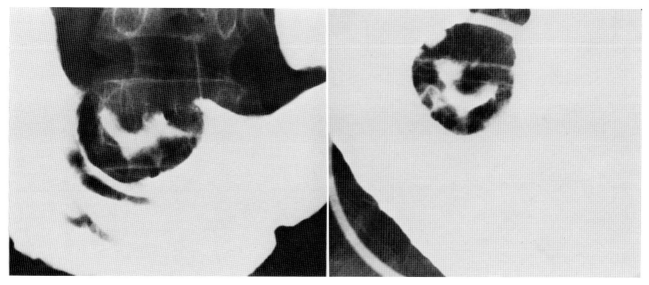

Fig. 14   Compresion radiograph in the prone position.   Fig. 15   Compression radiograph in the upright position.

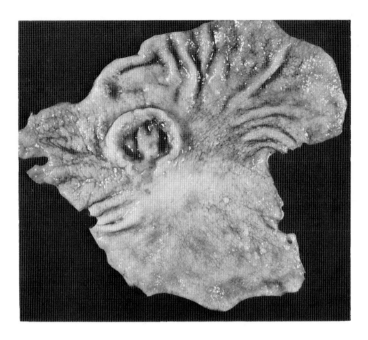

Fig. 16 Photograph of the resected specimen. The lesion is at the incisura, measuring 40 × 40 mm with invasion into the subserosa. Adenocarcinoma acinosum without lymph node metastasis.

Case 3 Typical Borrmann Type 3 Advanced Cancer.
A 35-year-old woman (CIH). (Figs. 17-19)

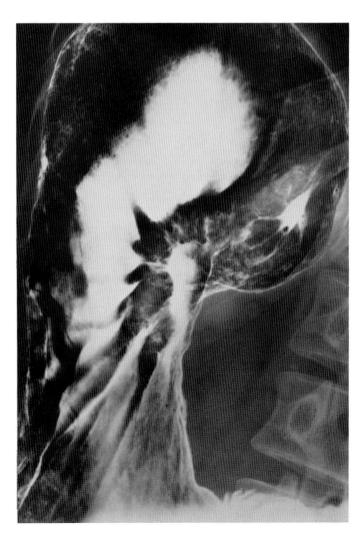

Fig. 17 Prone double contrast radiograph in the semi-upright position.

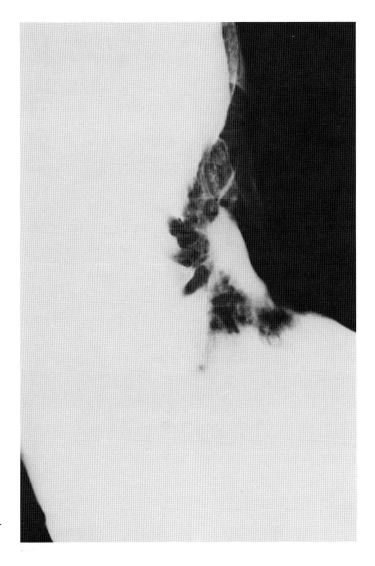

Fig. 18 Compression radiograph in the prone position.

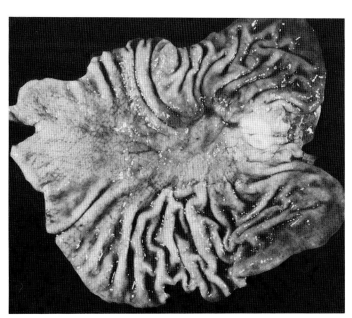

Fig. 19 Photograph of the resected specimen. The lesion is located from the cardia to the incisura, measuring 80 x 60 mm with penetration through the serosa. Adenocarcinoma scirrhosum, with lymph node metastasis (1/29).

Case 4   Typical Borrmann Type 4 Advanced Cancer.
A 57-year-old man (CIH). (Figs. 20 and 21)

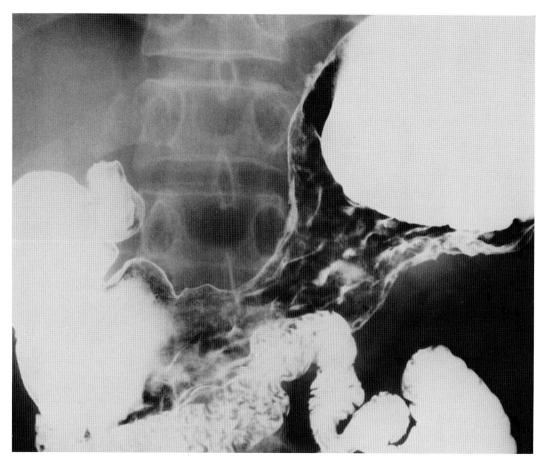

Fig. 20   Supine frontal double contrast radiograph.

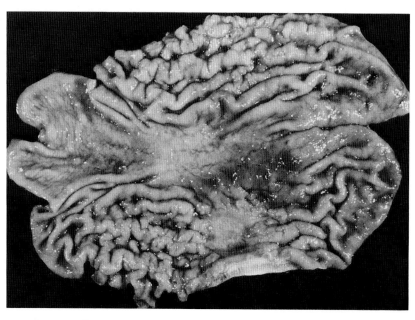

Fig. 21   Photograph of the resected specimen. The stomach is extensively involved by the scirrhous infiltration. Adenocarcinoma scirrhosum (linitis plastica type). The primary focus (UI-III) is completely surrounded in the fundic gland mucosa (refer to Chapter 11). Cancer is exposed to the serosa in most part, with lymph node metastasis (3/9).

Describing the Surgical Specimen

A thorough understanding of the correlation between marcoscopic evidence and radiologic findings is essential to the radiologist attempting to diagnose early gastric cancer. In order to better understand the cases presented in this book, some surgical specimen description is necessary, specifically how we have prepared, positioned and measured the lesions presented as part of our cases. The specimen is incised along the anterior wall aspect of the greater curvature just above the attachment of the omentum. After opening the specimen, it is positioned with the distal side on the left and the proximal side on the right. Consequently the anterior wall is superior and the posterior wall inferior, with the lesser curvature in the center (Fig. 22).

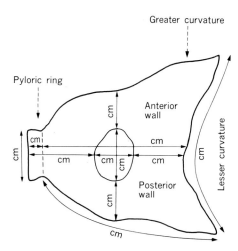

Fig. 22 The incised stomach and the method of estimating the size of lesion (From Japanese Research Society for Gastric Cancer: *The General Rules for the Gastric Cancer Study in Surgery and Pathology*, 9th ed., Kanehara Shuppan, Tokyo, 1974).

When a lesion is discovered on the radiograph, it should be oriented with the incised specimen arranged as in Figure 22. However, when the center of a lesion is located on the greater curvature side, the incision is made on the lesser curvature side of the specimen. In this case, the specimen is arranged with posterior wall superior and anterior wall inferior, with the greater curvature in the center.

A lesion is measured by the largest diameter and perpendicularly to the largest diameter. Its area is the product of its two largest diameters. The resected specimens presented in this book are described according to this rule.

Notes on the Histological Description of the Presented Cases

Histological classification of gastric cancer was instituted by the Japanese Research Society for Gastric Cancer (Table 11). As this classification is based upon a pure morphological standpoint, it is sometimes not best suited for correlating the histological finding with the clinical features. Thus, Nakamura's classification (Table 12) which was originally derived from the Oota's classification (Table 13) is used in this book because it is convenient for the clinicopathological correlation of gastric cancer. The common type in Table 11

Table 11 Histological classification of gastric cancer.

1. Common type;
   Papillary adenocarcinoma (pap)
   Tubular adenocarcinoma (tub)
   　Well differentiated type (tub-1)
   　Moderately differentiated type (tub-2)
   Poorly differentiated adenocarcinoma (por)
   Mucinous adenocarcinoma
   Signet-ring cell carcinoma
2. Specific type;
   Adenosquamous carcinoma (as)
   Squamous cell carcinoma (sq)
   Carcinoid tumor (cd)
   Undifferentiated carcinoma (ud)
   Miscellaneous (ms)

(From Japanese Research Society for Gastric Cancer: *The General Rules for the Gastric Cancer Study in Surgery and Pathology*, 9th ed., Kanehara Shuppan, Tokyo, 1974)

Table 12 Classification of histological types of gastric cancer by Nakamura.

Histologically	Morphologically
Undifferentiated cancer	Mucocellulare
	Scirrhosum
	Muconodulare
	Acinosum
Differentiated cancer	Papillotubulare
	Tubulare
	Muconodulare
	Acinosum
	Adenoacanthoma

(From Nakamura, K.: *Pathology of Gastric Cancer*, Kimpo-do, Kyoto, 1972)

17

Table 13 Classification of histological type of gastric cancer by Oota (1964).

Papillotubulare
Tubulare medullare
Acinosum
Scirrhosum
Gelatinocellulare
Gelatinonodulare
Adenoacanthoma

(From Oota, K.: *Trans. Soc. Pathol. Jap.*, 53: 3, 1964)

Table 14 Description of depth of invasion of gastric cancer.

Depth of invasion	Involved layer	Popular name
m	mucosa	intramucosal ca m-ca
sm	submucosa	ca. with submucosal involvement, sm-ca
pm	propria muscle	pm-ca
ss	subserosa	ss-ca
s	serosa	s-ca

(Arranged from Japanese Research Society for Gastric Cancer: *The General Rules for the Gastric Cancer Study in Surgery and Pathology*,

Table 15 Histological classification of common type gastric cancer.

Papillary adenocarcinoma (pap)	→ Adenocarcinoma papillotubulare
Tubular adenocarcinoma (tub)	
Well differentiated type (tub-1)	→ Adenocar. tubulare, Broders 1, 2.
Moderately differentiated type (tub-2)	→ Adenocar. tubulare, Broders 3
Poorly differentiated adenocarcinoma (por)	→ Adenocar. scirrhosum, acinosum
Mucinous adenocarcinoma	→ Adenocar. muconodulare
Signet-ring cell carcinoma	→ Adenocar. mucocellulare

(From Japanese Research Society for Gastric Cancer: *The General Rules for the Gastric Cancer Study in Surgey and Pathology*, 9th ed., Kanehara Shuppan, Tokyo, 1974)

corresponds with the Nakamura's classification if the Broders' classification (1925) is partly added to the latter, as shown in Table 14.

Depth of invasion of cancer is described with abbreviations of the terms representing each layer of the gastric wall (Table 15, The Japanese Research Society of Gastric Cancer, 1974).

In the last of the descriptions of the cases, the diagnosis was summarized by combining the histological diagnosis, macroscopic diagnosis (early or advanced), depth of invasion, depth of ulceration (if present), and finally the indication of lymph node metastasis (number of metastatic nodes/number of nodes examined).

Chapter 2

Principles and Application of Double Contrast Radiography

Basic Concepts of the Radiographic Examination of the Stomach

The basic concept of radiographic diagnosis is based on the assumption that any lesion which can be diagnosed macroscopically can be diagnosed radiographically. Accurate and exact reproduction of macroscopic findings is the foremost requirement for achieving this end. It first involves mapping the macroscopic findings on a radiograph. Then, a point on the macroscopic elevation or depression can be identified with a point on the corresponding radiographic image. The radiographic findings are a collection of these corresponding points. Thus, the main purpose of the detailed examination is to obtain radiographic findings in which a one-to-one correspondence to macroscopic findings is possible. In most cases, double contrast radiography is the most suitable procedure for this purpose, because it is easy and its result is always reproducible. But first the routine examination is performed. Once an abnormality is discovered, the detailed examination is done to obtain the radiographic findings necessary for a one-to-one correspondence to the macroscopic findings.

Principles of Double Contrast Radiography

Double contrast radiography is a method utilizing the shadows cast by two different contrast media, barium and air. Barium is a positive contrast medium which is impenetrable by X-ray and air is a negative contrast medium which allows X-rays to pass. These opposing contrast media present the mucosal pattern as a bouble contrast image.

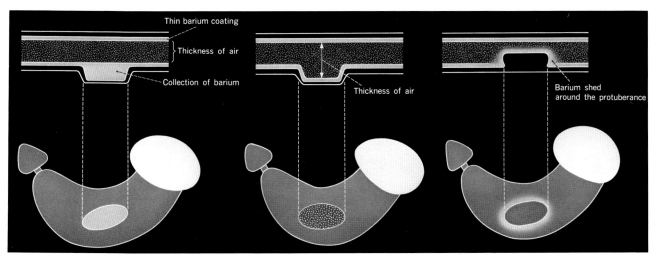

a. How a depression is delineated.   b. How a depression is delineated.   c. How a polypoid lesion is delineated.

Fig. 23   Principles of double contrast radiography.

Thus, a depression on the mucosal surface is usually visualized as a collection of barium in it (Fig. 23a), and its depth is measured by the thickness of the retained barium. In actual practice the retained barium may sometimes flow out of a depression by positional change, and in such a case the thicker layer of air reveals the depression as a radiolucency deeper than the surrounding double contrast shadow (Fig. 23b) (cf. Fig. 88). A type IIc lesion on the anterior wall may be visualized as a deep radiolucency. Contrary to a depression, an elevation of the mucosal surface is visualized as a localized radiolucency, because a layer of barium is spread over it, and the layer of air is relatively thinner. The thickness of the barium around the protuberance indicates its height, to some extent (Fig. 23c). Irregularities of a depressed surface in a type IIc lesion is visualized as a faint collection of barium, together with areas of radiolucency (Figs. 24, 25). The "areae gastricae" or "etat mamelloné" is delineated as a network.

Case 5 Type IIc Early Cancer.

A 46-year-old woman (NCCH). (Figs. 24 and 25)

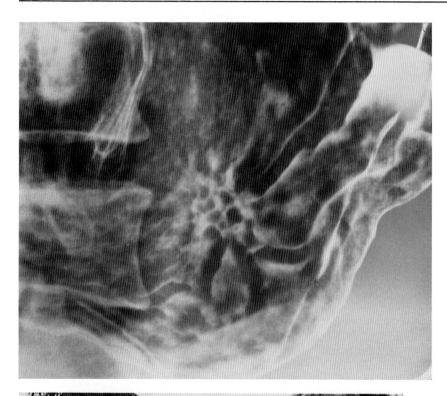

Fig. 24 Supine double contrast radiograph demonstrates small radiolucencies of various sizes in an irregular collection of contrast medium, which reveals an uneven cancerous erosion.

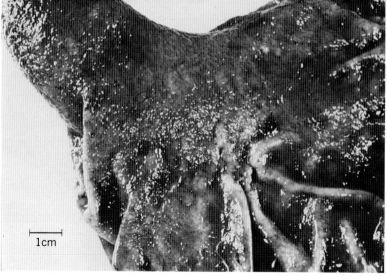

1cm

Fig. 25 Photograph of the resected specimen. The resected stomach is layed inside out to allow the lesion as it appers on the double contrast radiograph to be seen. This picture is somewhat different from that visualized in the double contrast study. Its shape and the nodularity of the erosion is not as well seen. The fold pattern also looks different from that of the double contrast radiograph, because the stomach is less distended.

Selection of the Contrast Medium

Although the quality of barium is important for obtaining good double contrast images, it is not crucial. The various preparations of contrast media differ in their viscosity, fluidity and coating properties, even at the same concentration. Barytgen de luxe* (120% w/v) is one of the most popular commercial products in Japan and gives stable mucosal coating under any condition. According to the author's experience in various countries, however, it is possible to obtain adequate mucosal coating for diagnosis with any product. It is most important to know the properties of the contrast medium, especially the concentrations which give the best mucosal coating.

Volume of Barium and Air

For double contrast radiography of the stomach, an adequate volume of barium and air, as well as frequent positional change of the patient, are the principal requirements. One must always use more than 200 ml of barium, except in some cases of gastric deformity. Less than 200 ml of barium does

* Available from EISAI CO. LTD. (Sole agent for overseas), 4 Koishikawa, Bunkyo-ku, Tokyo, 112 Japan.

not produce a good double contrast image, because it is unable to cover the entire mucosal surface. As a result, retained mucus and gastric juice may prevent adequate barium coating. Moreover, less than 200 ml of barium does not produce a uniform image of the filled stomach and it becomes difficult to interpret the lesser and greater curvatures, especially in the middle to upper third. Even with large amounts of barium, flow is directed along the lesser curvature side when the patient is turned to the right decubitus from the supine position and along the greater curvature side when the patient is returned to the left decubitus position (Fig. 26). The volume of air should be changed depending upon various circumstances. In the routine examination, however, the ideal amount is that which produces a double contrast image of the middle third in the supine position. This much air gives an impression that the stomach is overdistended, and delineation of a shallow depression such as type IIc around the incisura may be difficult (Fig. 27, 28) Otherwise, the entire stomach cannot be visualized as a double contrast image. At least 300 ml of air is required for this purpose. Frequent positional changes should be made to sweep the mucosal surface clean. By shifting the barium from the fundus to the antrum, adherent mucus is washed away and the gastric juice becomes mixed with the barium. Thus, good mucosal coating is obtained for each exposure. The speed of the positional change also may be varied to help detect some lesions.

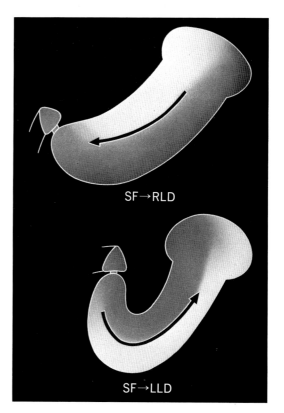

SF→RLD

SF→LLD

Fig. 26 Sketch showing flow of the barium by positional change in double contrast radiography.
SF: Supine frontal
RLD: Right lateral decubitus
LLD: Left lateral decubitus

Case 6   Type IIc Early Cancer.

A 28-year-old woman (NCCH). (Figs. 27 and 28)

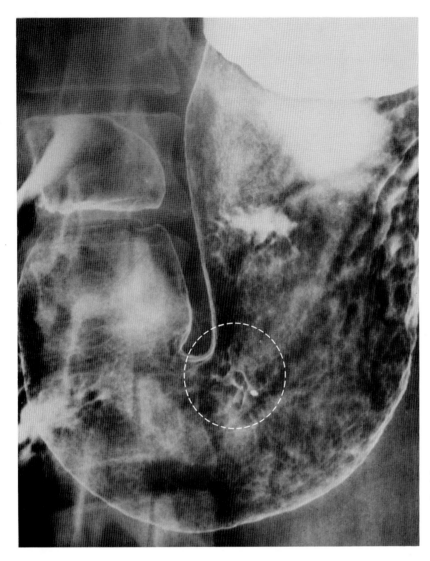

Fig. 27 Supine double contrast radiograph demonstrates an irregular barium-filled erosion, type IIc. The details of the erosion are almost the same as on the resected specimen. The fold pattern is effaced by over-distension of the stomach.

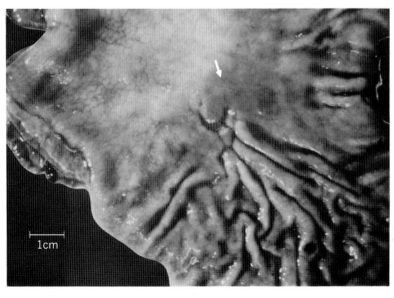

Fig. 28 Photograph of the resected specimen. A type IIc lesion with converging folds is seen on the posterior wall of the incisura region, measuring 18 × 15 mm. Adenocarcinoma mucocellulare with invasion limited to the mucosa (m).

Sequence of Radiographic Exposures in the Routine Examination

If possible, antispasmodic agents such as Coliopan* or Buscopan** should be administered intramuscularly 5 to 10 minutes before the examination. In

---

* Coliopan: Available through EISAI Co., Ltd., Tokyo (Japan)
** Buscopan: Available through Boehringer A. G., Ingelheim (West Germany)

countries where these drugs are not available glucagon (Laufer 1979) is recommended. These drugs diminish gastric peristalsis and make the examination easier to perform.

Figure 29 is a series of line drawings of each radiographic image and the corresponding diagnosable area used in the routine examination at the Cancer Institute Hospital. In most cases, we use a remote-controlled X-ray television apparatus. For the routine examination a total of 300 ml of barium is given. First, a mouthful or about 20 ml of the barium is swallowed and a mucosal relief picture of the stomach is taken in

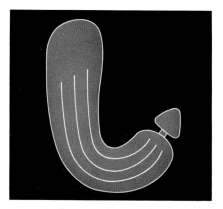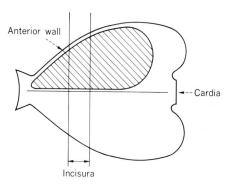

1. Diagnosable area by mucosal relief method in the prone frontal position.

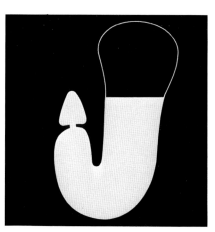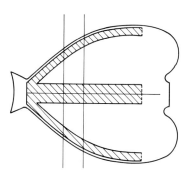

2. Diagnosable area by barium filling method in the upright frontal position.

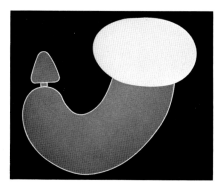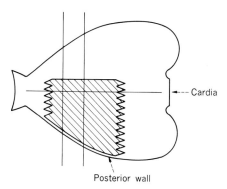

3. Diagnosable area in the supine frontal position.

Fig. 29-1   Line drawing of a sequence of exposures and the diagnosable areas in the routine examination of the stomach.

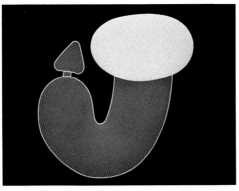 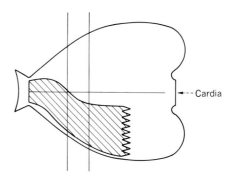

4. Diagnosable area in the supine right anterior oblique position.

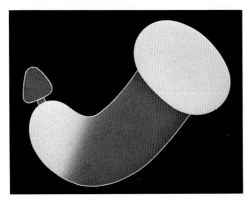 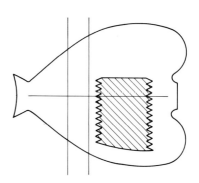

5. Diagnosable area in the supine left anterior oblique position.

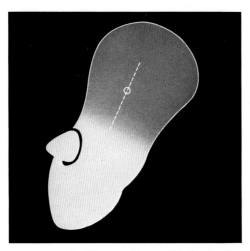 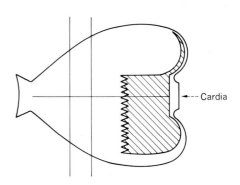

6. Diagnosable area in the semi-recumbent, left anterior oblique position.

Fig. 29-2 Line drawing of a sequence of exposures and the diagnosable areas in the routine examination of the stomach.

the prone position (No. 1). This is necessary for discovering anterior wall lesions* (Fig. 30).

---

* The mucosal relief picture in the prone position is sometimes replaced by the barium thin layer method (Shirakabe 1971), which is considered to be a simple method of prone double contrast radiography. For the barium thin layer method, 30–50 ml of balium with 50–60 %w/v is prepared. The barium is swallowed, and air is introduced into the stomach via a nasal or oral tube or an effervescent agent. 300–350 ml of air is desirable. Then, the patient is asked to perform abdominal respiration while moving the left hip up and down slightly or while the table is moved up and down in order to get uniform distribution of the layered barium.

Next, the esophagus is observed while the patient drinks the remaining barium in the upright right anterior oblique position. Spot films are obtained if necessary. Sometimes swallowed air gives an adequate double contrast image of the esophagus. A film of the barium-filled stomach is taken in the upright frontal position (No. 2). Next, effervescent tablets or granules (Fig. 31) are given in the upright position to achieve gaseous distension. These effervescent agents are designed to produce 300 to 400 ml of CO_2. The best gaseous dis-

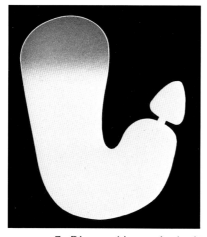 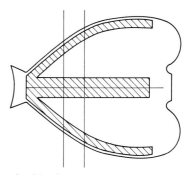

7. Diagnosable area by barium filling method in the prone position.

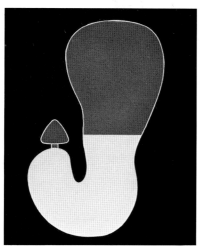 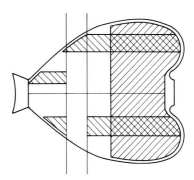

8. Diagnosable area in the upright, frontal position.

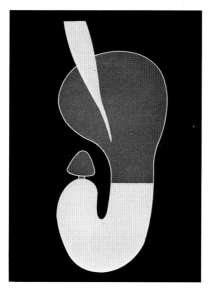 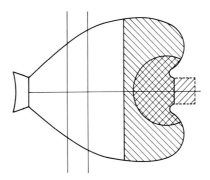

9. Upright, right oblique position for scrutinizing the esophagogastric junction and cardia.

Fig. 29-3   Line drawing of a sequence of exposures and the diagnosable areas in the routine examination of the stomach.

Case 7   Type IIc Early Cancer.
A 41-year-old woman (TH). (Fig. 30)

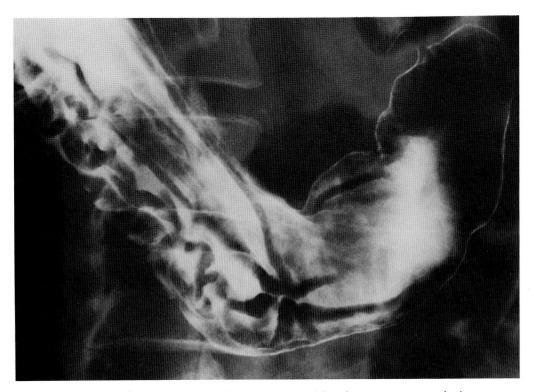

Fig. 30   Barium thin layer method in the prone position demonstrates a marked convergence of the folds at the anterior wall of the lower gastric body. Clubbing of the folds seems to be exaggerated at the interrupted ends. An erosion is not delineated effectively due to incomplete distension of the stomach.

tension is achieved through the use of a nasal or oral gastric tube. (If one has used the barium thin layer method as the first step, a barium-filled film is taken with the fundus distended, and additional air is not necessary.)

The table is tilted to the horizontal position and the patient is turned quickly to the right decubitus and then turned to the left decubitus position. A few seconds later, the patient is gently returned to the horizontal position. These are the basic positional changes for ,taking a double contrast radiograph in the supine frontal position (No. 3). The same positional changes are repeated for taking a double contrast radiograph in the right anterior oblique position (No. 4). For this exposure the patient is positioned under fluoroscopic control so that the antrum lies horizontal to the plane of the table or to the left side of the spine. A double contrast radiograph in the left anterior oblique position is taken by turning the patient to the right decubitus from No. 4 and then

returning him gently to the oblique position (No. 5). In this exposure the upper part of the gastric body, which is hidden by the contrast medium in the supine frontal position, is visualized.

Sequence No. 6 is taken by turning the patient to the right decubitus position in the horizontal or semi-upright position, or by maintaining a marked oblique position. It is important to bring the esophago-gastric junction to the central portion of the double contrast image under fluoroscopic control. This position itself is similar to that reported by Schatzki and Gary (1958), but the purpose of this exposure may be different, because Schatzki and Gary do not emphasize the importance of using a large volume of air. Following exposure No. 6, the patient is turned prone and a barium-filled film is taken (No. 7). The patient is then returned to the supine position, and a double contrast radiograph is taken in the upright position (No. 8) to further scrutinize the upper third of the stomach. Then, the patient is given another

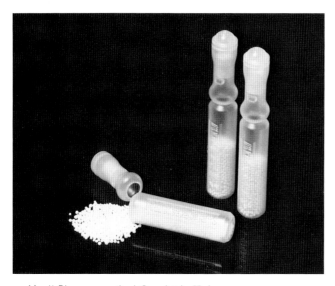
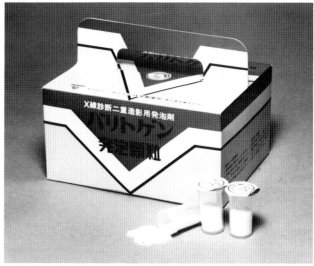

a. Horii Pharmaceutical Co., Ltd., Tokyo.   b. Fushimi-seiyaku Pharmaceutical Co., Ltd., Marugame.

Fig. 31 Photograph of effervescent granules.

mouthful of barium and flow through the cardia is observed and photographed (No. 9). I believe that sequence No. 9 is indispensable in order that cancer around the cardia not be overlooked. In countries where there is a high incidence of hiatal hernia, this procedure is performed at the beginning of the examination when the patient drinks the remainder of the barium through a large straw in the prone RAO position (Laufer and Kressel 1978), and two on one spot films are taken. For the final procedure of the routine examination, several compression pictures are taken of the stomach and duodenal bulb. The antrum and incisura are carefully examined. In the antrum attention is paid to the presence of any polypoid lesion, and two or three exposures are taken with an appropriate degree of compression for visualization of areae gastricae even when no definite abnormality is seen under fluoroscopy. Compression radiographs around the incisura are also necessary, because small ulcers or shallow depressions in this region sometimes are not visualized by double contrast radipgraphy.

Value of Fluoroscopy in the Routine Examination

It is not useful to spend much time in fluoroscopy. The sequence of exposures described above is designed in such a way as to visualize the entire stomach by the combination of a fixed number of films and positions of the patient. For this reason fluoroscopy should be used only for positioning of the patient. The emphasis in the routine examination should be placed upon interpretation of the radiographs. Modern radiographic examination of the stomach aims at film diagnosis, reducing skin dose to a minimum. However, if any abnormality is discovered, a detailed examination, including fluoroscopy is used.

Control of the Volume of Air

To obtain a good double contrast image, colonic gas should be eliminated by the preliminary administration of laxatives or by a cleansing enema early in the morning. Administration of antispasmodics usually yields good results, suppressing peristalsis and preventing outflow of barium into the duodenum. Drainage of the gastric juice is indispensable to obtain the best double contrast image (refer to the section on "Double Contrast Radiography in the Prone Position" in this chapter). If this is impossible, the examination should be started as early in the morning as possible.

Figure 32 shows the resected stomach which is incised along the greater curvature. There is a type IIc lesion measuring 30 × 30 mm on the posterior wall near the incisura. Various aspects of the lesion and the converging folds are visualized in the double contrast images (Fig. 33–35), which were taken by changing the volume of air and contrast medium through the oral gastric tube. A double

27

Case 8 Type IIc Early Cancer.

A 47-year-old man (CIH). (Figs. 32-35)

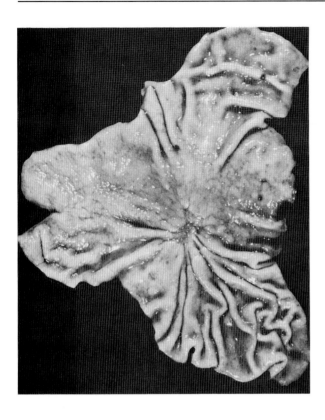

Fig. 32 Photograph of the resected specimen. Adenocarcinoma mucocellulare limited to the mucosa (m) with associated ulcer scar (UI-IIIs). The lesion is on the posterior wall of the incisura and measures 35 x 20 mm.

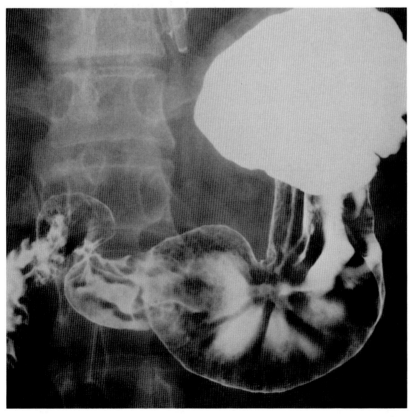

Fig. 33 Double contrast radiograph with 100 ml of barium and 200 ml of air.

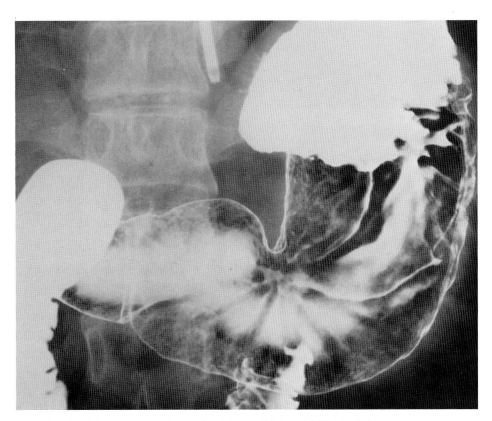

Fig. 34   Double contrast radiograph with an additional 100 ml of air.

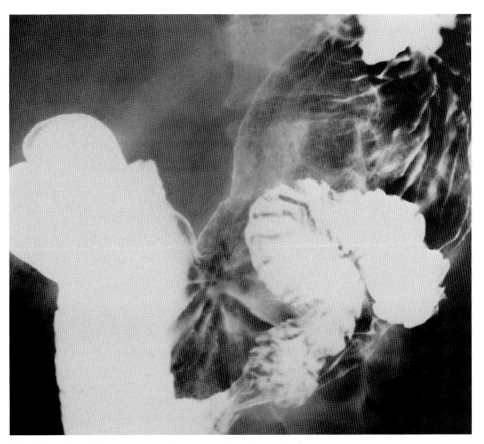

Fig. 35a   Double contrast radiograph with 200 ml of barium.

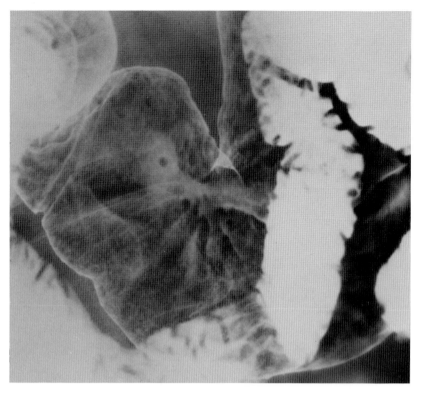

Fig. 35b Double contrast radiograph with an adtional 400 ml of air.

contrast radiograph with 100 ml of barium and 200 ml of air (Fig. 32) clearly reveals an irregular barium collection and converging folds. In this radiograph, however, the interrelationship between the depression and the converging folds is not clear due to insufficient distension of the gastric wall. Injection of an additional 100 ml of air has produced a double contrast radiograph which better demonstrates it (Fig. 34), but overdistension with 400 ml of air has almost effaced the converging folds (Fig. 35). For these double contrast radiographs different degrees of air distention, slight, moderate and extensive, are required for better visualization of the interrelationship between the converging folds and the depression itself (Frik 1973).

Double Contrast Radiography for Polypoid Early Cancer

As was emphasized by Shirakabe (1965), a polypoid lesion is best delineated by the compression method (Figs. 36, 40). Although the routine double contrast examination is able to delineate a polypoid lesion sufficiently to suggest its presence, it is not a reliable method for delineating all its aspects. The smaller the lesion the less reliable is the double contrast radiograph. On the other hand, the double contrast radiograph shows a wider diagnosable area, and includes the surrounding mucosal pattern of the polypoid lesion (Fig. 37). This becomes important in considering the histogenesis of cancer in relationship to intestinal metaplasia (Nakamura et al. 1971). At least two double contrast radiographs are taken. One in which the contrast medium is thick over protrusions (Figs. 37, 39) and the other in which the surrounding mucosal pattern is well delineated by only a slight mucosal coating (Kumakura 1969). In conclusion, the compression method and the double contrast method should always be employed together for the diagnosis of polypoid lesions. One must also pay attention to positioning when delineating a polypoid lesion by double contrast examination. In Figure 41 the proximal border of a type IIa + IIc lesion is not delineated clearly by the surrounding barium. In such a case the left anterior oblique position is best suited for delineation of the proximal border. Even the distal border becomes obscure, because the surrounding barium flows up due to the marked right anterior oblique positon shown in Figure 42.

Case 9   Type IIa + IIc Early Cancer.
A 64-year-old man (CIH). (Figs. 36-38)

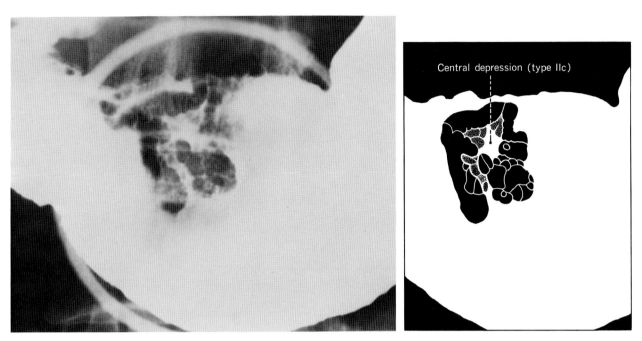

Fig. 36 Compression radiograph in the upright position is successful in demonstrating the relationship between mucosal elevation and depression.

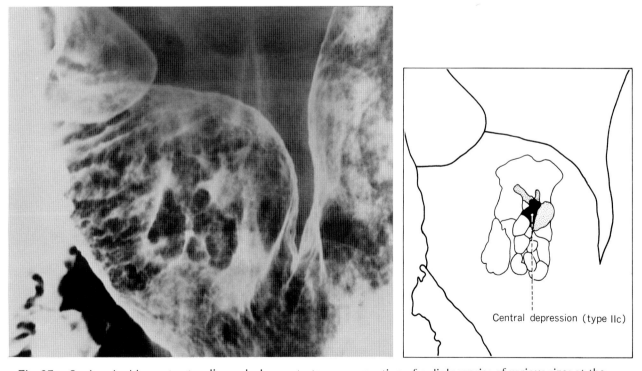

Fig. 37 Supine double contrast radiograph demonstrates an aggregation of radiolucencies of various sizes at the posterior wall of the antrum constituting a relatively large prominence of the mucosa. A faint irregular collection of barium, demonstrating a shallow depression is visualized at the right upper portion of the mucosal elevation.

31

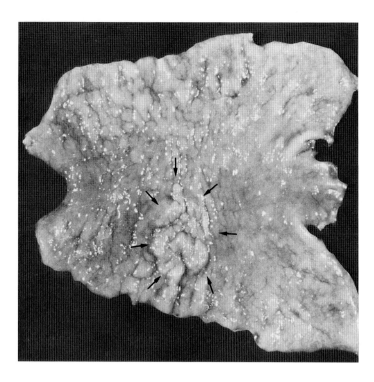

Fig. 38 Resected specimen. The lesion measures 40 x 25 mm with invasion of the submucosa (arrows). Adenocarcinoma tubulare (sm).

Case 10 Type IIa + IIc Early Cancer.
A 52-year-old man (JU). (Figs. 39 and 40)

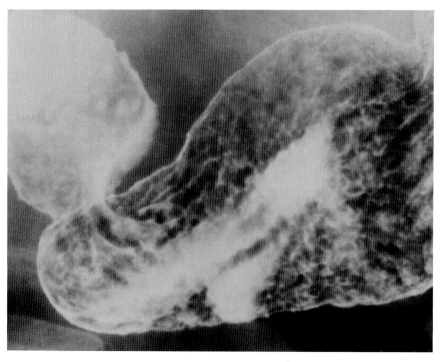

Fig. 39 Supine double contrast radiograph demonstrates an irregularly outlined radiolucency surrounding retained thin barium coating at the greater curvature aspect of the antrum. The distal margin of the posterior wall is obscure by an excess amount of retained barium and the outer, more radiolucent area seems to be prominent. The extent of the whole lesion does not correspond to the image demonstrated by compression (Fig. 40).

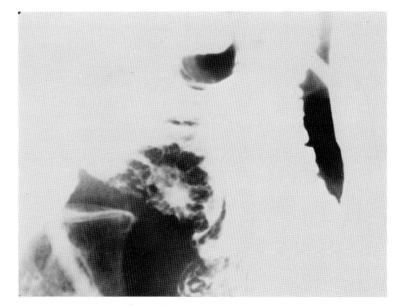

Fig. 40 Upright compression radiograph clearly demonstrates the size and the surface pattern of this lesion. The surrounding nodularity reveals an abnormal elevated mucosa and a central collection of barium which varies in density, revealing unevenness of the mucosal depression. The lesion measures 15 × 13 mm with invasion limited to the mucosa. Adenocarcinoma tubulare (m).

Case 11   Type IIa Early Cancer.
A 62-year-old man (NCCH). (Figs. 41-43)

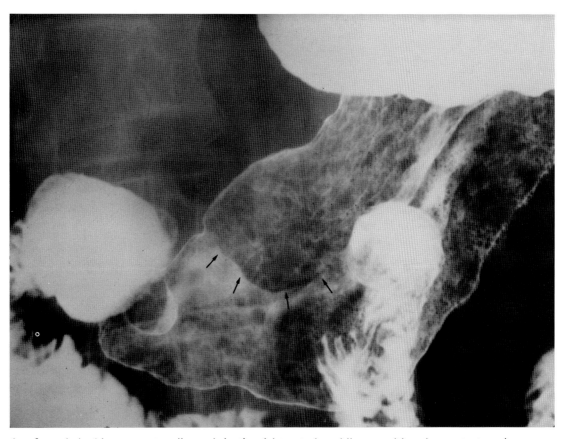

Fig. 41 Supine frontal double contrast radiograph in the right anterior oblique position demonstrates a large radiolucency on the posterior wall of the incisura. Its distal margin is outlined by thin retained barium (arrows), and its proximal margin is obscure. The surface configuration of the radiolucency is not visualized clearly.

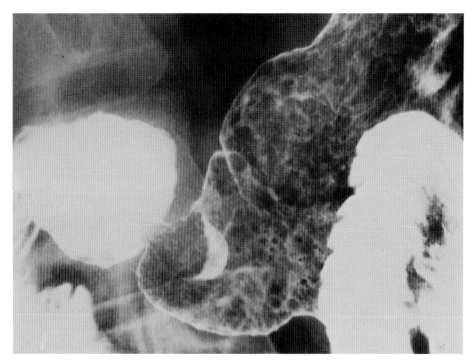

Fig. 42 In an additional double contrast radiograph of the same position as in Figure 50, even the outline of the radiolucency is obscure. The surface pattern, consisting of irregular nodularity, is demonstrated.

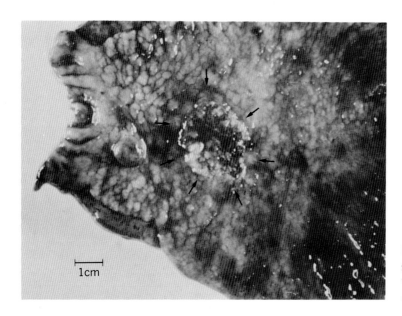

1cm

Fig. 43 Photograph of the resected specimen. The lesion measure 32 x 22 mm, with invasion into the submucosa (arrows). Adenocarcinoma mucocellulare (sm).

Double Contrast Radiography for Depressed Early Cancer

For delineation of a depression it is necessary to collect as much barium in it as possible. One must be careful to prevent the barium from spilling from the depression, which usually results from unnecessary postural change (Fig. 45). This frequently oc-

curs in depressions on the posterior wall of the incisura and the lower gastric body when a large volume of air is used and when the patient is quickly returned from the right to left decubitus position or from the supine to the left decubitus position. Accordingly, different positional changes should be performed for a depressed lesion located in this region. One double contrast radiograph is taken after the patient has been returned to the supine from the right decubitus. By this procedure the contrast medium is retained in the depression.

Case 12 Type IIc Early Cancer.

A 56-year-old man (CU). (Figs. 44 and 45)

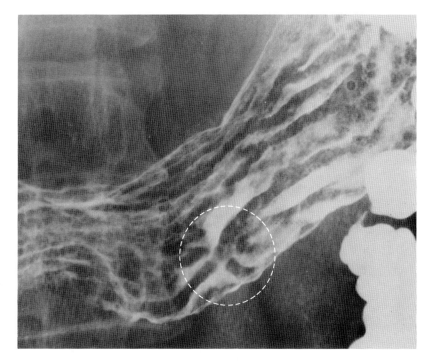

Fig. 44 Supine double contrast radiograph with a minimum amount of air demonstrated a small barium-filled erosion of type IIc with prominent converging folds. Their interrupted ends outline the erosion.

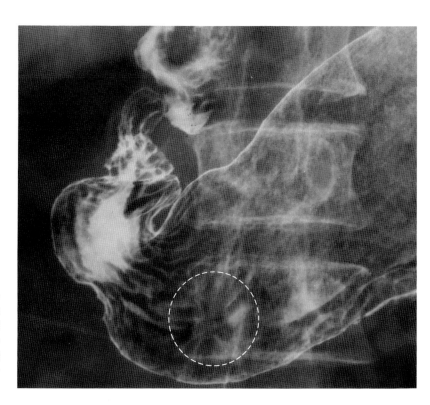

Fig. 45 Supine double contrast radiograph with moderate distension of the stomach. Distension of the stomach and superimposition upon the vertebral shadow, obscures the lesion. The converging ends of the folds are visualized as rounded translucencies.

Double Contrast Radiography in the Prone Position

This method was developed by Kumakura et al. in 1955. Kumakura succeeded in delineating two cancerous erosions (type IIc) which were located in the anterior wall of the gastric body. Before this method appeared, the mucosal relief method and the compression method were the only tools for visualization of anterior wall lesions, which nevertheless often escaped detection. Moreover, the mucosal relief method merely suggested the presence of a lesion and failed to adequately depict it. The compression method can delineate anterior

wall lesions effectively, but it cannot distinguish the anterior from the posterior wall. Moreover, the compression method cannot cover a whole lesion if it is larger than 50 mm in diameter.

The first step in prone double contrast radiography begins by the introduction of a naso-gastric or orogastric tube. After it has been confirmed that the tip of the tube is in the antrum, the patient is placed in the prone horizontal position. About 30 to 40 ml of barium is injected with a syringe and the table is tilted to a slightly head-down position. Then, the gastric contents mixed with barium drain spontaneously through the tube by a siphon effect. Deep abdominal respiration enhances this drainage. Since gastric contents interferes with the visualization of a

---

Case 13   **Type IIc Early Cancer in the Anterior Wall.**
A 43-year-old woman (CIH). (Figs. 46-51)

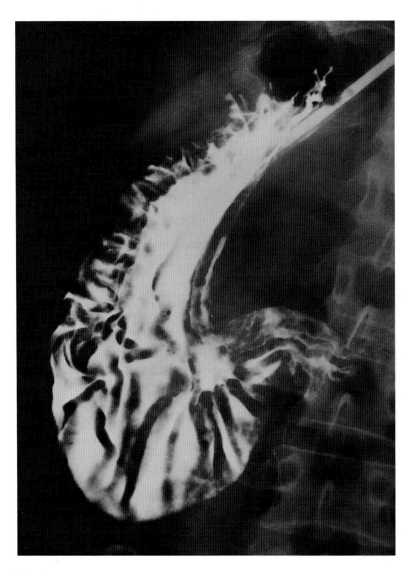

Fig. 46 Mucosal relief picture in the prone position taken just after aspiration of the gastric juice.

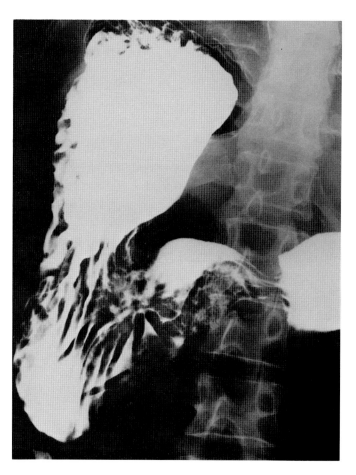

Fig. 47   Compression radiograph in the prone position with a cotton pad. 150 ml of barium was injected.

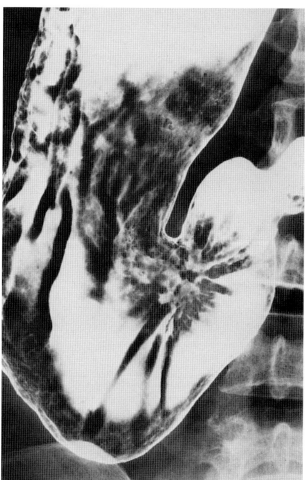

Fig. 48   Double contrast radiograph in the prone position. About 400 ml of air was injected.

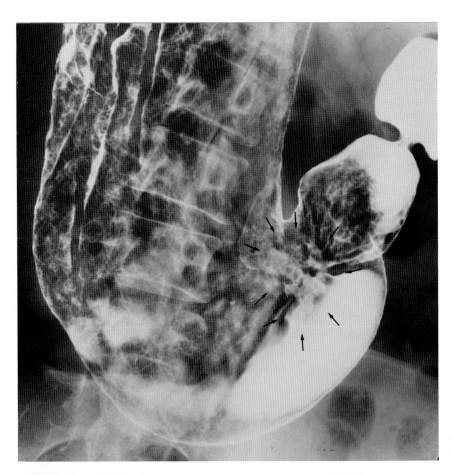

Fig. 49 Double contrast radiograph in the prone position. An additional 300 ml of air was injected.

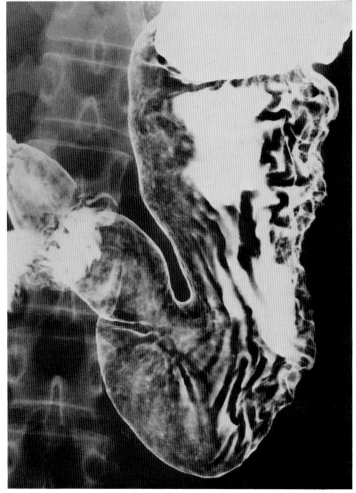

Fig. 50 Supine double contrast radiograph. About 400 ml of air was aspirated from that shown in Figure 58.

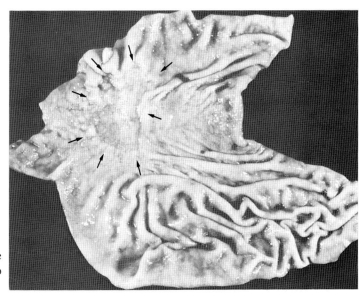

Fig. 51 Photograph of the resected specimen. The lesion measures 50 × 38 mm with invasion limited to the mucosa. Adenocarcinoma mucocellulare (m).

Case 14 Type IIc Early Cancer.
A 28-year-old man (CIH). (Figs. 52-55)

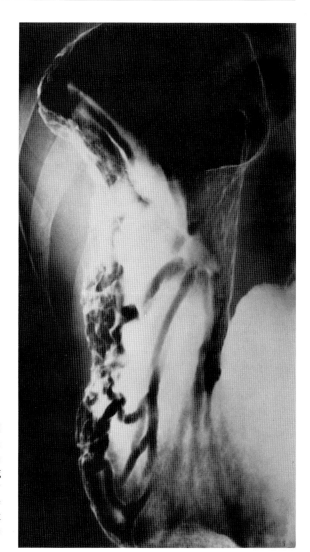

Fig. 52 Prone double contrast film with 40 ml of barium and about 300 ml of air. A faint, irregular collection of barium with convergence of the thick mucosal folds is visualized. Delineation of a barium-filled erosion and the irregular pattern of converging folds (tapering, clubbing and fusion) makes the diagnosis of early cancer easy in this image. Accordingly, this image may be satisfactory for the correct diagnosis of malignancy and, in fact, it is considered to be very effective for the first step of a routine examination which aims at picking up lesions in the anterior wall.

39

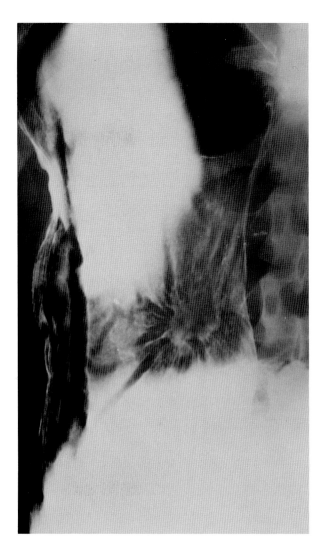

Fig. 53 Prone double contrast film with about 600 ml of air, and about 200 ml of barium, and a small cotton pad.

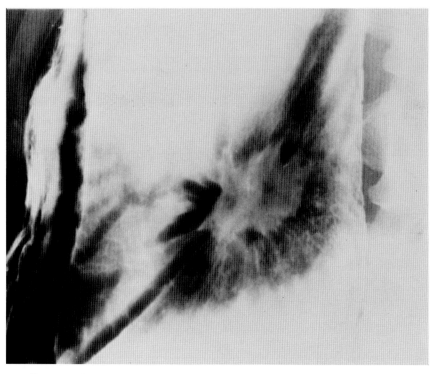

Fig. 54 Prone double contrast film with an additional 100 ml of barium, which reveals a slight difference in the quality of the image.

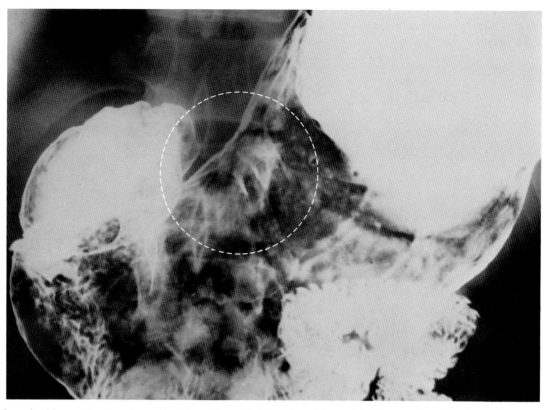

Fig. 55 Supine double contrast radiograph taken, immediately after Figure 64. It was taken in the supine frontal position and reveals a faint shadow of barium with a trace of a converging fold in the anterior wall. A slight deformity of the lesser curvature suggests long axis rotation of the stomach, bringing a part of the lesion on the line of the lesser curvature into this position.

lesion, this procedure is very important. This is especially true in the prone position, as less barium is used than in the supine position. The barium produces changing aspects of mucosal relief image in the prone position so the drainage can be observed. If the barium drains out almost completely, about 20 to 30 ml is added. A mucosal relief image is first taken in order to confirm the location of a lesion (Figs. 46—51). One must then change the volume of barium and air, depending upon the location of the lesion. If the lesion is in the anterior wall of the antrum, not more than 100 ml of barium is desirable. Air should be injected until the antrum is distended to such an extent that the anterior wall is separated from the posterior wall. Generally, 400 to 500 ml of air is necessary. The head-down position approximately 15 degrees from the horizontal and the right posterior oblique position (the right side to the patient is slightly elevated) are useful in obtaining adequate mucosal coating of the antrum.

If the lesion is located near the incisura and the body, more than 200 ml of barium gives a clear visualization. Air should be injected until both walls are completely separated. Usually, more than 600 ml of air is necessary. If the site of the lesion is higher than the middle third of the body, the semi-upright position is always effective (Figs. 52—55). If the lesion is near the incisura and in the lower body, the head-down position gives better visualization than the horizontal one. A cotton pad placed under the abdomen is very effective in obtaining a double contrast detail of the wider area around the lesion (Figs. 56, 57). Ballottement of the patient's abdomen also produces a uniform mucosal coating. Sometimes, in obese patients with cascade stomachs, a clear double contrast image is not obtained (Fig. 58). In such cases, deep abdominal repiration occassionally releases the cascade stomach. Notice the complete difference in technique between supine and prone double contrast radiography. In the former, simple positional change leads directly to an adequate mucosal coating of the posterior wall. In the latter, however, it is necessary to thin the barium layer by extensive distension of the gastric wall and by the effect of compression with a cotton pad.

41

Case 15   Type IIc Early Cancer.
A 51-year-old woman (JU). (Figs. 56 and 57)

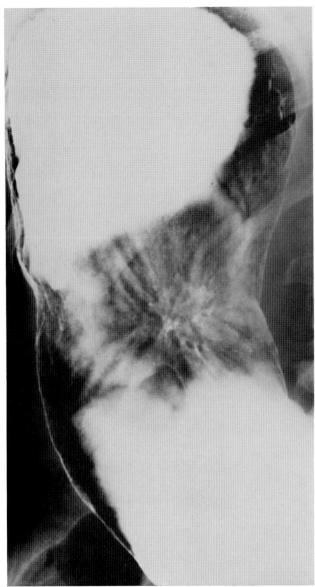

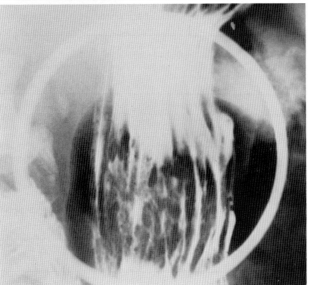

Fig. 56   Prone double contrast radiograph with compression. An irregularly barium-filled erosion is delineated effectively by a sufficient volume of barium and air. Extensive distension of the stomach by air in the presence of a moderate volume of barium has produced correct delineation of an irregular erosion, type IIc.

Fig. 57   Compression radiograph in the upright position demonstrates the erosion superimposed on the folds of the posterior wall.

Case 16   Type IIc Early Cancer.
A 53-year-old woman (JU). (Fig. 58)

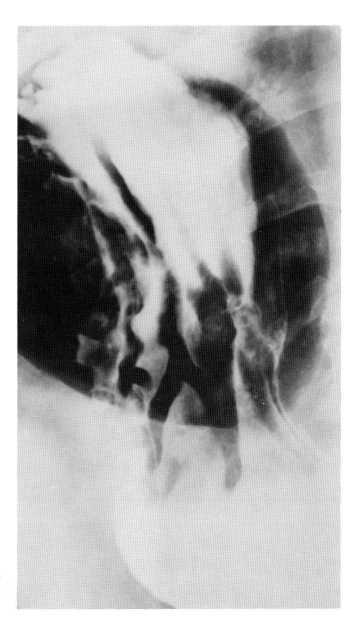

Fig. 58 Prone double contrast radiography is not effectively performed in the cascade stomach, as shown in this image.

Chapter 3

Diagnosis of Gastric Cancer

The Routine X-Ray Examination

The routine X-ray examination is performed either by darkroom fluoroscopy or by X-ray image intensification with TV. The image intensifier can either be maneuvered in the same room as the patient or remotely controlled from another room. Based upon the type of equipment, the following three methods are used clinically.

Darkroom fluoroscopy

A light-weight fluoroscopic screen makes maneuvering easy, but a poor image decreases the ability to detect lesions. X-ray image intensification with TV is better in this regard. Fluoroscopy is more effective in producing films with good radiographic detail, rather than in detecting the presence of lesions. This method is suitable for the detailed examination to reveal the nature of the lesion once its location has been identified. The compression method is easily applied to obtain sharp delineations on the films. Low-priced equipment and uncomplicated facilities are the other merits of fluoroscopy.

X-ray image intensification with TV

Maneuvering the equipment is not very different from that of darkroom fluoroscopy, but this method is now replacing it because a brighter image on the TV monitor is excellent in detecting lesions.

The advantage of these two methods is that the equipment is maneuvered at the side of the patient. Thus the patient's position is easily changed, good double contrast radiographs are obtained, and compression is readily applied. A disadvantage is the need to change film.

Remote-controlled X-ray TV method

The equipment employed in this method can be set up either in the same room as the patient or in another room and it is operated automatically. Quick positional changes of the patient are impossible, and good compression films are not obtained. Its advantages are that film changing is unnecessary (a hundred-sheet film or a roll film is used), the ability to detect lesions is excellent, and the examiner is not exposed to X-rays. Recently, darkroom fluoroscopy has gradually been replaced by X-ray TV equipment that can operate in a bright room.

1. Barium thin layer method* or mucosal relief method in the prone position for anterior wall lesions.

   ↓

   (Filming of the esophagus in the upright right anterior oblique position)

   ↓

2. Barium-filled film of the stomach in the upright frontal position.

   ↓

3. Barium-filled film in the prone position.

   ↓

4. Double contrast film in the supine position.

   Frontal

   ↓

   Right anterior oblique

   ↓

   Left anterior oblique

   ↓

5. Double contrast film in the semi-upright left anterior oblique position.

   ↓

6. Upright, right anterior oblique position.

   ↓

7. Compression film in the upright position.

   *Refer to footnote in Chapter 2 (see page 24).

Fig. 59   Sequence of radiographic filming in the routine examination of the stomach.

Aside from the advantages and disadvantages mentioned above, the two types of X-ray equipment show no significant difference in detecting lesions. If there is any difference, it lies in the quality of the radiograph, which is influenced by the skill of the examiner. In other words, sensitivity in detecting lesions depends on the skill of the examiner.

Figure 59 shows the method of filming the stomach, beginning with the thin-layer method or mucosal relief method for the anterior wall. Some 10 to 12 films are taken, including films of the esophagus. The filming proceeds in the order shown by the arrows (the details on the sequence of X-ray exposure are described in chapter 2).

Detection of Early Gastric Cancer by the Routine X-ray Examination

Figure 60 shows 740 cases (806 lesions) of histologically proven early gastric cancer detected and operated on in four institutions in the period from 1959 to 1977. The result of the study is shown in Figure 61. In 695 lesions of single early gastric cancer, 72 lesions (10.4%) were not detected by the X-ray examination. The X-ray examination also failed to detect 39 of 111 lesions (35.1%) that were subsequently detected by endoscopy or on the resected specimens. Table 16 is the analysis

Table 16 Detection of early gastric cancer in four institutions* (1959–1977).

	Single early cancer	Multiple early cancers	Total
Detected by radiographic examination	623 (89.6%)	72 (64.9%)	695 (86.2%)
Detected by endoscopy	55 (7.9%)	16 (14.4%)	71 (8.8%)
Overlooked by both methods	17 (2.5%)	23 (20.7%)	40 (5.0%)
Total	695 (100%)	111 (100%)	806 (100%)

*First Department of Internal Medicine, Chiba University.
 Department of Gastroenterology, Juntendo University.
 Chiba Prefectural Cancer Center.
 Tokyo Metropolitan Cancer Detection Center.

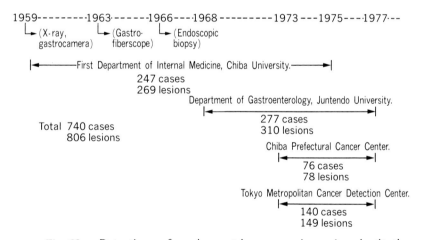

Fig. 60 Detection of early gastric cancer in various institutions.

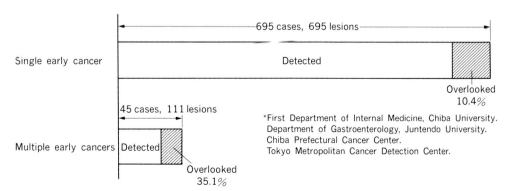

Fig. 61 Number of early gastric cancers overlooked in the routine radiographic examination in four institutions* (1959–1977).

of those cases in which the sites of the lesions were correctly identified. In 695 lesions of single early gastric cancer the X-ray examination detected 623 lesions (89.6%) and endoscopy detected another 55 lesions (7.9%). Seventeen lesions (2.5%) were undetected by both the X-ray and endoscopic examinations but were discovered incidentally during surgery for other reasons and confirmed histologically. The detection rate of multiple gastric cancers is worse. Seventy-two of 111 lesions

(64.9%) were detected by the X-ray examination and 16 lesions (14.4%) by endoscopy. Both examinations failed to detect 23 lesions (20.7%).

Of the total 806 lesions, 695 (86.2%) were detected by the X-ray examination and another 71 (8.8%) by endoscopy. Forty lesions (5.0%) were undetected by either examination. In summary, about 10 to 15 per cent of early gastric cancers are undetected by the X-ray examination.

Case 17   Type IIc Early Cancer.
A 38-year-old man (TH). (Figs. 62 and 63)

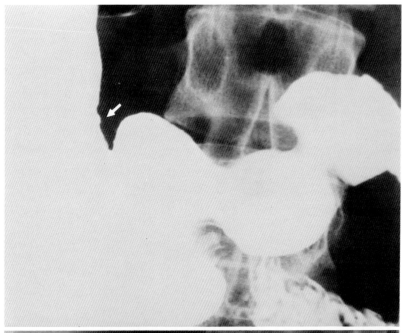

Fig. 62   Barium-filled film shows an irregularity of the incisura.

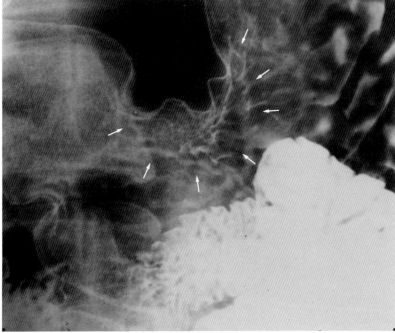

Fig. 63   Double contrast film shows mucosal abnormality around the deformed incisura.

Double contrast radiography is most important in the routine X-ray examination because of its ability to detect early gastric cancer. Figures 62 and 63 show early gastric cancer detected by the routine X-ray examination. In this case the lesion is situated on both sides of the lesser curvature. On the barium-filled film (Fig. 62) there is an irregularity of the margin. On the double contrast radiograph (Fig. 63) appears an irregular granularity, radiolucency on the proximal side, interrupted mucosal folds and irregularity of the incisura. Early gastric cancer saddling the incisura, as in this case, can often be found as an irregularity of the marginal contour on the barium-filled film, and can be detected by interpreting the marginal findings carefully. But double contrast films are more important than barium-filled films, since quite often the marginal contour of the lesion is not well delineated.

The greater and the lesser curvatures are infrequently involved in early gastric cancer.

The case shown in Figures 64 and 65 is detected only by double contrast radiography in the supine position. The marginal contour does not reveal the lesion, which is limited in the posterior wall, but is easily detected on the double contrast film. Both the barium-filled film and the double contrast films are unsuccessful in disclosing a lesion in the anterior wall. The size and location of lesions of single early cancer which were undetected by the routine X-ray examination but detected by endoscopy are shown in Figure 66. Twenty-seven of 55 lesions were located in the anterior wall. Lesions situated along the lesser curvature side of the antrum near the pylorus are frequently missed. Appreciable numbers of early cancer cases will become detectable by utilizing compression to the antrum as part of a routine examination.

The lesions undetected by both X-ray examination and endoscopy are shown in Figure 67. They were undetected because they were multiple lesions associated with a larger one such as advanced gastric cancer, which overshadowed them. This is

---

Case 18 **Type IIc Early Cancer.**
A 42-year-old woman (NCCH). (Figs. 64 and 65)

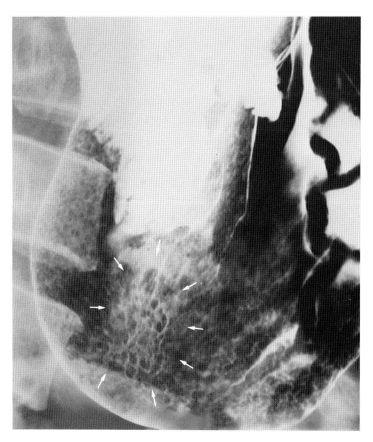

Fig. 64   Double contrast radiograph demonstrates granularity of the mucosa.

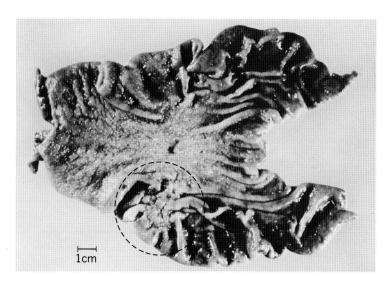

Fig. 65 Resected specimen.

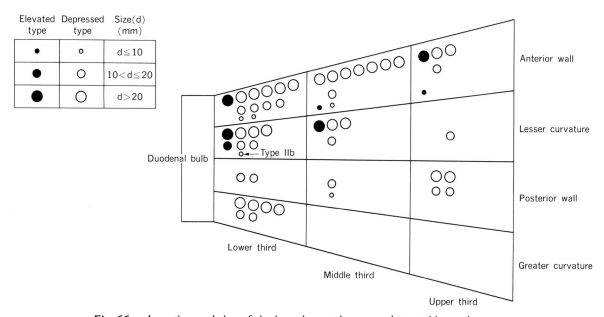

Fig. 66 Location and size of single early gastric cancer detected by endoscopy.

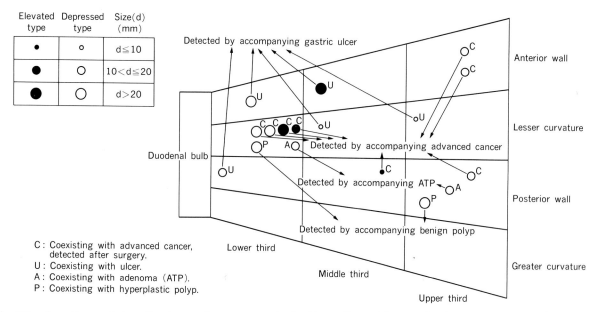

C : Coexisting with advanced cancer, detected after surgery.
U : Coexisting with ulcer.
A : Coexisting with adenoma (ATP).
P : Coexisting with hyperplastic polyp.

Fig. 67 Location and size of early gastric cancer overlooked by radiographic examination and endoscopy (17 lesions).

48

proved by the fact that 8 of the 17 lesions were resected for advanced cancer.

An early cancer detected by the barium thin-layer method in the prone position is shown in Figures 68–72. Neither the barium-filled film (Fig. 68) nor the double contrast radiograph on the supine position (Fig. 69) could reveal the lesion. Figure 70 is the film taken with the thin layer method in the prone position. When light compression was applied, the lesion appeared clearly. Frequently a supine double contrast radiograph with good barium coating discloses a lesion on the anterior wall. Figures 73–76 show such a lesion on the anterior wall detected on the double contrast radiograph in the supine position. The configuration of the converging folds in the lower portion of the gastric body (Fig. 73) is discernible as thinly

coated barium shadows. They are not as clear as the folds of the posterior wall. There is a collection of barium in the center which is the shadow of barium-coated erosion at the center of the converging folds of the anterior wall. The detailed examination of the double contrast radiograph in the prone position revealed a prominence in the center of the depressed lesion, as shown in Figure 74. The lesion is surrounded by a shallow collection of barium (erosion), from where the converging folds start. The folds are interrupted in an irregular shape. A comparison of the X-ray films with the resected specimen demonstrates that the films reproduced the precise macroscopic findings. The diagnosis established by the histological examination was of an early cancer limited to the mucosa.

Case 19   Type IIc Early Cancer.
A 34-year-old man (JU). (Figs. 68-72)

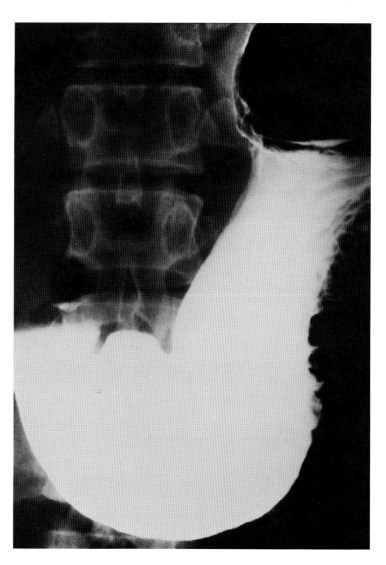

Fig. 68   Barium-filled film.

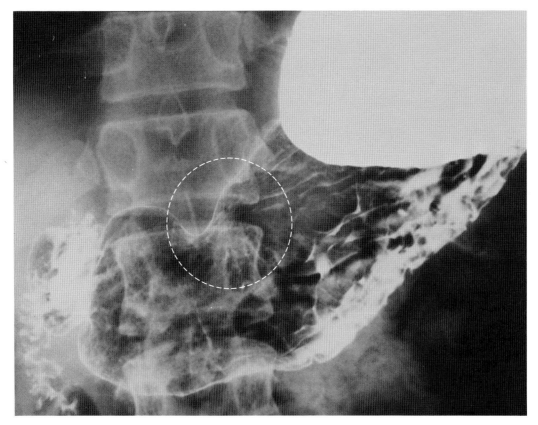

Fig. 69   Supine double contrast film.

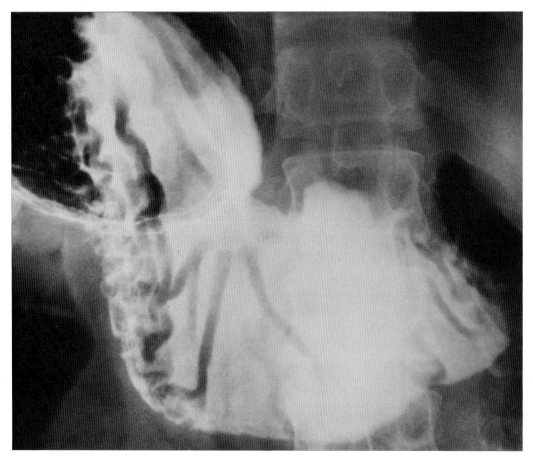

Fig. 70   Radiograph in the prone position using the thin layer method.

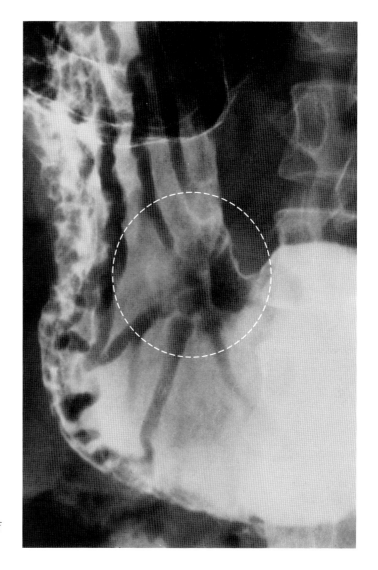

Fig.71 Prone double contrast radiograph of type IIc early cancer.

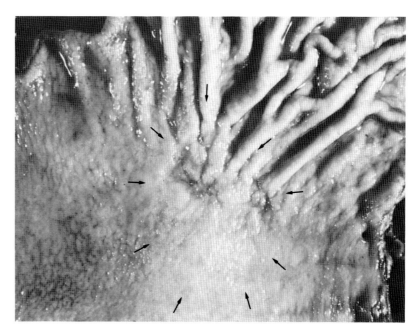

Fig. 72 Resected specimen.

Case 20   Type IIc Early Cancer.
A 57-year-old man (CPCC). (Figs. 73-76)

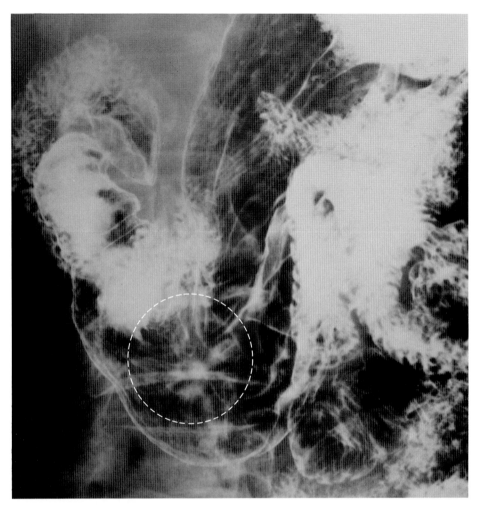

Fig. 73   Double contrast film shows converging folds.

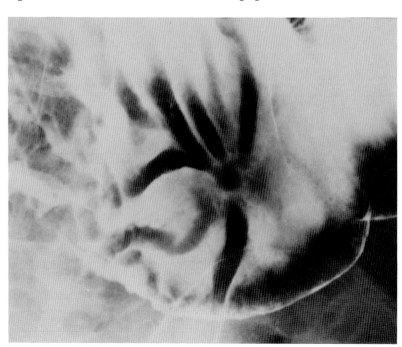

Fig. 74   Prone double contrast film shows a prominence in the center of the depression.

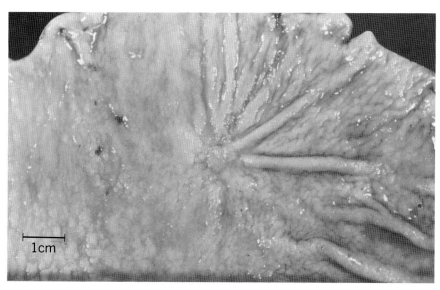

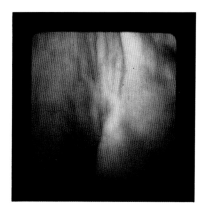

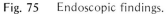

1cm

Fig. 75   Endoscopic findings.   Fig. 76   The resected specimen.

Detailed X-ray Examination

As soon as a lesion is discovered by fluoroscopy, the detailed examination is performed. The detailed examination is often necessary when endoscopy or biopsy reveals a lesion which is malignant or malignant-suspect, and gastric endoscopy is performed when lesions are detected or suspected by the routine X-ray examination. Detailed X-ray films can be obtained because the location of the lesion has already been identified. According to the location and the configuration of a lesion, the concentration of barium, the volume of air and barium for double contrast radiography, application of compression and changing the body position are adjusted individually in order to produce good radiographic details. Sometimes, such high-quality films reveal subtle changes better than macroscopic examination of a resected specimen. They are especially helpful in deciding the extent of infiltration and the depth of invasion, and they can delineate minute early cancers, as small as 5 mm in diameter, as an elevation or a depression of the surface. Endoscopic diagnosis is based upon changes in color, but radiographic diagnosis is based upon the elevation or depression of the surface. Since better delineation of a subtle elevation or depression is produced on an X-ray film, it gives better comparison with the resected specimen. Its superiority is attested to, for example, by the fact that endoscopy is able to detect changes in "areae gastricae" only with the help of the dye-spraying method (see Chapter 14).

The use of antispasmodics aids in the detailed examination of the stomach. Usually 20 to 40 mg of Coliopan (commercial name in Japan) is given 5 minutes prior to the examination except to patients for whom such medicine is contraindicated.

Elevated lesions and depressed lesions

Most of the elevated lesions (types I, IIa, IIa + IIc) measure less than 50 mm in diameter. The majority is between 20 and 30 mm in diameter. The compression method can reveal the entire aspect of a lesion. Although a large diagnosable area of the double contrast radiograph suffices for the detection of an elevated lesion, it is easily discovered by X-ray TV when compression is applied at the end of routine filming. Sometimes the compression method successfully detects a small lesion in the anterior wall or in the antrum and is qualitatively superior to double contrast radiography.

The compression method is effective with elevated lesions in the antrum, which is a frequent site of occurrence, while lesions in the upper portion of the stomach are better evaluated by the double contrast method, providing a good barium coating is present.

A good film of elevated lesions should be produced to disclose the size, height, configuration (broad based or pedunculated), and the nature of the mucosal surface (Yamada-Fukutomi's classification, see Fig. 140 in Chapter 4).

Differential diagnosis is possible with high-quality radiographs; it can determine whether the

53

lesion is benign, ATP (refer to Chapter 5), or malignant; epithelial or non-epithelial; polypoid, type I early cancer or flat, type IIa early cancer; small Borrmann type 2 or type IIa + IIc early cancer with central depression or ulceration. Depth of invasion can be determined as well.

Type IIa early cancer of a flat elevation is shown in Figures 77–79. Located on the posterior wall, it is well delineated on both the compression film and the double contrast radiograph. The contour of the elevation and the shallow central depression, however, are better delineated on the compression film. The nature of the depressed lesions is best described by double contrast radiography. As most of the cases of depressed early cancers are associated with the erosive area affected by type IIc cancer, its shallow depression must be delineated by double contrast radiography. An exception is ulcerating cancer of Hauser type (type III early cancer), which is a large area covered with open ulcer (see page 129). Compression method is effective in this case.

In order to produce high-quality films for the diagnosis of a depressed lesion, the following procedure is observed. Gastric juice and mucus should be removed from the mucosal surface by a quick change of the body position; at the same time the surface should be well coated by barium while double contrast radiographs are taken. Two kinds of double contrast radiographs, one with a fairly large amount of air to extend the mucosal surface and the other with a moderate amount of air to delineate the mucosal folds, are most helpful. A compression film is indispensable when the lesion has a large open ulcer, especially when the major area of the lesion is occupied by a deep depression.

Case 21   Type IIa Early Cancer.
A 41-year-old man (CU). (Figs. 77-79)

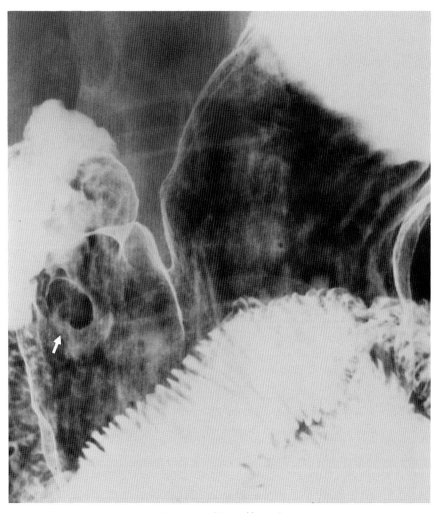

Fig. 77   Double contrast radiograph of type IIa early cancer.

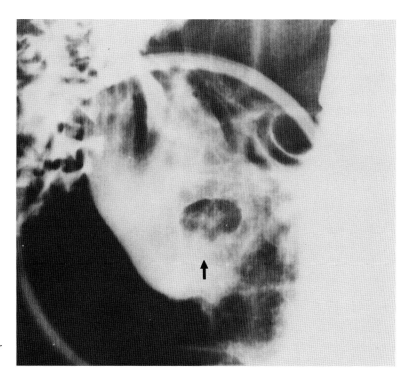

Fig. 78 Compression film shows the contour of the elevation.

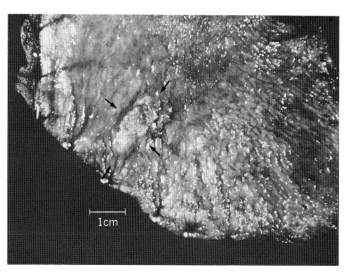

Fig. 79 Resected specimen. The lesion measures 15 × 27 mm.

The differential diagnosis of a depressed lesion is based upon the following findings: the form and the size of the lesion, its depth, the granularity in its depression and the nature of its borders and of the mucosal folds surrounding of the lesion, as well as of the remaining normal mucosa. With deep depressions, the nature of the contour, the nature of the mucosal folds and a shallow erosion surrounding the ulcer should be studied carefully on the compression film. Once the lesion is diagnosed as malignant, the extent of infiltration and depth of invasion should be studied. This is vital for the surgeon, who, without this information, sometimes cannot determine the proximal incision line of the stomach. Lesions with a deep depression (types III, III + IIc) are not easily differentiated from benign peptic ulcer. X-ray films with characteristic findings are most reliable for diagnosing depressed early cancer.

Figures 80 and 81 show type IIc early cancer. A benign ulcer scar coexists in the gastric body. It is essential to differentiate malignancy and benignancy of the upper lesion (arrow) and to define the extent of infiltration of the lower lesion in early cancer. The double contrast radiograph is better able to reveal the extent of infiltration than the resected specimen in this case.

Case 22 Type IIc + III Early Cancer and Ulcer scar.
A 56-year-old woman (JU). (Figs. 80 and 81)

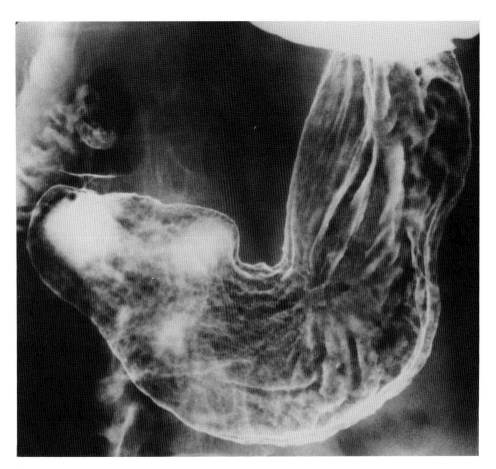

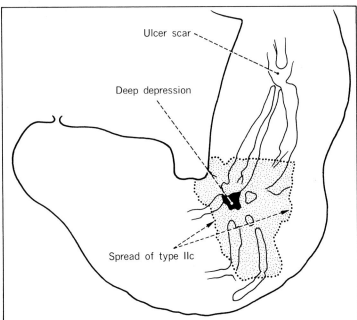

Fig. 80 Double contrast film of type IIc cancer.

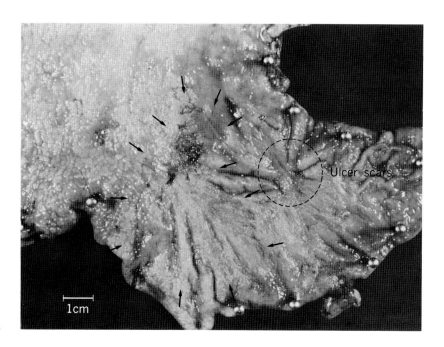

Fig. 81   Resected specimen.

Location of the lesion and its diagnosis

In order to obtain films of good quality, careful filming technique is important. Attention should be paid to the lesions in the upper third (the cardia and fundus), to those in the greater curvature, and to those in the pylorus. Early cancer, when comparatively small, is not easily diagnosed in these locations. When the lesion has extended toward the posterior wall, diagnosis is easily made only by the double contrast radiograph in the supine position.

Lesion in the anterior wall (see also Chapter 2)

In the routine examination, the patient takes 30 to 50 ml of barium (50 % w/v), and filming is started in the prone position with a slight compression. In the detailed examination a better anterior wall picture is obtained with barium of higher density. Effervescent powder is not as good as air injected through a gastric tube. If a tube is used it is introduced into the antrum and excessive gastric juice is removed. The patient is turned prone, and 50 to 70 ml of barium, with a concentration of 100 to 120 % w/v and a fairly large amount of air (300 to 400 ml), is introduced. A good film will be produced to reveal the lesion, but slight compression with a thin pillow will improve the detail. Administration of antispasmodics is indispensable. The barium-filled compression film in the upright or the prone

position reveals the lesion well. Even if a definitive diagnosis is made by this film, the double contrast radiograph of the anterior wall is necessary, since it provides a larger diagnosable area and effectively reveals type IIc lesions without converging folds, which the compression method often cannot do. It also produces a picture similar to the macroscopic findings of the resected specimen, just as do lesions in the posterior wall on the double contrast radiograph in the supine position.

Figures 71, 72 and 73–76 show type IIc early cancer in the anterior wall. The nature of the lesion is very well revealed on the double contrast radiograph in the prone position.

Type IIc early cancer in the anterior wall of the antrum is shown in Figures 82–85. Figure 82 is the double contrast radiograph in the prone position with a large amount of air. Figure 84 was filmed with a small amount of air and compression. The erosive area and the extent of the lesion are better discernible on the former film, as are posterior wall lesions, while the nature of the folds is better discernible on the latter, as slight compression improves visualization of minute elevations and depressions. When the resected specimen is well distended, it is identical to the former picture; and when it is fixed with minimal distension to present the nature of the folds, it is identical to the latter. The former is suited to visualization of depression, and the latter to analysis of the changes of the folds.

Case 23   Type IIc + III Early Cancer.
A 57-year-old man (JU). (Figs. 82-85)

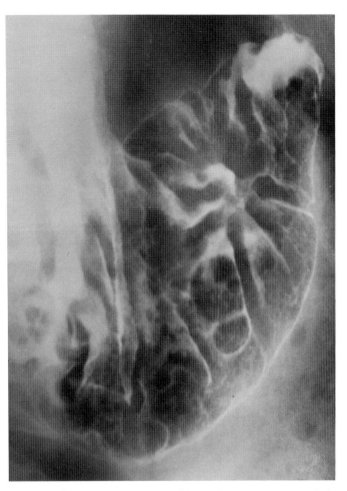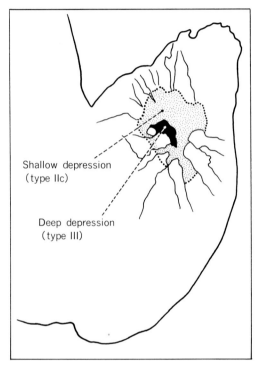

Shallow depression
(type IIc)

Deep depression
(type III)

Fig. 82   Prone double contrast film with a large amount of air.

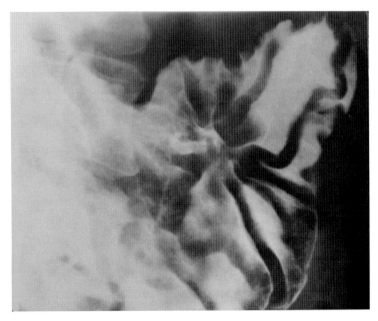

Fig. 83   Radiograph taken with a small amount of air and compression.

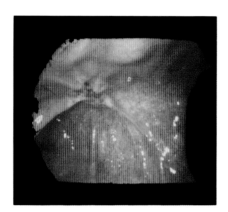

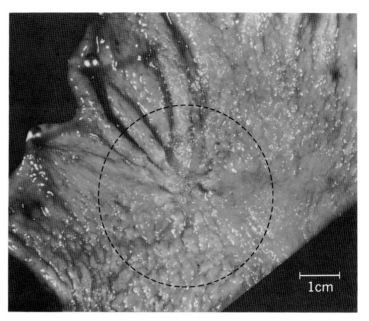

Fig. 84   Endoscopic findings.

Fig. 85   Resected specimen (type IIc Early Cancer). Peptic ulcer (type III portion) healed at the time of surgery.

Lesion in the pylorus

Early cancer near the pylorus is often undetectable, except for cases associated with a marked change such as pyloric stricture. This is because lesions near the pylorus are difficult to visualize as a double contrast image, because anatomic location and changes near the pyloric ring are perplexing, and because an associated ulcer often narrows the antrum.

The barium-filled film of Figure 86 reveals the changes of pyloric stenosis. The compression film is better than the double contrast image in visualizing the lesion. Figures 86—90 show type IIc early cancer in the anterior wall of the pylorus. The lesion is easily detected on the barium-filled film in the upright position (Fig. 86). The finding of deep, irregular erosion suggests malignancy on the double contrast radiograph in the prone position with compression (Fig. 87). The approximate extent of the lesion is discernible on the double contrast radiograph in the supine position (Fig. 88). Each of these three different findings are shown on the three radiographs.

Lesion in the greater curvature

There is a tendency not to pay much attention to the greater curvature because of a lower incidence of lesions compared with the lesser curvature. Also, lesions in the body pass undetected due to prominent mucosal folds, which make visualization extremely difficult.

It still holds true that lesions on the greater curvature are more likely to be malignant (see page 285).

A markedly lower incidence of benign ulcer is found on the greater curvature compared with the lesser curvature. Recent diagnostic developments have made ulcers in the greater curvature (mostly a small ulcer or a scar) detectable. Still, the high incidence of malignancy persists.

When a lesion is situated in an area of prominent mucosal folds on the greater curvature side, the folds should be distended with a large volume of air to produce a diagnostic double contrast radiograph. Unless the lesion is in the uppermost portion of the stomach, a compression film should be taken to reveal its nature.

Differential diagnosis between type IIc early cancer and linitis plastica without contraction of the stomach is not easily made in the thick folds of the greater curvature of the body, which is a favorite site for the latter. Attention must be given to the analysis of the nature of the mucosal folds and the pliability of the contour.

Figures 91—94 show a type IIc early cancer in the antrum on the greater curvature. The compression image reveals its nature well.

Figures 95—98 show a type IIc early cancer in the body on the greater curvature. The barium-filled film of Figure 95 discloses a small indentation of the greater curvature. This film alone suggests the lesion's malignancy. The lesion

Case 24 Type IIc Early Cancer.
A 52-year-old man (CU). (Figs. 86-89)

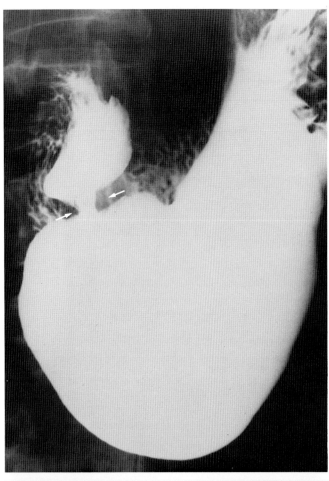

Fig. 86   Upright barium-filled film of type IIc cancer.

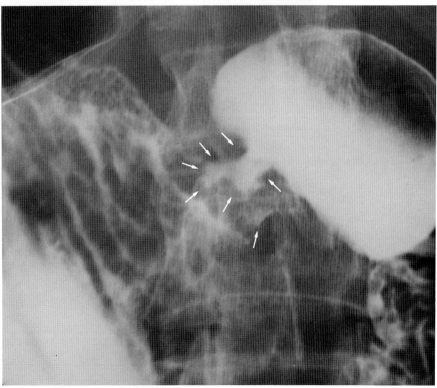

Fig. 87 Prone double contrast film with compression.

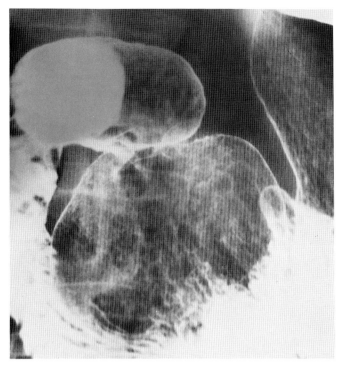

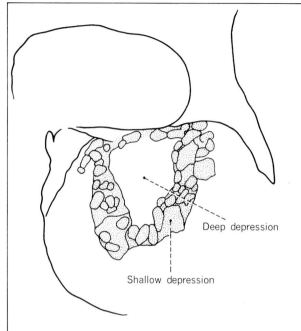

Fig. 88   Supine double contrast film.

Deep depression

Shallow depression

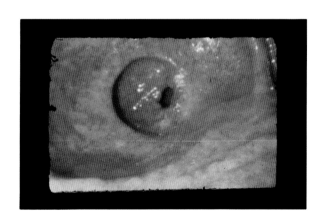

Fig. 89   Endoscopic findings.

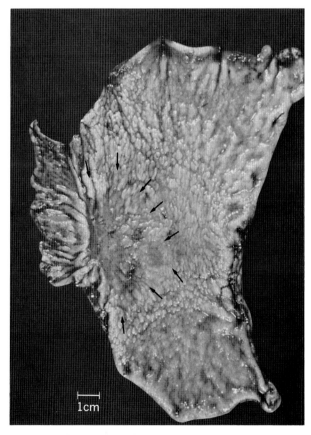

1cm

Fig. 90   Resected specimen.

Case 25 Type IIc Early Cancer.

A 70-year-old woman (JU). (Figs. 91-94)

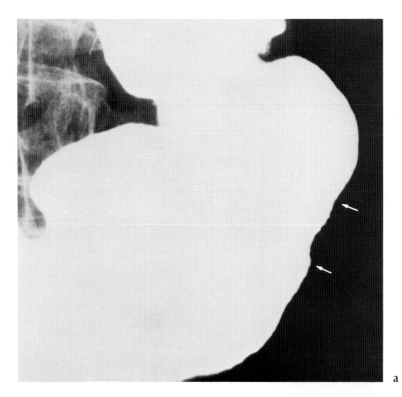

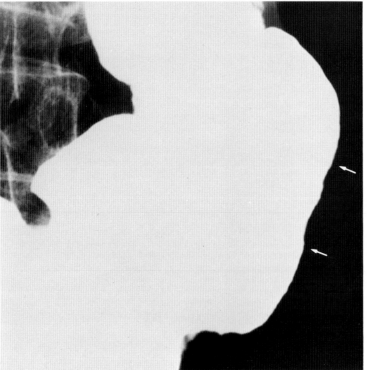

Fig. 91 a and b Prone barium-filled radiographs of type IIc early cancer.

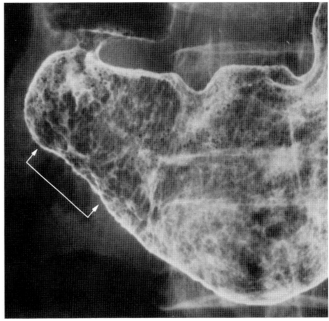

Fig. 92   Double contrast film.

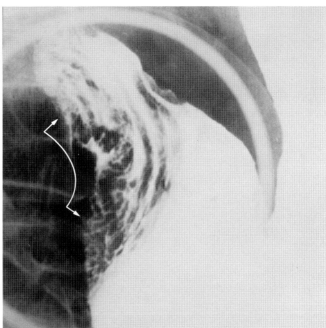

Fig. 93   Compression film.

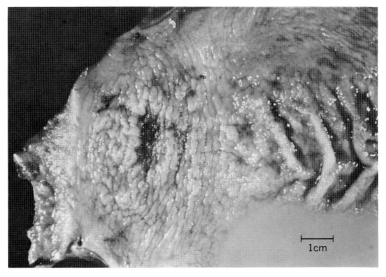

Fig. 94   Resected specimen.

Case 26   Type IIc Early Cancer.
A 44-year-old man (NCCH). (Figs. 95-98)

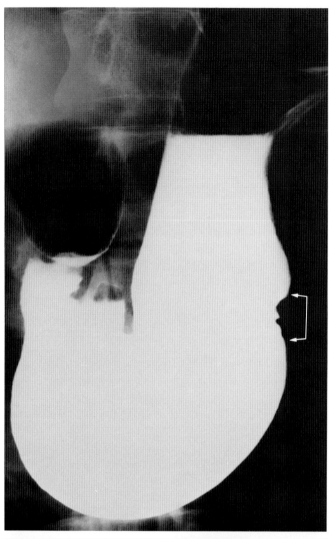

Fig. 95   Barium-filled film reveals a small indentation on the greater curvature (type IIc cancer).

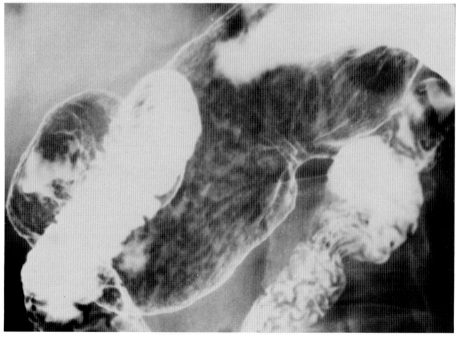

Fig. 96   Left anterior oblique double contrast film.

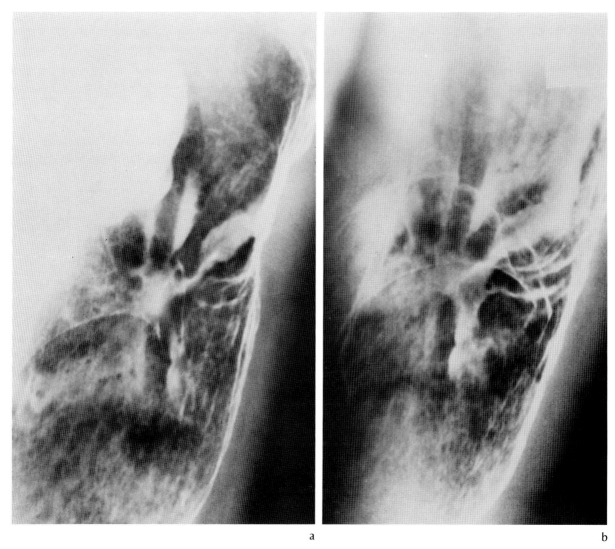

a   b

Fig. 97 a and b Right anterior oblique double contrast radiographs.

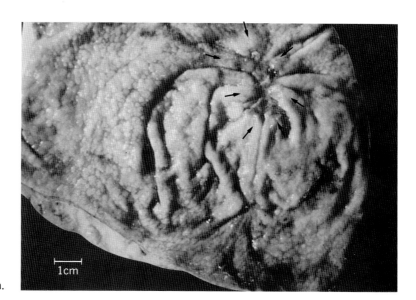

Fig. 98 Resected specimen.

shifts a little toward the anterior wall on the double contrast radiograph in the left anterior oblique position, as shown in Figure 96. It is demonstrated en face on the posterior wall as shown in Figure 97a and b in the right anterior oblique with head-down position, revealing the nature of the lesion and the extent of the infiltration. The diagnosis is easily made on the basis of these findings.

Lesions in the upper portion of the stomach

The poor demonstrability of a lesion in the upper portion of the stomach makes it difficult to detect cancer in its early stage in this location.

The following procedure is suggested to obtain good radiographs: Change the patient's body position frequently to wash the mucosal surface with barium; take the double contrast radiographs in the upright right anterior oblique position and in the semi-upright left anterior oblique position. Filming of the esophagus after the passage of barium is also necessary to study the relation between the cardia and the lesion.

Figures 99—103 show a type IIa elevated early cancer in the anterior wall of the cardia. Figures 104—108 show a type IIc early cancer in the anterior wall of the fundus. The nature of an elevated lesion is revealed easily, providing there is good barium coating, while the nature of the folds of a depressed lesion varies according to the volume of air or the degree of compression. With a large volume of air the mucosa is distended, as shown in Figure 104, to reveal the elements of cancerous ulcer. With a smaller volume of air, as shown in Figure 106, the nature of the folds is well demonstrated.

Case 27　Type IIa Early Cancer.
A 60-year-old man (CU). (Figs. 99-103)

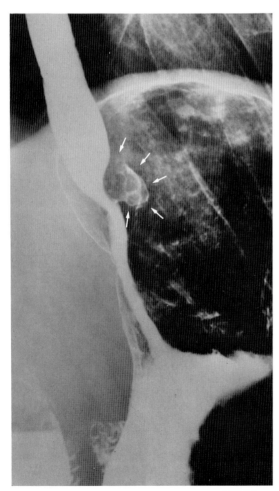

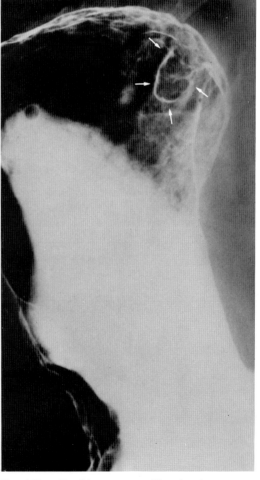

Fig. 99　Double contrast film of type IIa early cancer.

Fig. 100　Double contrast film in the prone position.

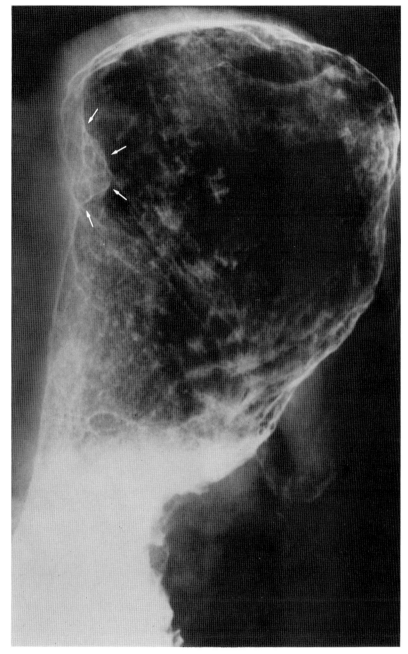

Fig. 101   Double contrast film in the upright position.

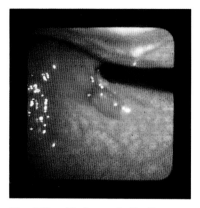

Fig. 102   Endoscopic findings.

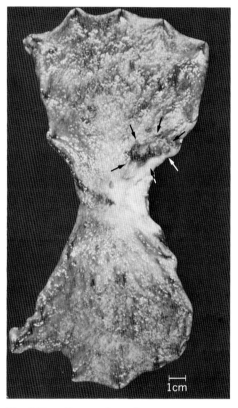

Fig. 103   Resected specimen.

Case 28 Type IIc Early Cancer.
A 65-year-old man (JU), (Figs. 104-108)

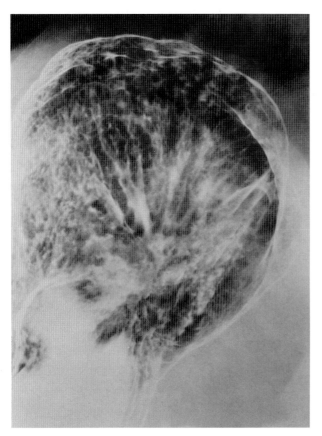

Fig. 104 Double contrast film in the prone position with a large amount of air.

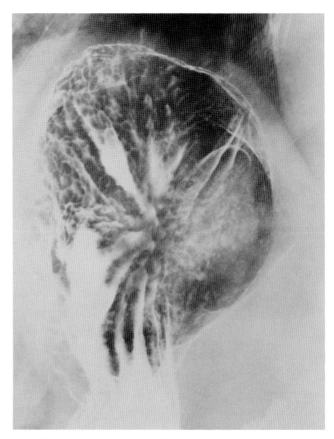

Fig. 105 Double contrast film in the prone position with a moderate amount of air.

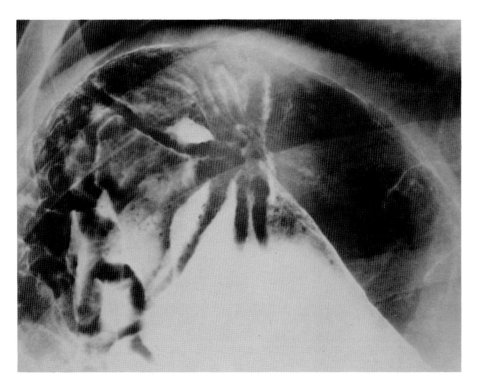

Fig. 106 Double contrast film in the prone position with a small amount of air.

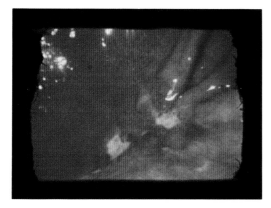

Fig. 107   Endoscopic findings.

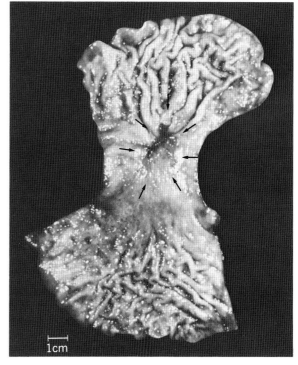

Fig. 108   Resected specimen.

Diagnosis according to the size of the lesion

A lesion's size, type and site affect its detectability. Lesions measuring 10 mm or more in diameter generally can be detected. An exception is the superficial flat type of cancer (type IIb), which will be discussed below. Detailed examinations can detect superficial lesions (types IIa and IIc) as small as 5 mm in diameter. Not only the size but also the height or depth of elevation or depression determines the lesion's demonstrability at the routine and the detailed examination (Refer to the section on Detection of Early Gastric Cancer by the Routine X-ray Examination in this chapter).

Case 29   Type IIa Early Cancer.
A 55-year-old man (CU). (Figs. 109-112)

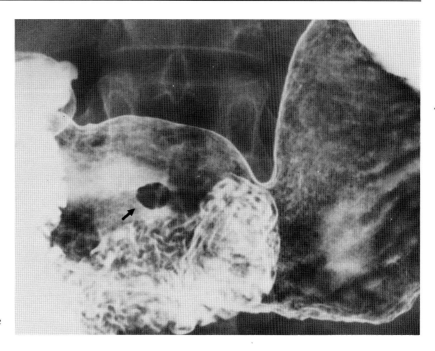

Fig. 109   Double contrast film of type IIa early cancer.

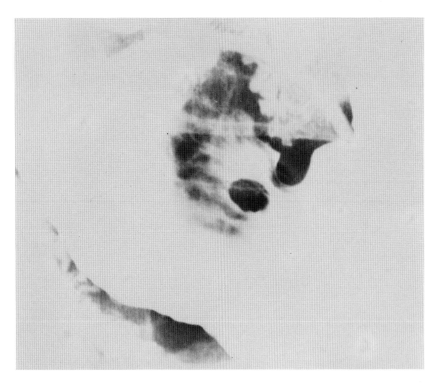

Fig. 110   Compression film.

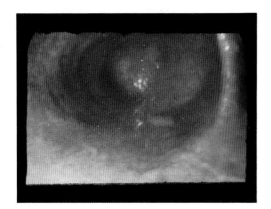

Fig. 111   Endoscopic findings.

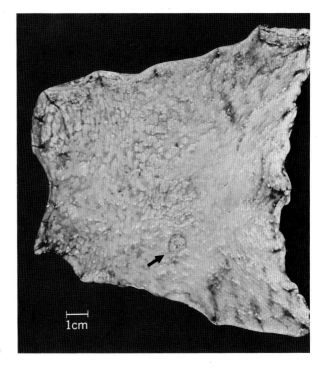

1cm

Fig. 112   Resected specimen.

Figures 109–112 show a type IIa early cancer measuring less than 10 mm in diameter. This is an example in which the differential diagnosis of malignancy and benignancy is difficult.

Figures 113–116 show a type IIc early cancer measuring about 7 mm in diameter. Macroscopic findings of the resected specimen barely reveal the lesion. It was detected by endoscopy and demonstrated only on the compression film.

As seen above, it is not difficult to reveal elevated lesions, even if they are less than 10 mm in diameter. On the contrary, depressed lesions (type IIc) having very shallow erosive changes without mucosal convergence or elevation around the lesion may be difficult to demonstrate when they measure less than 10 mm in diameter.

Case 30 Type IIc Early Cancer.
A 38-year-old man (CU). (Figs. 113-116)

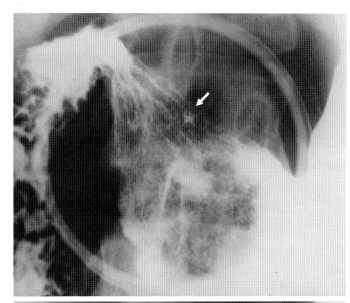

Fig. 113 Compression film demonstrates 7mm type IIc early cancer.

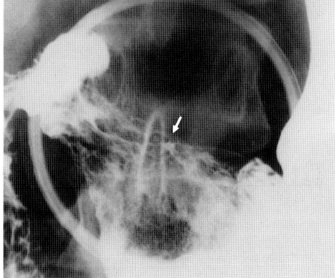

Fig. 114 Compression film

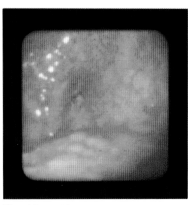

Fig. 115 Endoscopic findings.

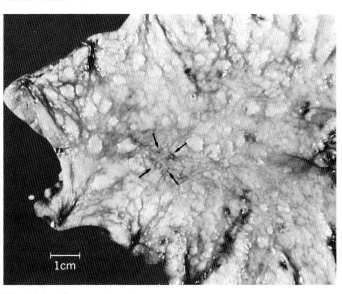

1cm

Fig. 116 Resected specimen.

Combined Diagnosis

Whenever a lesion or any abnormality is detected by the routine X-ray examination, endoscopy is performed as the next step, followed immediately by biopsy.

If necessary, the detailed X-ray examination should be performed again to reveal the exact nature of early gastric cancer.

As stated above, approximately 90 per cent of single cancer was accurately detected by the X-ray examination (Fig. 61). The result of total diagnosis made by a combined examination of X-ray and endoscopy on 596 cases of single early cancer is shown in Figure 117.

The X-ray examination accurately detected 91.1 per cent of the lesions, and endoscopy 95.6 per cent. 70.8 per cent were diagnosed as malignant or malignancy-suspect by X-ray and 86.4 per cent by endoscopy, the latter being somewhat more diagnostic. 46.3 per cent were radiographically diagnosed as malignant, and 65.1 per cent endoscopically. Biopsy is necessary to make the differential diagnosis between malignancy and benignancy. In other words, about 35 per cent of the detected early gastric cancers could not be accurately diagnosed and were labelled malignancy-suspect or benign. Biopsy was needed to establish the final diagnosis as malignant.

These figures vary, depending on what criterion one uses to establish the diagnosis of a lesion as malignant or malignancy-suspect. If one overdiagnoses, the number of malignant or malignancy-suspect lesions increases, and the number of cases of benignancy that become malignancy-suspect increases. If one underdiagnoses, choosing only certain cases as malignant, the number of cases of benignancy that become malignancy-suspect decreases, but increases the chance of diagnosing gastric cancer as benign. Figure 117 gives the

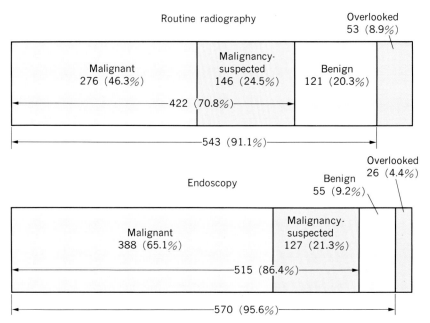

Fig. 117 Comparison of radiography and endoscopy in the diagnosis of early gastric cancer in 596 operated cases.

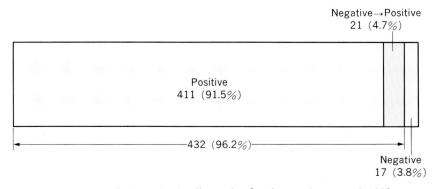

Fig. 118 Results of biopsy in the diagnosis of early gastric cancer in 449 cases.

numbers of malignancy-suspect lesions showing suspicious findings after biopsy. A considerable number of benign lesions which were diagnosed as malignancy-suspect were negated by biopsy. Biopsy under direct visualization enhances the value of endoscopy.

Efficient utilization of resources uses the X-ray examination for detection of lesions and endoscopy with biopsy for definitive diagnosis.

Figure 118 shows the result of biopsies in 449 lesions. 91.5 per cent were positive at the first examination, and 4.7 per cent were negative initially but were changed to positive after two or more specimens were received. This totalled 96.2 per cent in which the presence of cancer was proved. Negative cases operated on comprise 3.8 per cent. A few cases are negative by biopsy but suspicious of malignancy by X-ray examination and endoscopy. Follow-up study should be made in these cases until a final diagnosis is established. A yearly examination should be performed on cases that are diagnosed as benign ulcer or ulcer scar.

Chapter 4

Theoretical Basis for the Radiographic Diagnosis of Polypoid Early Cancer

General Considesations

The radiographic diagnosis of early gastric cancer presumes that by comparing a more detailed analysis of radiographic findings to macroscopic. pathology, polypoid lesions of different histologic types will have different characteristics. This contrasts to large bowel polyps in which the distinguishing features are only size and shape. (Maruyama 1978).

The radiologic diagnosis of early cancer starts with recognition of size, form and surface configuration. Most lesions are 10 to 40 mm in largest diameter, with few exceptions. The height of the polypoid lesion is next estimated either by compression or by a double contrast image if

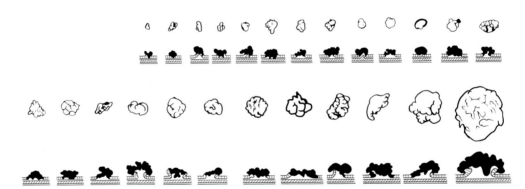

Fig. 119   Macroscopic form and surface pattern of type I early cancer (25 lesions) (Courtesy of Dr. N. Sugiyama 1971)

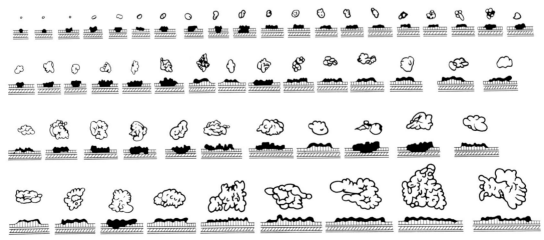

Fig. 120   Macroscopic form and surface pattern of type IIa early cancer (55 lesions) (Courtesy of Dr. N. Sugiyama 1971).

possible. Estimation of the height roughly distinguishes type I from type IIa (malignant).

The surface pattern of the lesion is vital in distinguishing benign from malignant polyps. Several malignant lesions smaller than 10 mm have a smooth surface pattern but most larger than 10 mm have the granular surface pattern characteristic of early cancer (Figs. 119–121). They also have a notched contour (Figs. 119–121). The granularity

is similar to the mucosal surface surrounding the lesion but is irregular and enlarged (Fig. 122). As was indicated by Nakamura et al. (1971), a stomach harboring polypoid cancer is usually lined with intestinal metaplasia in a moderate to severe degree. Radiographically, this condition is visualized as uniform granularity, or "areae gastricae," which vary in degree, depending upon the intensity of the intestinal metaplasia. In most cases of

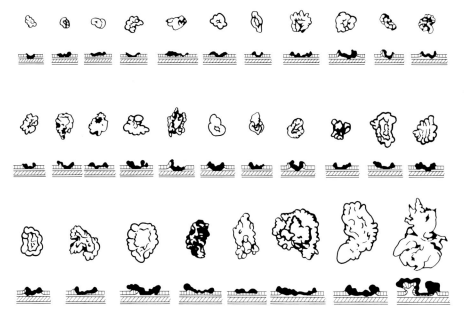

Fig. 121 Macroscopic form and surface pattern of type IIa + IIc early cancer (31 lesions) (Courtesy of Dr. N. Sugiyama 1971)

Case 31 Macroscopic Findings of a Typical Type IIa Early Cancer.
A 51-year-old man (JU). (Fig. 122)

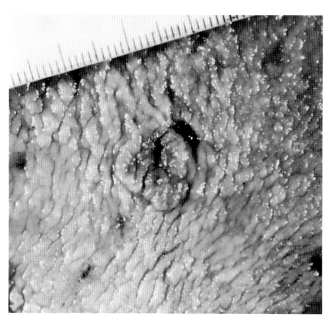

Fig. 122 Typical surface pattern of type IIa, which simulates surrounding mucosa (areae gastricae).

early polypoid cancer the surface pattern is comparable to the surrouding "areae gastricae" (Figs. 119, 120). In other words, a tendency of imitating the pattern of "areae gastricae" is still preserved in polypoid cancer whose invasion is limited to the submucosa. This observation is the most reliable radiographic sign for establishing the diagnosis of "early cancer." It is obvious that double contrast radiography is best able to visualize a background where polypoid cancer has originated.

As the cancerous infiltration goes deeper than the submucosa, such a similarity of the surface pattern disappears and is replaced by a marked erosion or ulceration in most cases. Even a large polypoid cancer preserves the similarity, as long as the depth of invasion is limited to the submucosa (Figs. 123, 124). In any case, the surface pattern of early polypoid cancer reveals one of the developing phases of differentiated cancer (Nakamura et al. 1971).

Case 32   Type IIa + IIc Early Cancer.
A 61-year-old man (CIH). (Figs. 123 and 124)

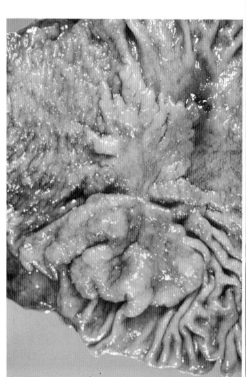

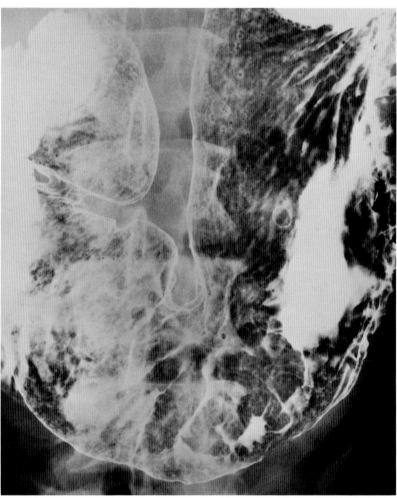

Fig. 123   Fig. 124

Fig. 123   Macroscopic findings of a large type IIa + IIc. The surface pattern of the lesion, though large (60 × 90 mm), is similar to the surrounding normal mucosa and to the mucosal folds. Cancer was limited to the submucosa (sm).

Fig. 124   Double contrast radiograph. The surface pattern is not delineated satisfactorily due to overdistension of the stomach, but it appears to consist of several enlarged mucosal folds.

Histogenesis of Epithelial Polypoid Lesions

The gastric mucosa is broadly divided into gastric mucosa proper and intestinalized mucosa. The gastric mucosa includes foveolar epithelium, pyloric gland mucosa and the fundic gland mucosa. As shown in Table 17, there is a similarity of the gastric mucosa in the histological component of the polypoid lesions. Most polypoid lesions with a similarity to the gastric mucosa proper consist of hyperplasia of the foveolar epithelium and rarely to hyperplasia of the pyloric and fundic gland mucosa. Usually, there is a central depression in sessile polypoid lesions which consists of hyperplasia of the pyloric gland mucosa. This form resembles an octopus sucker and when multiple is regarded as a healing process of erosions, so-called "gastritis verrucosa." Polypoid lesions consisting of hyperplasia of the fundic gland mucosa are often observed in cases of familial polyposis coli (Watanabe 1976, 1978) (Figs. 125, 126). Most polyps of the stomach consist of foveolar epithelium or intestinalized mucosa. They show various degrees of atypia, from normal mucosa to cancer. Those lesions without atypia and with a similarity to the foveolar epithelium are most frequently encountered (Figs. 127, 128). And those with atypia and with a similarity to the intestinalized mucosa are next in frequency.

Lesions without atypia and with a similarity to the intestinalized mucosa and those with atypia and with similarity to the foveolar epithelium are exceedingly rare. Most polypoid cancers are differentiated and have a similarity to the intestinalized mucosa, whereas polypoid cancer of the undifferentiated type is quite rare.

A polypoid lesion of the stomach is a localized elevation of the epithelium, having macroscopic and histological characteristics. It is named according to its frequency, rarity or clinical importance (Table 18). The most frequently encountered lesion is pedunculated, with a smooth surface pattern and a histological similarity to the foveolar epithelium without atypia. This is called adenomatous polyp by Stout (1953), regenerative hyperplastic polyp by Evans (1964), regenerative polyp by Ming and Goldman (1965) or adenomatous polyp of foveolar epithelium by Oota (1964).

Recognition of regenerative hyperplasia is relatively easy in most cases, because there is an

Table 17 Histologic components of gastric polyps.

		Atypicality		Carcinoma
		Absent	Present	
Gastric mucosa proper	Foveolar epithelium	Many	Few	Undifferentiated carcinoma is extremely rare. Carcinoma cells sometimes may take a form simulating pyloric gland mucosa. And malignant parietal cell rarely appears.
	Pyloric gland mucosa	Gastritis verrucosa or polyposa	(−)	
	Fundic gland mucosa	Familial polyposis	(−)	
Intestinalized mucosa		Few	So-called ATP	Differentiated carcinoma, malignant goblet cell; rarely malignant Paneth cell.

(From Nakamura, K. et al.: *Nippon Rinsho*, 34: 1341−1349, 1976)

Table 18 Macroscopic form and histologic findings of gastric polyps.

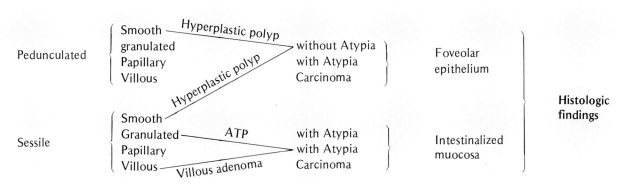

(From Nakamura, K. et al: *Nippon Rinsho*, 34: 1341−1349, 1976)

Case 33   Polyposis of the Stomach in Familial Polyposis Coli.

A 26-year-old woman (Courtesy of Dr. H. Watanabe* and Dr. T. Yao**)
(Figs. 125 and 126).

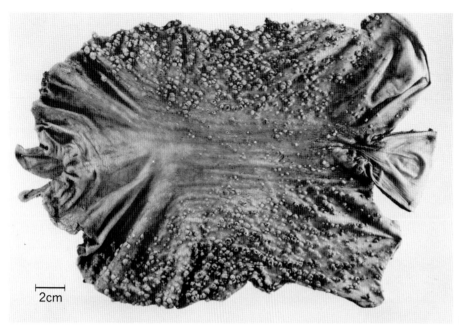

Fig. 125   Polyposis of the stomach in a case of familial polyposis.

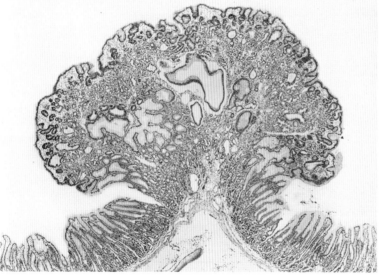

Fig. 126   Histologic findings showing hyperplasia of the foveolar epithelium in the fundic gland mucosa.

*First Department of Pathology, Niigata University School of Medicine, Niigata.
**First Department of Medicine, Fukuoka University School of Medicine, Fukuoka.

erosion on its surface with normal surrounding mucosa, whereas in malignancy a polypoid lesion is formed from epithelium which has severe atypia. However, there are some benign polypoid lesions which are difficult to recognize definitively as regenerative or neoplastic. For instance, a large polypoid lesion which consists of hyperplasia of the foveolar epithelium is regarded as a benign neoplasm due to its excess proliferation, but it cannot be locally distinguished from the foveolar epithelium of regenerative change because of the absence of atypia. Thus, a large polyp which is regarded as a benign neoplasm is not classified as adenoma histologically, but rather as a hyperplasia due to regenerative change. This is because adenoma is defined histologically as a lesion having atypia.

Atypical epithelium (ATP, cf. Chapter 5) is a polypoid lesion which must be clinically and histologically differentiated from differentiated cancer. ATP is the most popular name in Japan, but it is also called adenoma of the stomach (Ming

Table 19 Histologic order of gastric polyps.

Order	Atypicality		
	Absent ———————————————————————————————→		Marked
Foveolar epithelium	Hyperplastic polyp	Foveolar type polyp with atypia	Undifferentiated carcinoma
Intestinalized mucosa	Hyperplastic polyp	So-called atypical epithelium	Differentiated carcinoma

(From Nakamura, K.: *Nippon Rinsho*, 34, 1341—1349, 1976)

and Goldman 1965). Histologically ATP demonstrates cystic dilatation of the glands of the lower half. It is usually less than 20 mm in greatest diameter (cf. Chapter 5).

Gastric polypoid lesions can be divided into two groups: those with similarities to normal appearing mucosa and those having various degrees of atypia (Table 19). Polypoid lesions consisting of foveolar epithelium range from hyperplastic polyp without atypia to undifferentiated cancer, and lesions consisting of intestinalized mucosa range from hyperplasia of the intestinalized mucosa without atypia to differentiated cancer. There are many cases of polyps consisting of foveolar epithelium whose histology borders between hyperplasia and neoplasia. This is similar to polyps consisting of intestinalized mucosa having histology between atypical epithelium and differentiated cancer.

Actually, the incidence of polypoid lesions of the stomach consisting of foveolar epithelium with atypia is very low and their malignant transformation (Figs. 127—136) is also considered to be extremely rare (Fig. 136). It may be better to call those lesions without atypia adenomatous polyp, and further investigation should be done as to whether they are regenerative or neoplastic in origin.

Case 34 Malignant Transformation of Adenomatous Polyp of Foveolar Epithelium.
A 66-year-old woman (CIH). (Figs. 127–136)

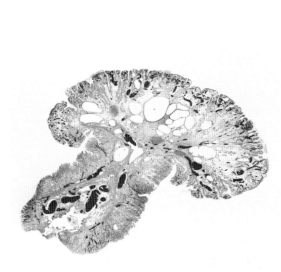 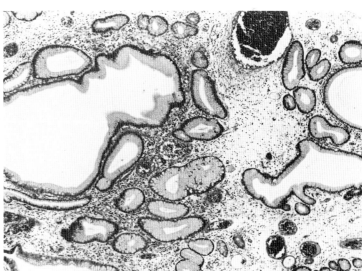

Fig. 127 Cross section of the hyperplastic polyp. **Fig. 128** Histologic findings of the hyperplastic polyp.

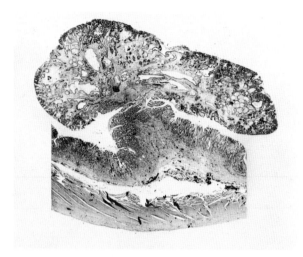

Fig. 129 Cross section of the lesion showing a hyperplastic polyp without malignant transformation.

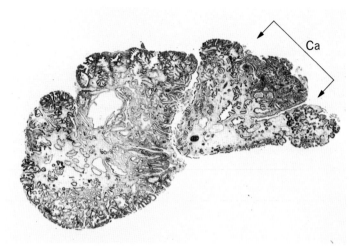

Fig. 130 Another cross section of the lesion with an area of malignant transformation. The lesion consists mostly of hyperplastic foveolar epithelium but contains a small adenocarcinoma (arrow-line).

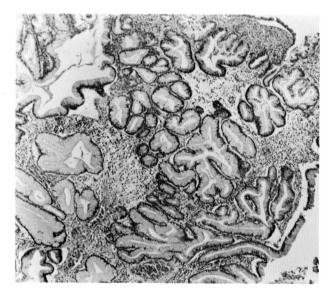

Fig. 131 Histologic findings of the hyperplastic polyp.

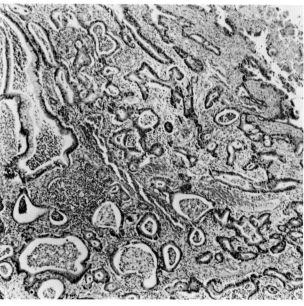

Fig. 132 Histologic findings of adenocarcinoma tubulae (well-differentiated adenocarcinoma).

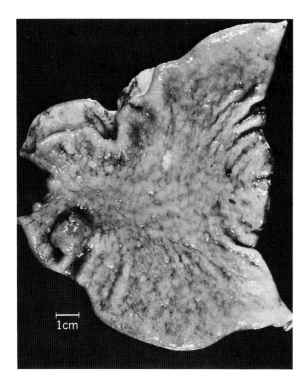

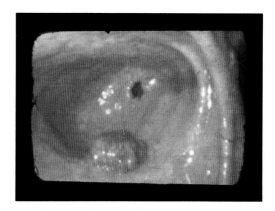

Fig. 134   Endoscopic findings.

Fig. 133   Resected specimen. The lesion, measuring 18 × 16 × 8 mm, is located in the antrum.

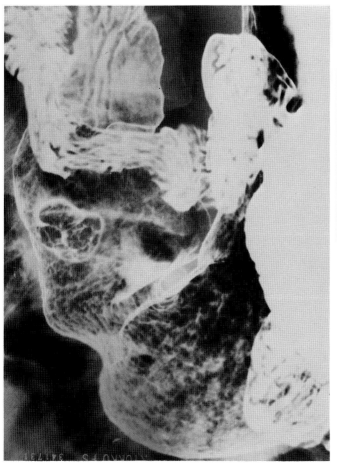

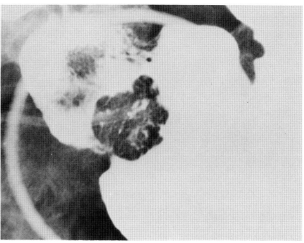

Fig. 136   Compression radiograph. The lesion is diagnosed radiographically as malignant, based on the diagnostic criteria for polypoid lesions of the stomach.

Fig. 135   Double contrast radiograph.

A polypoid early cancer of undifferentiated type is not an imaginary figure, as such a lesion, though rare, exists (Figs. 137–139). This lesion may be lined by foveolar epithelium. On the other hand, there is also a case of focal, differentiated cancer in a lesion of hyperplastic foveolar epithelium, as was shown in Figures 127–136. A rare case, however, does not contradict the histogenetic theory of gastric polypoid lesions.

Malignant transformation of polypoid lesions consisting of foveolar epithelium is considered to be very rare, and such a case is shown in Figures 127–136. It is the presence of the atypical epithelium that is questioned. Incidence of malignant transformation of atypical epithelium is regarded to be high in lesions larger than 20 mm (Nakamura and Takagi 1975). But, most lesions do not become that large. Therefore, the distinction between malignant and benign lesions is more important than a problem of malignant transformation as far as atypical epithelium is concerned.

Case 35   Type IIa Early Cancer of Undifferentiated Type.
A 76-year-old woman (CIH). (Figs. 137-139)

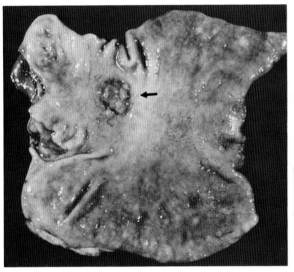

Fig. 137   Macroscopic findings of type IIa undifferentiated adenocarcinoma (adenocarcinoma mucocellulare), measuring 24 × 20 mm (arrow).

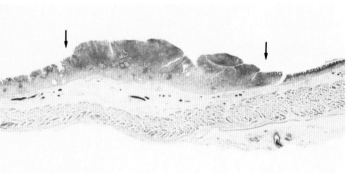

Fig. 138   A cross section of the lesion. Cancer was limited to the mucosa (m).

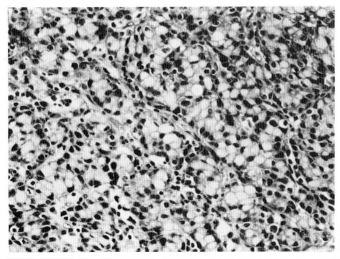

Fig. 139   Histologic findings of adenocarcinoma mucocellulare.

Macroscopic Classification of Polypoid Lesions

Several macroscopic classifications have been proposed for the purpose of facilitating the differential diagnosis of polypoid lesions of the stomach (Yamada and Fukutomi 1966, Furusawa 1966, Kosaki et al. 1967, Fukuchi and Mochizuki 1967, Utsumi et al. 1967, Takagi et al. 1967, Nishizawa et al. 1968, Nishizawa 1977) (Fig. 140). Yamada-Fukutomi's classification (Fig. 142) has been widely used as one that roughly defines the form of polypoid lesions endoscopically as well as radiographically. It can easily be used because all polypoid lesions of the stomach are classified into the four categories. But, it seems to be inadequate for distinguishing polypoid early cancer, especially type IIa, from other polypoid lesions. The profile form of type IIa is better represented as a flat elevation of the mucosa with slight constriction at

of the stomach, as demonstrated by Nishizawa et al. (1968).

Generally, a classification with more than 6 categories is very confusing and is not useful for practical purposes. Macroscopic appearance should be defined as pedunculated, subpedunculated and sessile (Table 20). Subpedunculated is comparable to narrow-base sessile polyp and sessile to wide-base sessile polyp. Sessile lesion (wide-base sessile) should be divided into two subclassifications, those with constriction at the base and the other with gradual sloping (Takagi 1968). Most lesions of type IIa and atypical epithelium belong to those with constriction at the base, while benign lesions, including epithelial and submucosal, belong to those with gradual sloping (Takagi 1968, Fig. 142).

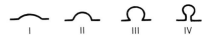

Fig. 140 Morphological classification of polypoid lesions of the stomach (Yamada and Fukutomi 1966).

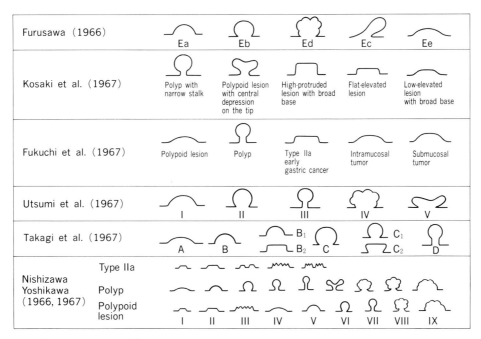

Fig. 141 Morphologic classification of polypoid lesions of the stomach according to various authors.

Table 20 Macroscopic form of gastric polyps.

Pedunculated
Subpedunculated .... Narrow base sessile
Sessile .... Wide base sessile

its base, which may fall in between type II and type III in the Yamada-Fukutomi's classification (Fig. 141). This classification is useful for defining the macroscopic form of bebign polypoid lesions

Endoscopically		
Radiographically	○	◯
Pathologically	Benign	ATP* cancer

Fig. 142 Macroscopic classification of polypoid lesions of the stomach (From Takagi 1968).
*ATP: Atypical epithelium

Pedunculated lesions

The radiographic diagnosis of polypoid early cancer begins with recognition of the size, form and surface pattern. According to Nishizawa's series (Fig. 143), there was no malignancy in lesions with a definite stalk (classifications 4, 5, 6) and smaller than 20 mm. In Sugiyama's series (Fig. 144) there were several malignancies in lesions larger than 10 mm. In the range of 10 mm 12 per cent (4/33) were malignant, and of the lesions

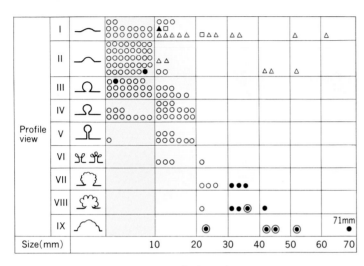

- ◉ Borrmann type I
- ● Early cancer type I
- ▲ Early cancer type IIa
- ○ Benign polyp
- △ Submucosal tumor
- □ Localized thickening of the mucosa

Fig. 143 Size and profile view of polypoid lesions of the stomach (From Nishizawa et al. 1968).

Largest diameter	5mm or <			6–10mm			11–20mm			21mm or >		
Profile view	Smooth	Intermediate	Irregular	Smooth	Intermediate	Irregular	Smooth	Intermediate	Irregular	Smooth	Intermediate	Irregular
Type I	○○○○○○ ○○ ○○○○○ ○○	○		○○○○○○ ○○	○							
Type II	○○○○○○ ○○○○○○ ○○○○○○	○		○○○○○○ ○○○○○○ ○○○	○○○○		○○	○				
Type III	○ / △△	△ / △		○○○○○○ ○○ / △	○○○○○○ / △	■■	○○	○○○ / △	■■■■	○○○○		■■■■■ ■■■■ / △
Type IV				○○○○○○	○○○○○○ ○○○		○○○○○○ ○○○○○○	○○○○○○ ○○○○ / ■	○ / ■■■	○○○○○ ○○○	○○○○○○ ○○○○ / ■	○ / △△ / ■■■■■
	● / △△△△△△ △△△	●● / △△△		●● / △△△△△△ △△△△	●● / △△	●●●● / △△△ / ▲	●●●●● ●●● / △	●●●● / △△△△△△ △△ / ▲▲	●●●● / △△△ / ▲	●●●●●● / △△ / ▲▲	△△	●●●●●● ●●●●●● ●●●●● / △△ / ▲▲▲▲▲▲ ▲▲▲▲▲▲ ▲▲▲▲▲ ▲▲
				△△	△		△△					

- ○ Benign
- △ Atypical epithelium (ATP)
- ● Early cancer, type IIa
- ▲ Early cancer, type IIa + IIc
- ■ Early cancer, type I

Fig. 144 Size and profile view of polypoid lesions of the stomach (Courtesy of Dr. N. Sugiyama 1971)

larger than 20 mm 29 per cent (7/24) were malignant. Those malignancies larger than 10 mm were all irregular in their contour (Figs. 119 and 120), while the other benign lesions were smooth (Fig. 145). Therefore, a pedunculated lesion is most probably malignant if its size is more than 20 mm and its surface pattern is irregular (Figs. 146–151).

On the other hand, hyperplastic polyps almost always have a smooth surface pattern and contour as opposed to the granular surface and lobulation of ATP and polypoid early cancers. Hyperplastic polyps are almost always smaller than 20 mm in diameter (Figs. 152 and 153) and pedunculated or subpedunculated.

Endoscopic polypectomy is the treatment of choice for pedunculated lesions. Results of endoscopic polypectomy reveal that almost all these lesions are benign hyperplastic polyps (Fujii and Funada 1979, Table 21).

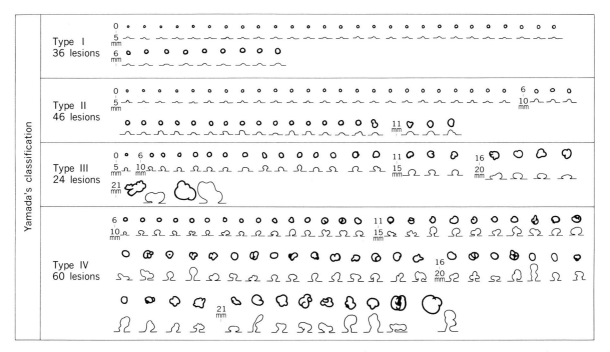

Fig. 145　Macroscopic findings of benign polypoid lesions (Courtesy of Dr. N. Sugiyama, 1971).

Table 21　Histologic diagnosis of polypectomized specimens.

Macroscopic form	Histologic diagnosis				Total
	Carcinoma	Adenoma (Atypical epithelium)	Hyperplasia	Cyst	
⌒	0	2	1	1	4 Foci
Ω	0	0	25	0	25
Ω̨	2	0	58	0	60
Total	2 (2.2)	2 (2.2)	84 (94.5)	1 (1.1)	89 Foci (100)

( ): %　　　　　(From Fujii, A. and Funada, A.: *Progr. Digest. Endosc.*, 14: 19-23, 1979)

Case 36   Type I Early Cancer, Pedunculated.

A 70-year-old woman (CIH). (Figs. 146-151)

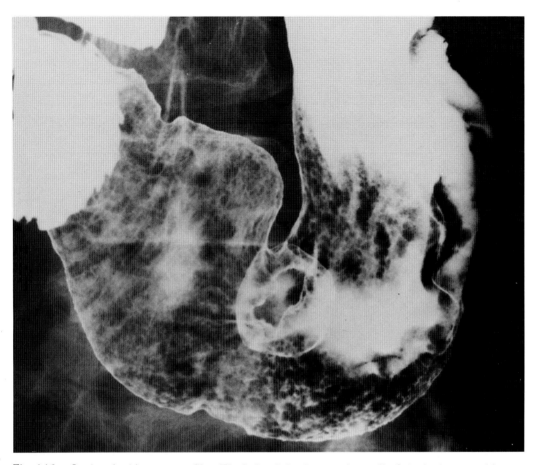

Fig. 146   Supine double contrast film. The lesion is in the anterior wall of the incisura, and has a short stalk.

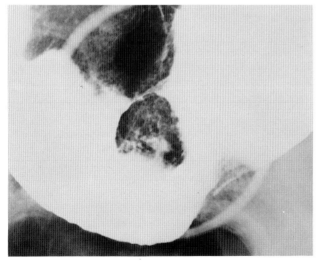

Fig. 147   Upright compression film. The surface pattern of the lesion is similar to the surrounding normal mucosa. Barium flecks reveal a slight depressions in its surface.

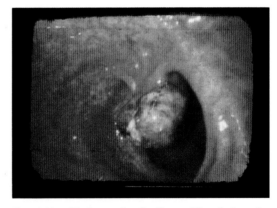

Fig. 148   Endoscopic findings. The lesion in the anterior wall is suspended by a short stalk.

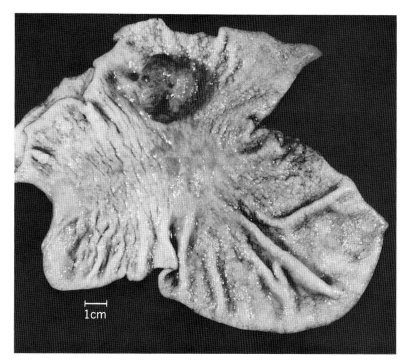

Fig. 149 Resected specimen showing an en face view of the lesion (30 x 30 mm).

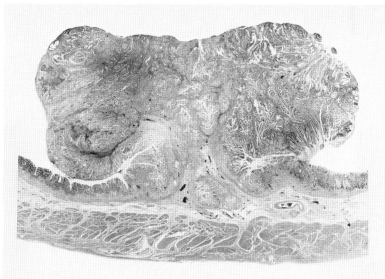

Fig. 150 Cross section of the lesion. The submucosa was only slightly involved (sm).

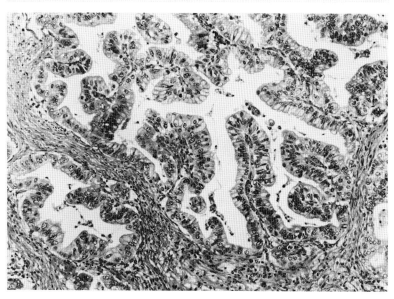

Fig. 151 Histologic findings showing adenocarcinoma papillotubulae (well differentiated adenocarcinoma).

Case 37 Benign Pedunculated Polyp (Hyperplastic Polyp).
A 64-year-old man (CPCC). (Figs. 152 and 153)

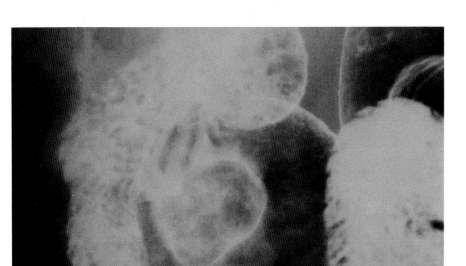

Fig. 152 Double contrast film. The contour and surface pattern appear smooth compared with polypoid lesions of the intestinal type (IIa, I).

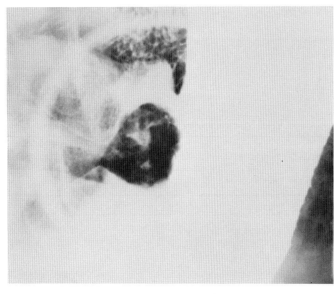

Fig. 153 Compression film of Figure 152. The head and stalk are delineated effectively. Barium flecks reveals slight surface depression.

Subpedunculated lesions

In Nishizawa's series (Fig. 143) all subpedunculated lesions were benign hyperplastic polyps (Figs. 154–156) and no lesion was more than 20 mm in its largest diameter (Fig. 143). Sugiyama et al. (1971) reported several malignancies in subpedunculated lesions (Fig. 144) and these were more than 20 mm. However, Sugiyama used the Yamada-Fukutomi's classification, which has no separate category type IIa and therefore forces these lesions to be classified as type III. This may account for the difference between Nishizawa and Sugiyama. Since these malignancies are macroscopically wide-base sessile, they cannot reasonably be classified by the Yamada-Fukutomi's classification.

Case 38   Benign Subpedunculated Polyp.
A 64-year-old woman (CPCC). (Figs. 154 and 155)

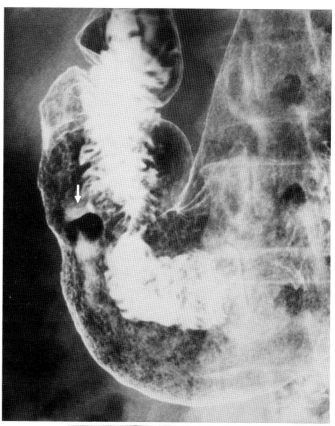

Fig. 154 Supine double contrast film of a benign subpedunculated polyp.

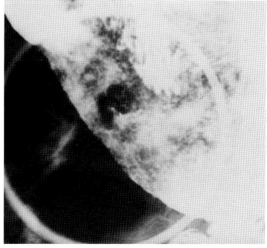

Fig. 155 Upright compression film of the same case as Figure 154.

Case 39 Benign Subpedunculated Polyp (Hyperplastic Polyp).
A 52-year-old woman (CPCC). (Fig. 156)

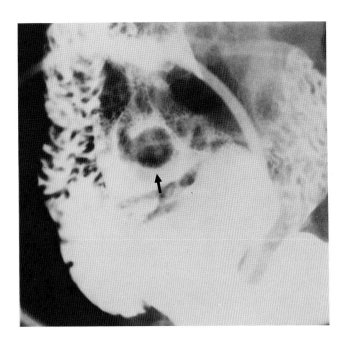

Fig. 156 Compression film of a benign subpedunculated polyp.

Sessile lesions

It is very rare for a gradual sloping lesion (Yamada-Fukutomi type I and type II) to be malignant. Malignant lesions are mostly flat and angular in profile (Fig. 142). If such an elevation is not higher than 5 mm it is most probably type IIa (Figs. 157–161 and 162–166). If an elevation is higher than 5 mm, it may be diagnosed as type I (Figs. 167–172). The surface pattern of the lesion is most important for differential diagnosis between ATP and type IIa or between type IIa and advanced cancer, as was mentioned above.

Case 40 Type IIa Early Cancer.
A 60-year-old woman (JU). (Figs. 157-161)

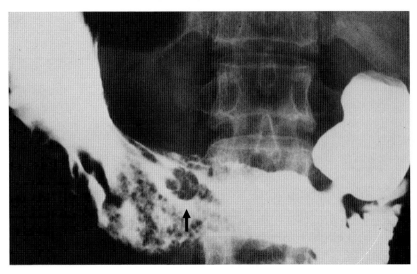

Fig. 157 Mucosal relief film in the prone position demonstrates an irregular radiolucency with small, uniform nodules.

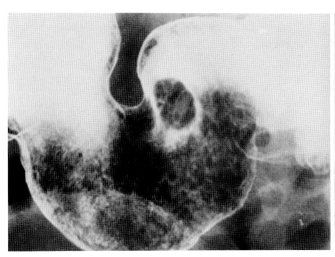

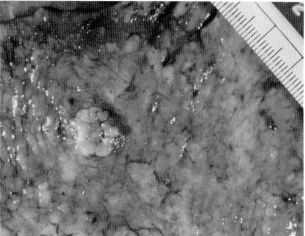

Fig. 158   Fig. 159

Fig. 158   Double contrast film in the prone position demonstrates similar finding to that of Figure 157. The thickness of the barium outlining the radiolucency enables one to estimate the height of the polypoid lesion (type IIa).

Fig. 159   Resected specimen. There is a flat, nodular elevation of the mucosa, measuring 12 x 11 mm, on the anterior wall near the incisura. It is of nearly uniform nodularity. Macroscopically, the lesion is most likely an early cancer, type IIa.

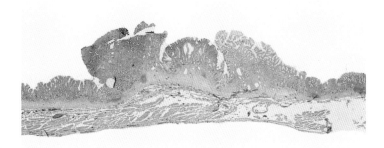

Fig. 160   Cross section of the lesion.

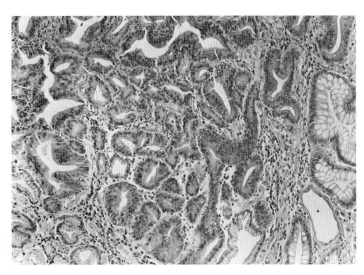

Fig. 161   Histologic findings of adenocarcinoma tubulare (well differentiated adenocarcinoma). Cancer was limited to the mucosa (m).

Case 41 Type IIa Early Cancer.
A 60-year-old woman (CIH). (Figs. 162-166)

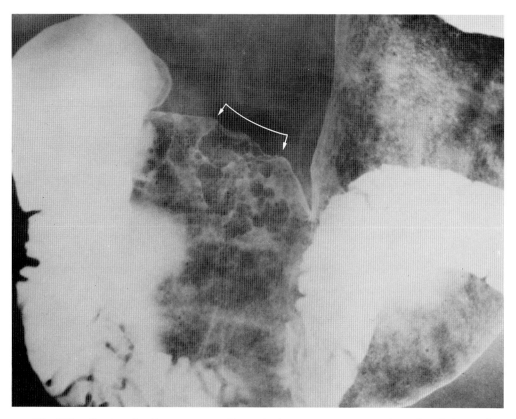

Fig 162 Supine double contrast radiograph demonstrates aggregation of radiolucencies of various sizes on the posterior wall of the lesser curvature of the antrum, which gives the impression of general polypoid elevation of the mucosa (arrow line).

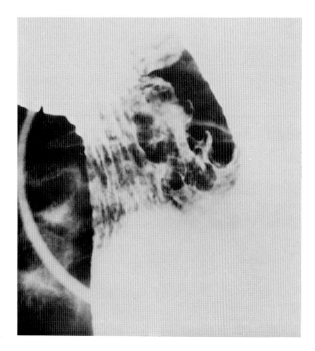

Fig. 163 Upright compression film demonstrates radiolucencies of various sizes, with a flattened, lobular elevation of the mucosa.

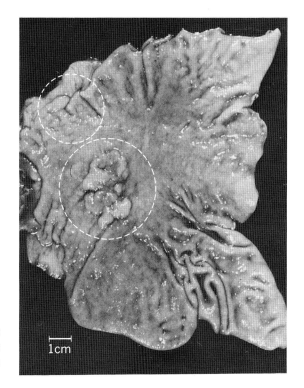

Fig. 164 Resected specimen. The lesion, measuring 33 × 23 mm, is located at the lesser curvature of the antrum. The size of the nodules varies, but still preserves a similarity to the antral mucosa (compare with the encircled area).

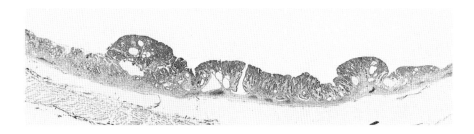

Fig. 165 Cross section of the lesion.

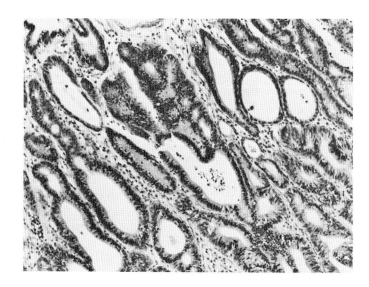

Fig. 166 Histologic findings of adenocarcinoma tubulae (well-differentiated adenocarcinoma). Cancer was limited to the mucosa (m).

Case 42   Type I Early Cancer.
A 74-year-old man (JU). (Figs. 167-172)

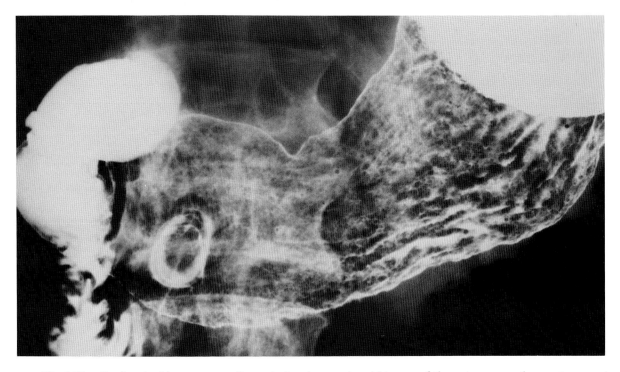

Fig. 167   Supine double contrast radiograph showing a polypoid tumor of the antrum near the greater curvature which appears smooth in outline and oval. A double-contoured shadow of the tumor suggests that it may be located on the anterior wall.

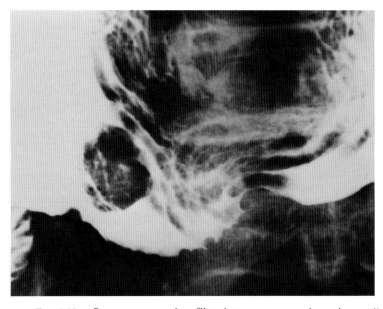

Fig. 168   Prone compression film demonstrates an irregular outline of the tumor with tiny flecks of barium on its surface.

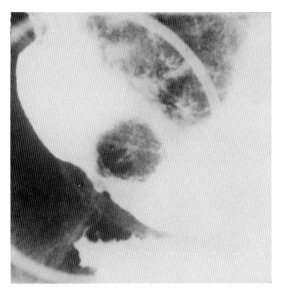

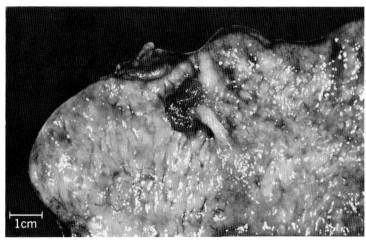

Fig. 169   Fig. 170

Fig. 169 Upright compression film demonstrates findings similar to those in Figure 168. In this case the double contrast image does not reveal the fine details of the tumor, but helps localize it. Fine details are visualized clearly in the mucosal relief and compression images.

Fig. 170 The lesion is located at the anterior wall of the antrum and measures 15 x 15 x 10 mm.

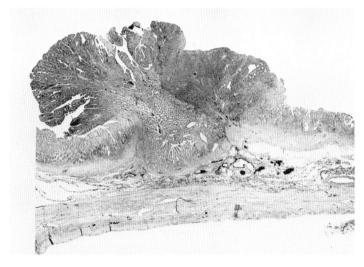

Fig. 171 Cross section of the lesion.

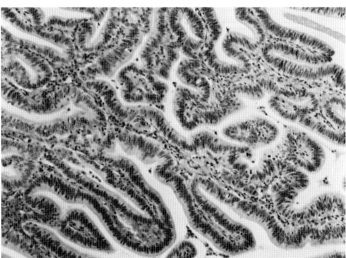

Fig. 172 Histologic findings of the lesion, showing adenocarcinoma tubulae (well-differentiated adenocarcinoma). Cancer was limited to the mucosa (m).

95

Sessile Lesions with Central Depression

When a central depression which is recognizable macroscopically is present on surface of a flat polypoid lesion, it is diagnosed as type IIa + IIc. When a central depression is predominant, the lesion is diagnosed as IIc + IIa. Even if a central depression is irregular in form, it is still considered a type IIc lesion. Actually, there are various kinds of type IIa + IIc, according to macroscopic form and spreading pattern, as shown in Figure 173. Rarely, the depression is not in the center of a polypoid lesion but adjacent to it (form d in Fig. 173; and Fig. 3 in Chapter 1). The size of type IIa

+ IIc usually ranges from 10 to 20 mm, but sometimes it is larger than 30 mm.

There is a close relationship between the depth of a central depression and cancerous invasion (Nishizawa 1977). The larger and the deeper the depression, the deeper the invasion of cancer is suspected. There is also a risk of lymph node metastasis in this form (refer to the section on Prognosis of Early Gastric Cancer in Chapter 1).

On the other hand, a slight central depression is sometimes observed in an atypical epithelium (see Figs. 195, 196; 215, 216 in Chapter 5). Or, sometimes, the trough between nodules looks like a depression (see Fig. 162).

Radiologically, central depression is best delineated by the compression method (Figs. 174–180). Sometimes a simple mucosal relief image in the prone position may be effective, when a lesion is on the anterior wall (Fig. 181).

However, it may be difficult to make the differential diagnosis between type IIa + IIc (sm) and Borrmann type 2 (advanced), as far as these two cases are concerned. From the clinical point of view, they should be diagnosed as advanced cancer,

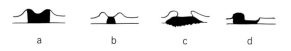

Fig. 173 Macroscopic appearance and pattern of the spread of early cancer, type IIa + IIc.

Case 43 Type IIa Early Cancer and ATP.
A 49-year-old man (JU). (Figs. 174-180)

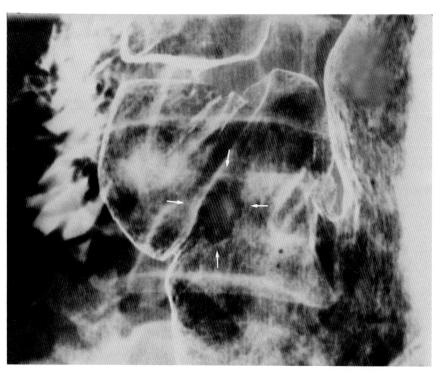

Fig. 174 Supine double contrast film demonstrates an irregular, elliptical radiolucency on the posterior wall of the antrum near the greater curvature with very faint barium retention (arrows).

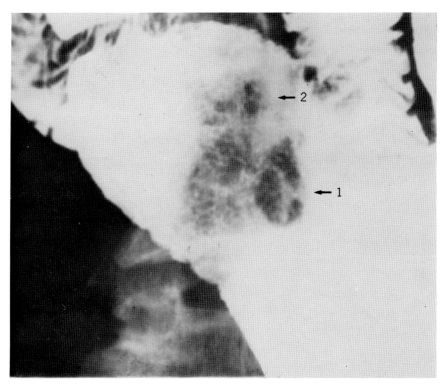

Fig. 175 Supine compression film demonstrates the lesion more clearly. In this view, a somewhat linear collection of barium, which is obscure on the double contrast image, is delineated (arrow 1). Another, smaller, radiolucency is visualized between the lesion and the lesser curvature (arrow 2).

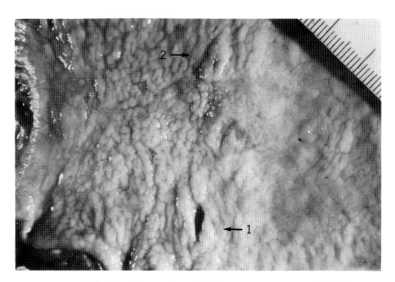

Fig. 176 Resected specimen. The lesion appears as a cleft-like depression of the mucosa surrounded by nodularity and measures 13 × 8 mm (type IIa + IIc) (arrow 1). Another lesion (shown in Figure 175) is on the anterior wall, and measures 12 × 6 mm (arrow 2). This lesion was diagnosed as ATP.

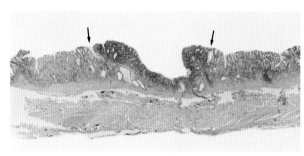

Fig. 177 Cross section of the lesion (type IIa + IIc).

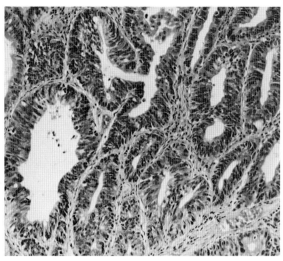

Fig. 178 Histologic findings of adenocarcinoma tubulae (well-differentiated adenocarcinoma). Cancer was limited to the mucosa (m).

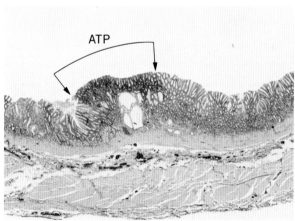

Fig. 179 Cross section of ATP.

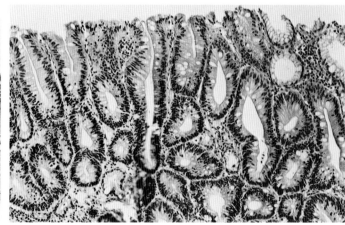

Fig. 180 Histologic findings of ATP.

because their size is larger than 20 mm and because the central depression is prominent.

Double contrast radiography is not as effective as compression in demonstrating the central depression. Especially an elevated portion is not well delineated in a double contrast radiograph taken in such a way as to visualize mucosal pattern (Figs. 182—185).

On the other hand, it becomes difficult to recognize the central depression macroscopically in a small lesion, though it is delineated clearly in the radiographic findings (Figs. 186—189).

Non-malignant sessile lesions with central depression always have the shape of submucosal tumor (see Chapter 15) and the radiographic diagnosis is easily made.

Case 44   Type IIa + IIc Early Cancer.

A 68-year-old man (CPCC, the same case as Figs. 442 to 445 in Chapter 10). (Fig. 181)

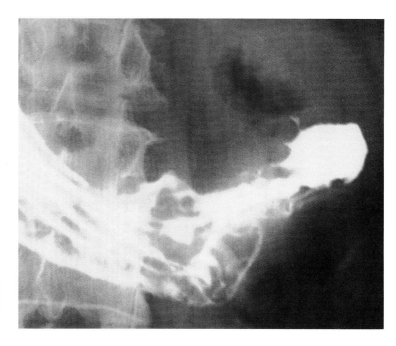

Fig. 181 Mucosal relief film demonstrates a large central depression surrounded by a raised margin. The lesion is large enough to permit the diagnosis of advanced cancer.

Case 45   Type IIc + IIa Early Cancer.

A 64-year-old man (NCCH). (Figs. 182-185)

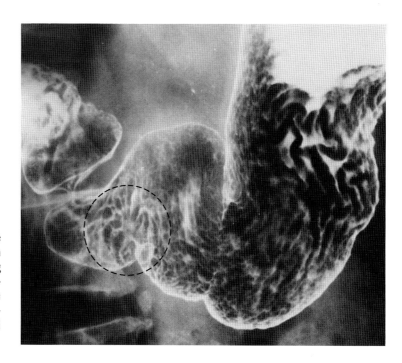

Fig. 182 Supine double contrast film in the right anterior oblique position demonstrates an irregular collection of barium. The surrounding mucosa is nodular. Radiographically it is diagnosted as early cancer, type IIc + IIa, because the nodularity surrounding the depression is distinguished from the normal appearing antral mucosa.

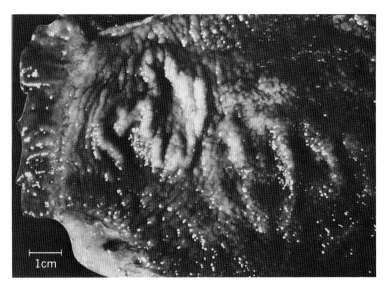

Fig. 183 Resected specimen. The resected stomach is incised along the lesser curvature. The lesion is on the posterior wall, and measure 32 × 18 mm. The depression is more prominent than the elevation (type IIc + IIa).

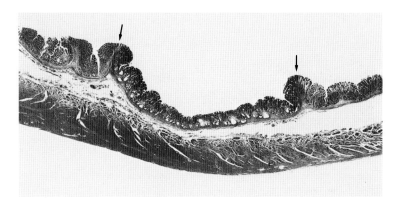

Fig. 184 Cross section of the lesion. Cancer was limited to the mucosa (m).

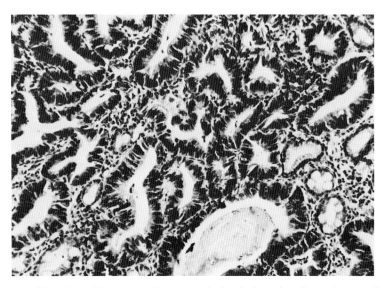

Fig. 185 Histologic findings of the lesion showing adenocarcinoma tubulae (well-differentiated adenocarcinoma).

Case 46   Type IIa + IIc Early Cancer.

A 65-year-old man (NCCH). (Figs. 186-189)

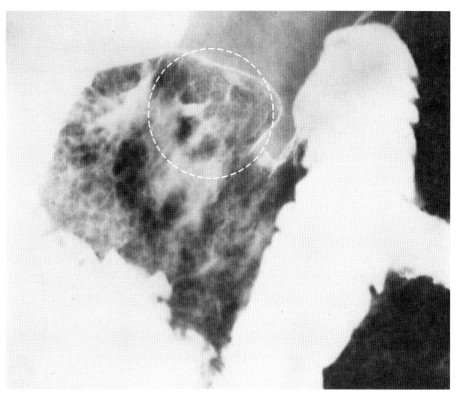

Fig. 186   Supine double contrast film demonstrates thinly retained barium framing a vague nodular lesion. Collections of barium in the nodularity suggest surface erosions.

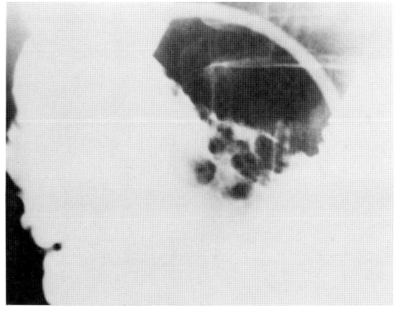

Fig. 187   Upright compression film demonstrates nodularity and intervening retention of barium.

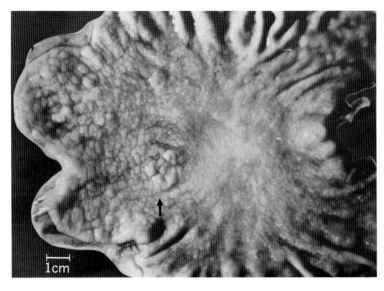

Fig. 188 Resected specimen. The lesion measures 18 × 18 mm. The erosion (arrows) is not clearly recognized.

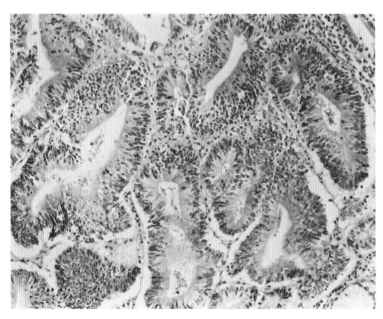

Fig. 189 Histologic finding showing adenocarcinoma tubulae (well-differentiated adenocarcinoma). Cancer was limited to the mucosa (m).

Chapter 5

The Concept of Atypical Epithelium (ATP) and Its Radiographic Characteristics

Atypical epithelium (ATP) is a lesion which histologically shows borderline atypia between benignancy and malignancy. It should be distinguished clinically from a differentiated adenocarcinoma. Various names are given to this lesion, whose histologic characteristics are diffent from hyperplasia of the foveolar epithelium, i.e. adenomatous polyp (Oota 1964), adenoma (Enjoji and Watanabe 1975, Ishidate 1975, Kino et al. 1969, Taniguchi et al. 1975), IIa-subtype (Fukuchi 1972), Nakamura's type III (T. Nakamura et al. 1962) and ATP (Takagi 1968, Nakamura 1969). In this book the name ATP is used.

Nakamura and Takagi (1975) defined ATP as follows: a localized lesion with cylindrical epithelium of many glands, showing varying degrees of atypia, and arising from intestinal type metaplasia of the gastric mucosa. The concept of ATP was developed to account for those cases of atypia which could not be classified as either benign or malignant but whose histology was somewhere in between (Fig. 190). This concept assumes that atypicality is a continuum. Intestinal metaplasia may play a very important role in the evolution of ATP. Fukuchi and Mochizuki (1972) described an association of severe atrophy of the surrounding gastric mucosa with ATP. Such atrophy markedly impairs the secretion of gastric acid. Nakamura T. (1976) emphasized that ATP has a two-layer structure (Fig. 191). The upper layer shows atypical epithelium and the lower one cyst formation and pyloric glands. Goblet cells are often observed in the surface portion of the upper layer and Paneth cells are observed in the deeper portion. Indeed, ATP has histologic similarity to an adenoma of the small intestine (Enjoji and Watanabe 1975).

ATP is frequently seen in the over-50-year age group and shows the highest incidence at the age of 60 (Sano 1975). Sex ratio (M/F) is reported to be 1.7 by Sano (1975) and 3.3 by Enjoji and Watanabe (1975).

The macroscopic form of ATP usually presents a flat mucosal elevation or polypoid lesion. It does not exceed 2.0 cm in most cases, and about 50 per cent of them are on the order of 1.0 cm. ATP measuring less than 1.0 cm are frequently seen in association with other lesions, including early and advanced cancer (Nakamura and Takagi 1975). The gastric antrum is a frequent site for ATP. It is rarely seen in the upper third of the stomach.

Long-term follow-up study discloses that an ATP does not change its size for several years, although there are exceptions. Enjoji and Watanabe (1975) described one case showing a slight increase in size 9 years after the initial examination. Fukuchi and Mochizuki (1975) observed no case of ATP increasing in size in follow-up studies by endoscopy. Most investigators admit that ATP is generally a stable lesion. Fukuchi and Mochizuki

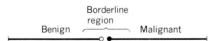

Fig. 190 One-to-one correspondence of atypical lesions (From Nakamura and Takagi 1975).

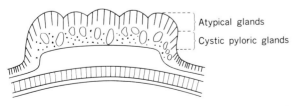

Fig. 191 Schema showing a two-layer structure of the type III polyp (ATP) (From Nakamura, T. and Nakano, G.: *Nippon Rinsho*, 34: 1368, 1976).

(1975) still insist upon calling it IIa-subtype, because further follow-up studies would be necessary to prove this as a distinct disease entity, although typical cases of ATP are distinguishable from type IIa cancer clinically as well as histologically.

Nakamura and Takagi (1975) estimated the incidence of malignant transformation of ATP as no higher than 0.4 per cent and emphasized the importance of selective follow-up study if biopsy revealed ATP (Group III) (Figs. 192—194). Otherwise, endoscopic polypectomy is recommended if it is technically possible for lesions less than 20 mm in diameter (Figs. 195—199). Sano reported that malignant foci were observed in 4.5 per cent of the ATP in his series, all of which were larger than 20 mm in greatest diameter. Enjoji and Watanabe (1975) also described that malignant focus is frequently observed in ATP with diameters larger than 20 mm.

Case 47 Malignant Focus in ATP.
A 65-year-old man (CIH). (Figs. 192-194)

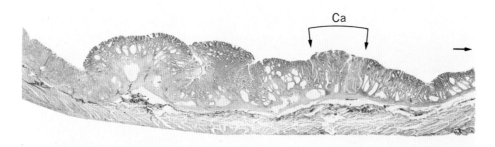

Fig. 192 Cross section of the lesion, showing the portion containing cancer (arrow line).

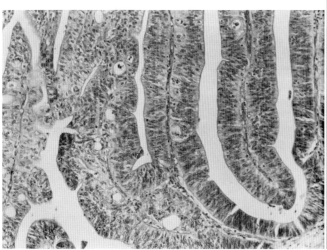

Fig. 193 Histologic findings of cancer.

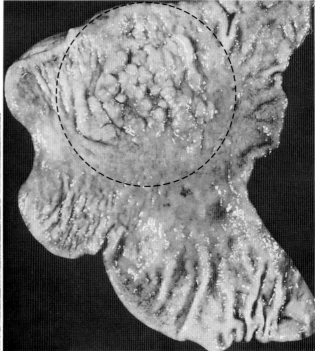

Fig. 194 A case of malignant transformation of ATP. Macroscopic findings show a nodular polypoid lesion, measuring 55 x 38 mm on the anterior wall of the incisura.

Case 48 ATP with Central Depression (Polypectomized Case).
A 61-year-old woman (CIH). (Figs. 195-199)

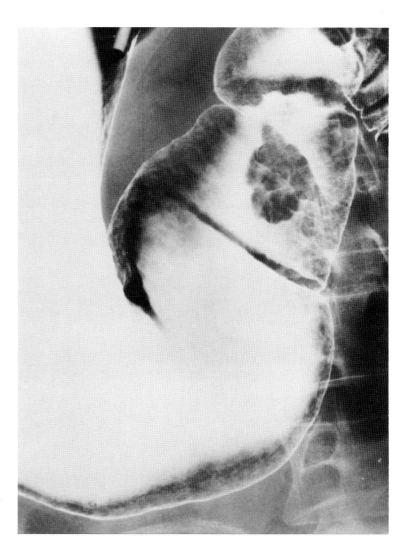

Fig. 195 Prone double contrast film demonstrates an irregular polypoid lesion with surface granularity on the anterior wall of the antrum.

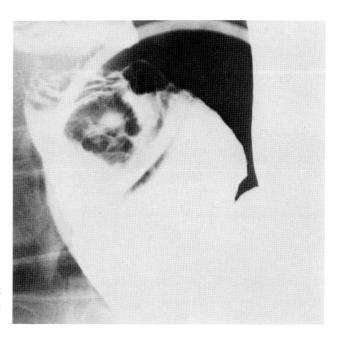

Fig. 196 Upright compression film demonstrates a slight central depression. The lesion measures about 20 mm in the greatest diameter.

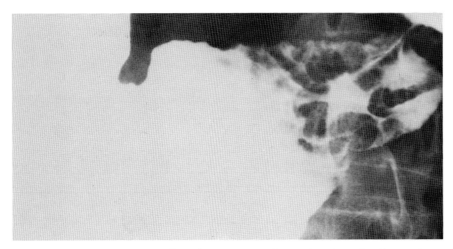

Fig. 197   Prone compression film demonstrates a large ulcer 2 weeks after endoscopic polypectomy.

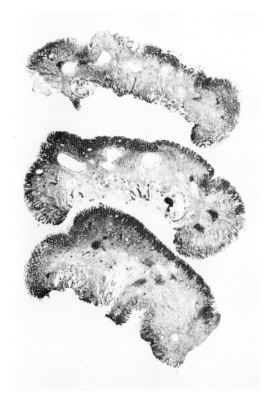

Fig. 198   Cross section of the poly-pectomized specimen.

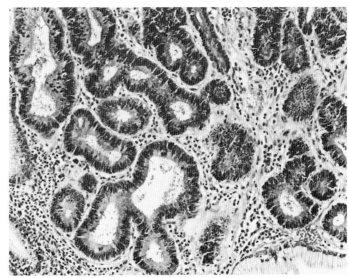

Fig. 199   Histologic findings of ATP.

Fukuchi et al. (1972) reported that correct diagnosis of IIa-subtype was established endoscopically in 62 per cent, but radiographically the definitive diagnosis of ATP could not be established because there was no marked difference in the surface configuration between ATP and type IIa. Yamada et al. (1975) stated that the surface configuration of ATP reveals a slightly enlarged but uniform granularity which is more similar to the surrounding "areae gastricae" than early cancer, type IIa (Figs. 200—204 and 205—208). ATP with a central depression is rare (Figs. 195—196 and 215—216). Therefore, the diagnosis of ATP is based upon a flat mucosal elevation with greatest diameter on the order of 10 mm and with a surface pattern similar to the surrounding "areae gastricae."

Case 49   ATP

A 54-year-old woman (JU). (Figs. 200-204)

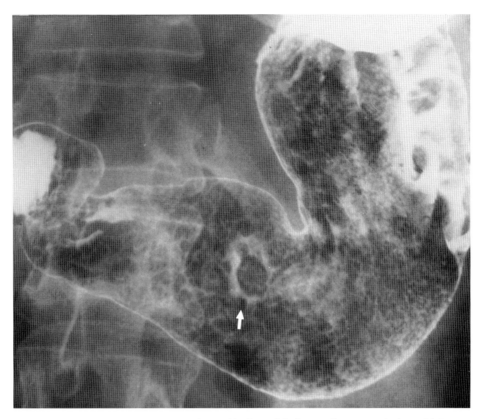

Fig. 200   Supine double contrast film demonstrates an oval polypoid lesion with fine surface granularity which is similar to the areae gastricae of the surrounding normal mucosa (arrow).

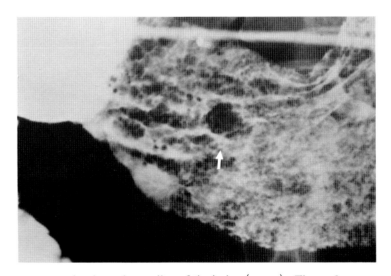

Fig. 201   Supine compression film demonstrates a somewhat irregular outline of the lesion (arrow). The surface pattern is nearly identical to that visualized in Figure 200.

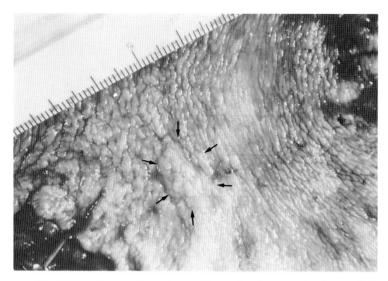

Fig. 202   Resected specimen. The lesion is recognized as a slight mucosal elevation on the posterior wall of the antrum, and measures 11 x 6 mm (arrows). Its surface pattern is nearly identical to that of the surrounding antral mucosa but the lesion is elevated.

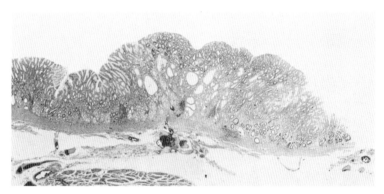

Fig. 203   Cross section of the lesion.

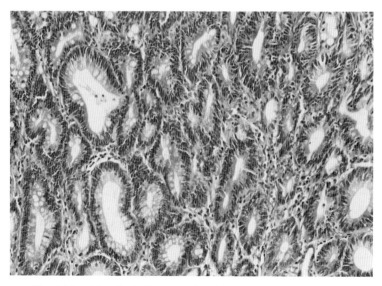

Fig. 204   Histologic findings showing ATP.

Case 50 ATP

A 51-year-old woman (JU). (Figs. 205-208)

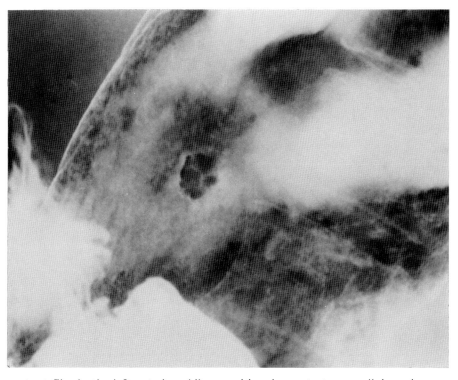

Fig. 205 Semi-upright double contrast film in the left anterior oblique position demonstrates a small, irregular polypoid lesion with a nodular surface on the posterior wall of the gastric body near the lesser curvature. In this case the granularity of the surface is irregular. The thinly coated barium frames the lesion and enables one to estimate its height. Double contrast radiography is the only method for this lesion, because the upper portion of the stomach cannot be compressed.

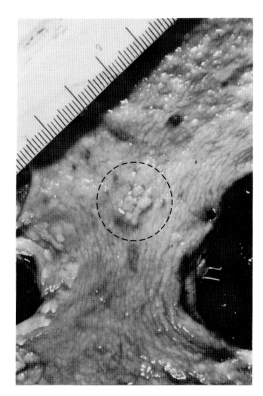

Fig. 206 Resected specimen (by cardiotomy). There is an elevation of the mucosa on the posterior wall of the upper gastric body near the lesser curvature, measuring 9 x 7 mm. The granularity of the surface appears somewhat irregular, compared with that of Figure 202.

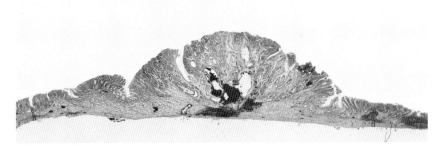

Fig. 207   Cross section of the lesion.

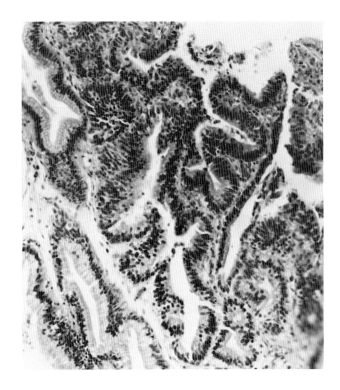

Fig. 208   Histologic findings of ATP.

Case 51   ATP

A 53-year-old man (CIH). (Figs. 209-214)

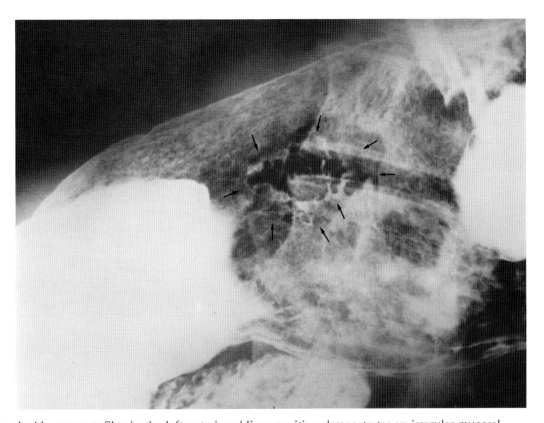

Fig. 209   Supine double contrast film in the left anterior oblique position demonstrates an irregular mucosal elevation on the mid-portion of the gastric body which is framed by thinly coated barium and is composed of fine, uniform granularity.

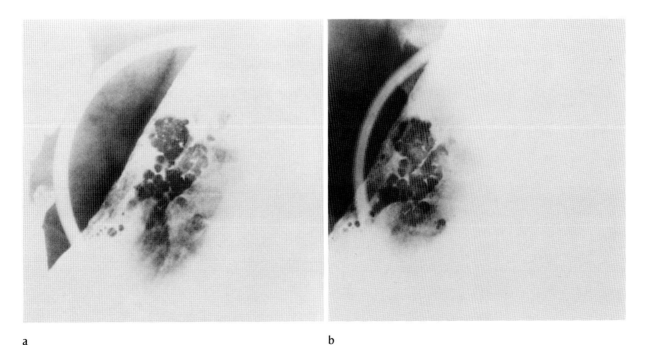

a   b

Fig. 210 a and b   Upright compression films reveal the surface configuration more clearly than does the double contrast image

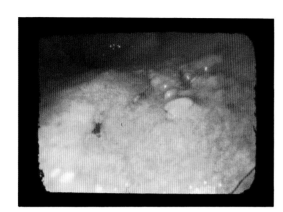

Fig. 211   Endoscopic findings.

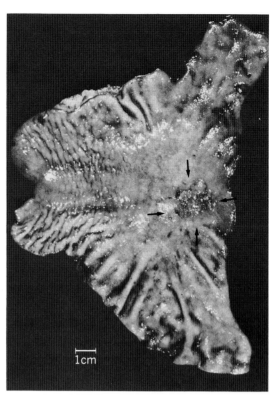

Fig. 212

Fig. 212   Resected specimen. The lesion (arrows) is located on the lesser curvature of the lower gastric body, and measures 23 x 15 mm. The surrounding normal mucosa appears rather atrophic. The surface granularity is similar to that of the antral mucosa.

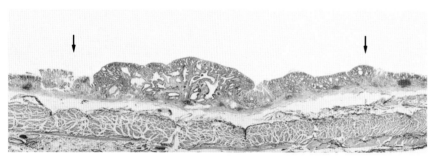

Fig. 213   Cross section of the lesion.

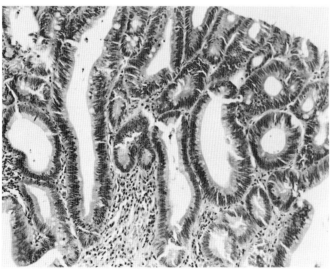

Fig. 214   Histologic findings of ATP.

Case 52   ATP with Central Depression

A 61-year-old woman (JU). (Figs. 215-216)

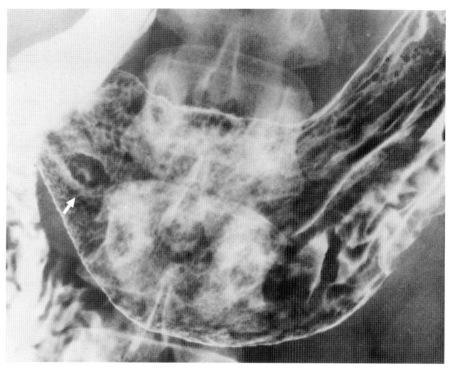

Fig. 215   Supine double contrast film demonstrates a small oval polypoid lesion on the posterior wall of the antrum (arrow). Faint barium collection on the surface reveals a slight depression.

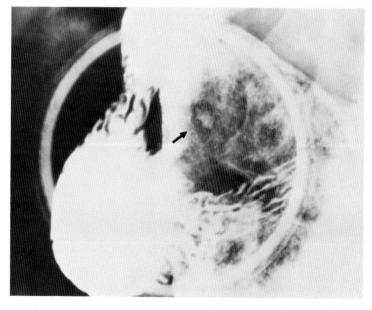

Fig. 216   Upright compression film demonstrates the central depression more clearly than does the double contrast image (arrow). The elevated portion has a surface pattern almost identical to the that of surrounding antral mucosa.

Chapter 6

Theoretical Basis for the Radiographic Diagnosis of Depressed Early Cancer

General Considerations

The radiographic diagnosis of depressed early cancer is based upon the analysis of the depression and of the converging folds. The depression is analyzed in terms of its shape, surface and depth. Generally, the shape of the depression is irregular with serrated or spiculated margins, compared with that of a benign ulcer (Fig. 217). However, irregular margins are sometimes visualized in cases of recurrent peptic ulcer and cannot be distinguished from those of early depressed cancer (Figs. 218–219). The margins of depressed early cancer usually are clearly distinguished from the normal

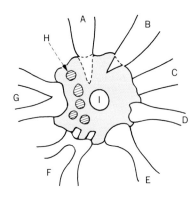

A : Gradual tapering   B : Abrupt tapering
C : Abrupt interruption   D, E : Clubbing
F : Fusion with abrupt tapering   G : Fusion (V-shaped deformity)
H : Unevenness   I : Regenerative epithelium

Fig. 217 Various appearances of converging folds and uneveness of depression in early depressed cancer (From Shirakabe and Maruyama 1981).

Case 53   **Peptic Ulcer with Irregular Niche.**
A 45-year-old man (CIH). (Figs. 218 and 219)

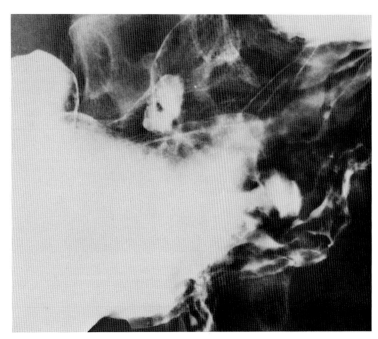

Fig. 218 Double contrast radiograph demonstrates an irregular niche in a case of recurrent peptic ulcer.

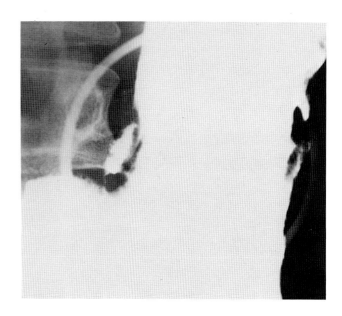

Fig. 219 Compression film demonstrates the irregular niche and the surrounding radiolucency, which also appears slightly irregular.

Case 54   Type IIc Early Cancer.
A 45-year-old women (CIH). (Fig. 220)

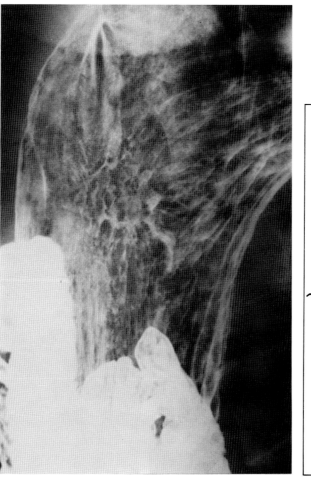
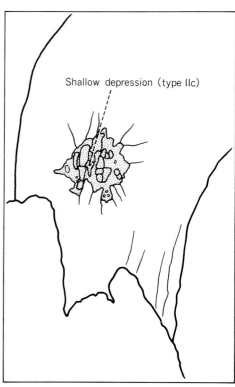

Shallow depression (type IIc)

Fig. 220 Double contrast film in the left anterior oblique position demonstrates typical unevenness of the depressed surface in a type IIc lesion.

mucosal surface, and sometimes gradually merges with it. In the latter case it is difficult to define the extent of a depressed lesion (refer to Chapter 11).

In most cases of depressed early cancer, the surface of the depression has unevenness caused by irregular proliferation of cancerous tissue (Fig. 220). Sometimes there remain a few island-like nodules in the depression which are more prominent than the unevenness of the depression. These consist of regenerative epithelium. Their presence strongly suggests the possibility of early cancer. Depth of depression varies depending upon the degree of cancerous erosion and of associated peptic ulceration. Usually, the depression of the cancerous erosion is no deeper than 2 to 3 mm.

The converging folds in depressed early cancer reveal characteristic findings such as tapering, clubbing, interruption and fusion (Fig. 217). The fusion of the folds is called "V deformity" (Shirakabe and Ichikawa 1973). These abnormalities of the fold pattern are signs of malignancy.

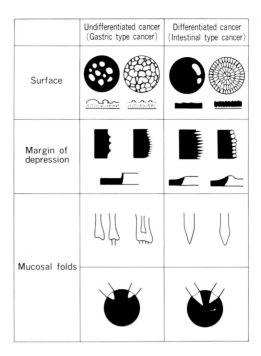

Fig. 221 Typical radiographic findings of early gastric cancer in each histologic type (Baba et al. 1977).

Radiographic Diagnosis of Depressed Lesions

Baba et al. (1977) has shown a close correlation of the radiographic findings with the histologic type of early cancer. As Nakamura et al. (1971) proposed, it is practical and reasonable to divide gastric cancer into two basic histologic types, namely, undifferentiated and differentiated cancer. It is widely acknowledged that undifferentiated cancer arises from the ordinary gastric mucosa (pyloric and fundic glands) and differentiated cancer from intestinal metaplasia. This is why the former is called gastric type cancer and the latter is called intestinal type cancer. Baba disclosed the significant difference in the radiographic findings of depressed early cancer between the two histologic types. In the undifferentiated cancer the surface is mostly uneven and coarse, while in differentiated cancer it is mostly fine and uniform. In many undifferentiated cancers and abrupt transition takes place from the normal surrounding mucosa to depression, while in differentiated cancer there is a gradual transition from the normal surrounding mucosa to a depression which tends to obscure its borders. The converging folds reveal sudden interruption or tapering in the undifferentiated cancer, while they reveal gradual tapering in the differentiated cancer. Club-shaped thickening and fusion of the folds are often visualized in the undifferentiated cancer (Fig. 221).

Clinically, the recognition of the difference in the histologic type of depressed early cancer helps determine the line of resection. Radiologists should report on a proximal border of a lesion when taking the histologic type into consideration.

Radiographic Diagnosis of Types IIc, III and IIc+III

The difference between type IIc and type III is radiographically recognized by the thickness of collected barium in a depression. A thick collection of barium in a depression in benign peptic ulcer can be regarded as that of type III (Figs. 222—225) but a thinner collection of barium is regarded as a depression of type IIc. Lesions having a combination of the two different depths is termed IIc + III (Figs. 226—228) or type III + IIc (Figs. 229—232). Usually the deeper part (type III) is in the center of the depression and is surrounded by the shallower part (type IIc).

A type IIc lesion does not show uniform density of barium in its depression. An ulcer scar with slight depression must be differentiated from type IIc lesion. Usually the depression of the ulcer scar is fainter than that of the type IIc lesion and reveals homogeneous density of the contrast medium (Fig. 233). Moreover, the converging folds show gradual tapering.

Case 55   Type III Early Cancer.

A 58-year-old man (CU). (Figs. 222-225)

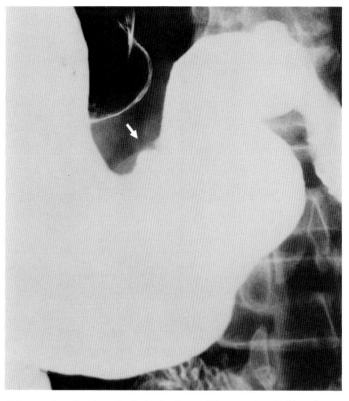

Fig. 222   Prone barium-filled film demonstrates a niche at the distal end of the incisura. The proximal side of the niche appears to be irregular (arrow).

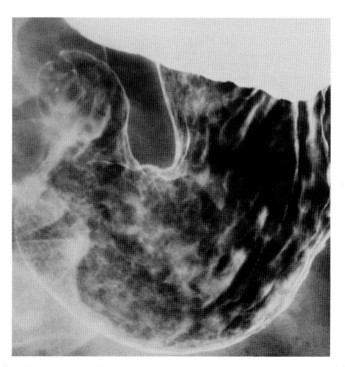

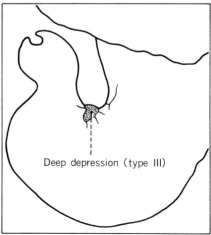

Deep depression (type III)

Fig. 223   Double contrast film in the supine right anterior oblique position demonstrates irregularity of the niche at the incisura. The barium is not thickly collected in the depression on the posterior wall.

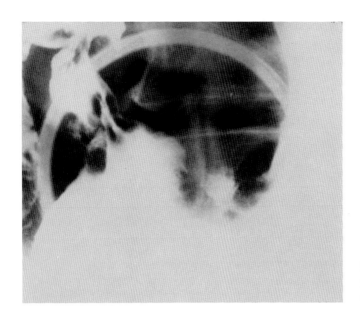

Fig. 224 Upright compression film demonstrates the irregular niche and the surrounding radiolucency, which is diagnosed as type III.

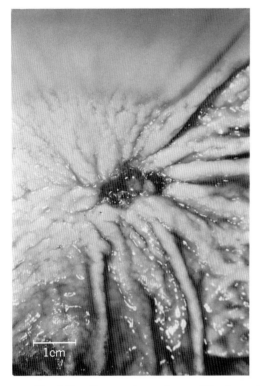
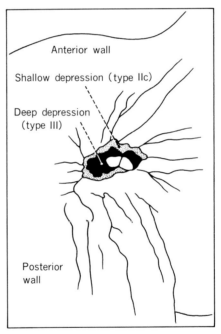

Fig. 225 Resected specimen. The irregular ulcer, measuring 18 x 13 mm is at the insura. It is diagnosed macroscopically as type III. Histological findings showed adenocarcinoma tubulare (well-differentiated adenocarcinoma). Cancer was limited to the mucosa (m). Schematic representation showing localization of cancer.

Type III is an extreme case with no macroscopically recognizable type IIc (Chapter 1). Cancer is indentified radiographically in these lesions by the slightest findings of type IIc or by irregularity partially or completely surrounding the niche (Figs. 234–240) (Kumakura et al. 1973, Maruyama 1979). Accordingly, close observation of a niche may lead to recognition of the partial irregularity of its margin. Sometimes, the surrounding radiolucency seems to be prominent in a type III lesion when an acute peptic change has taken place (Figs. 241–245).

Attention should be paid to a profile niche which does not reveal any irregularity. In such a case the diagnosis of a peptic ulcer should be made very carefully by confirming an absence of type IIc lesion around the niche. Hampton's line alone cannot be a sign of benign peptic ulcer. A frontal view of the niche and the surrounding mucosa is required in order to make sure that no type IIc part is present. Otherwise the diagnosis of type III + IIc is missed. With follow-up studies the niche

may decrease in size and the surrounding type IIc lesion become clearly recognized. The appearance and disappearance of the niche may be repeated in a type IIc lesion during a long clinical course. This phenomenon is called "malignant cycle" (Murakami 1966, see Chapter 12). Thus, simple disappearance of the niche by medical treatment cannot be used as a sign of benign peptic ulcer.

In certain phases of healing peptic ulcer, erosions may be visualized around a small niche simulating a type IIc + III lesion (Figs. 244, 245). Although the erosion may disappear in a short period, endoscopic biopsy is necessary to confirm its benign nature.

Case 56 Type IIc + III Early Cancer.
A 58-year-old man (CPCC). (Figs. 226-228)

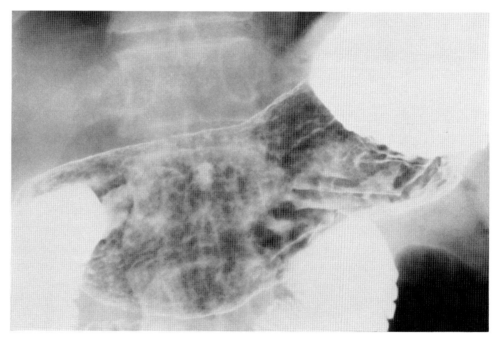

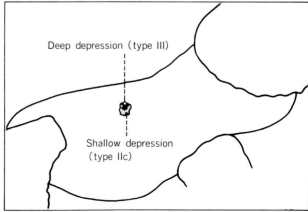

Fig. 226 Supine double contrast film demonstrates an irregular niche (type III) and a surrounding faint barium collection (type IIc) on the posterior wall of the incisura.

119

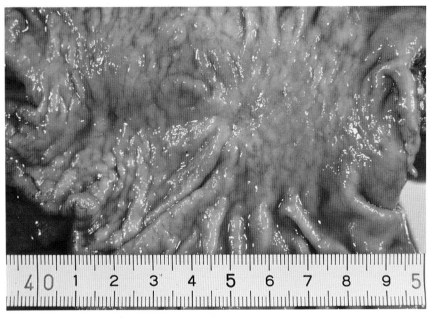

Fig. 227 Resected specimen. The depression measures 17 x 16 mm. The deeper part is diagnosed as ulcer and the surrounding shallow depression is diagnosed as type IIc. The entire lesion is diagnosed as type III + IIc.

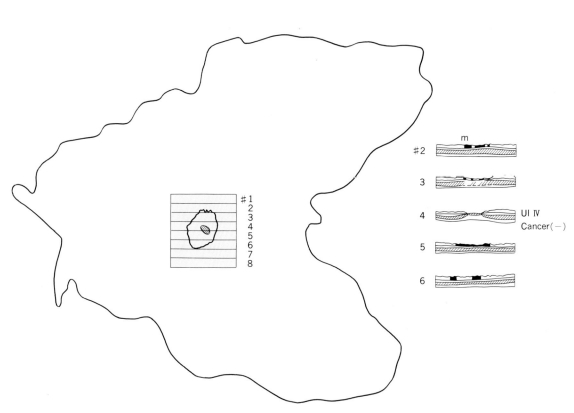

Fig. 228 Schematic representation of the macroscopic findings showing localization of cancer. Histologic examination revealed poorly adenocarcinoma scirrhosum (differentiated adenocarcinoma) limited to the mucosa (m). Depth of ulcer was Ul-IV.

120

Case 57   Type III + IIc + IIb (IIc) Early Cancer.
A 53-year-old woman (CPCC). (Figs. 229 -232) (See Chapter 1)

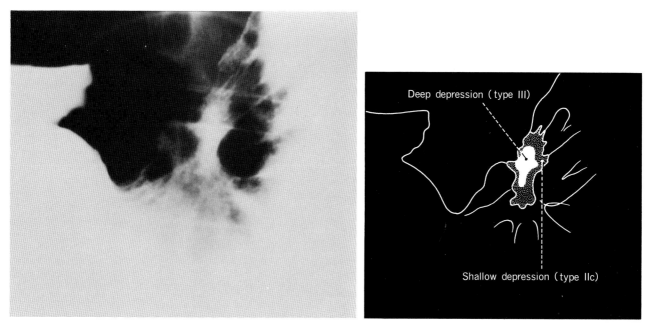

Fig. 229   Upright compression film demonstrates an irregular collection of barium at the upper part of the incisura near the lesser curvature. The thicker collection of barium indicates type III, and the surrounding thinner collection, type IIc.

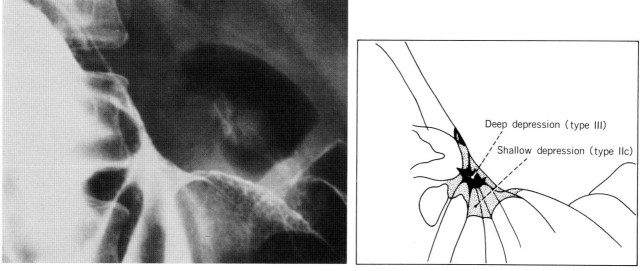

Fig. 230   Prone double contrast film demonstrates the same depression as was visualized in Figure 229. The mucosal convergence is typical of early depressed cancer.

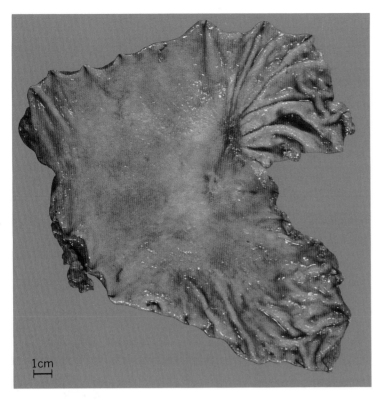

Fig. 231 Resected specimen. The depressive lesion measures 100 x 70 mm.

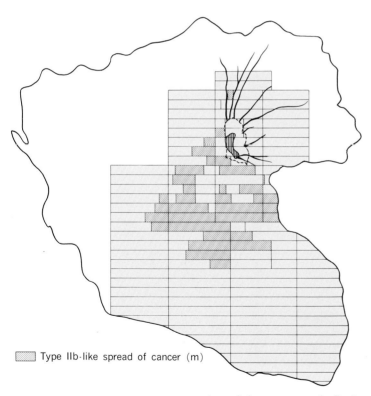

▨ Type IIb-like spread of cancer (m)

Fig. 232 Schematic representation of the macroscopic findings and localization of cancer. Histologic examination disclosed a large area of IIb-like spread of cancer extending to the posterior wall which could not be detected before surgery (refer to Chapter 11).

Case 58 Ulcer Scar with Slight Depression.
A 54-year-old man (CIH). (Fig. 233)

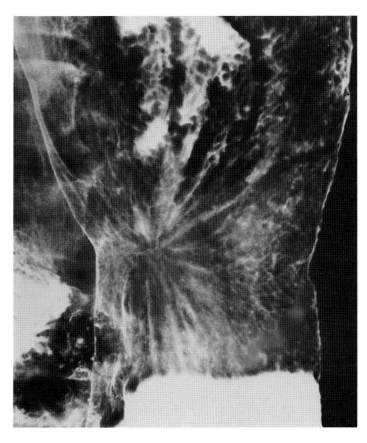

Fig. 233 Double contrast film showing benign ulcer scar with slight depression.

Case 59 Type III Early Cancer.
A 57-year-old man (CIH). (Figs. 234-240)

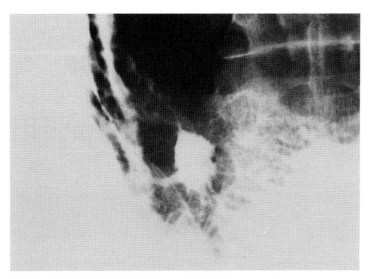

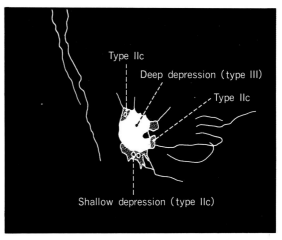

Fig. 234 Prone compression film demonstrates an irregular niche at the incisura. Irregularity is more pronounced on the antral side of the niche, where a thinner collection of barium indicates type IIc.

123

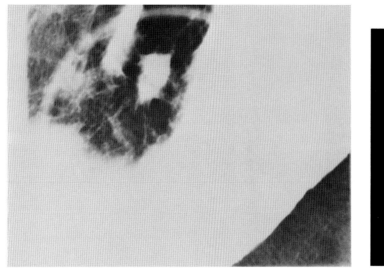
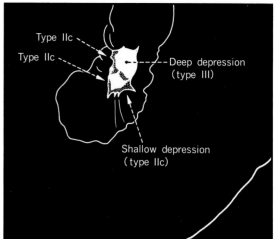

Fig. 235   Upright compression film demonstrates the irregular niche.

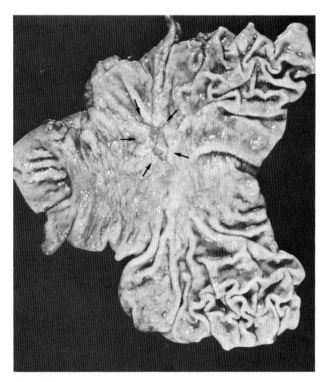
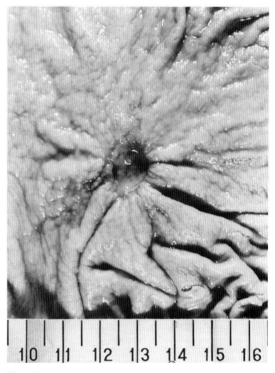

Fig. 236   Fig. 237

Fig. 236 and 237   Resected specimen. The depression, measuring 20 x 15 mm, is on the anterior wall near the incisura.

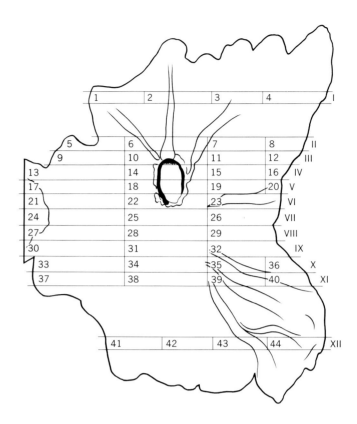

Fig. 238 Schematic representation of the macroscopic findings and localization of cancer.

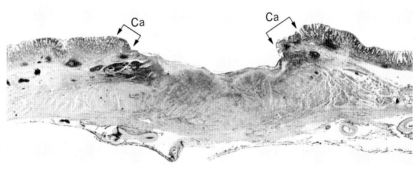

Fig. 239 Cross section of the lesion (UI-III).

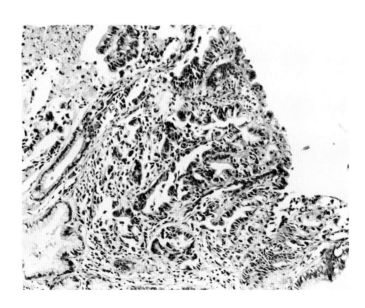

Fig. 240 Histologic findings showing adenocarcinoma tubulare (well-differentiated adenocarcinoma). Cancer was limited to the mucosa (m) and the depth of ulcer was UI-III.

Case 60 Type III Early Cancer.

A 67-year-old man (CIH). (Figs. 240-245)

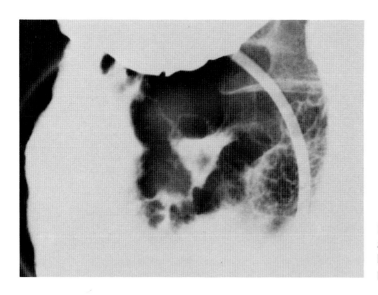

Fig. 241 Upright compression film demonstrates an irregular niche with marked surrounding radiolucency. It was felt that acute exacerbation of a peptic ulcer has taken place in the lesion.

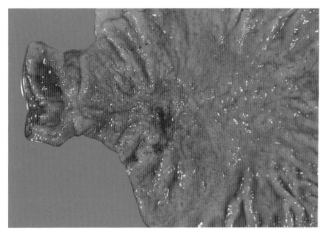

Fig. 242 Resected specimen. The lesion, measuring 40 x 25 mm, is on the anterior wall near the incisura.

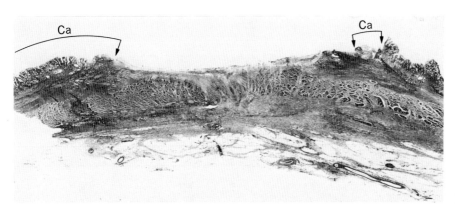

Fig. 243 Cross section of the lesion.

Case 61 Peptic Ulcer with Surrounding Erosion
A 34-year-old woman (CIH). (Figs. 244 and 245)

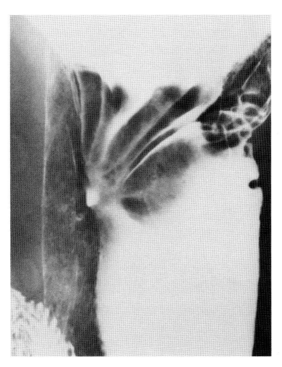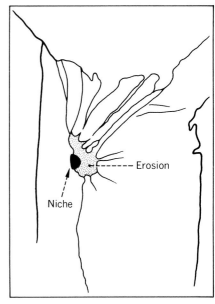

Fig. 244 Supine double contrast film demonstrating a small peptic ulcer surrounded by a benign erosion. The converging folds reveal a somewhat irregular interruption at the edge of the erosion.

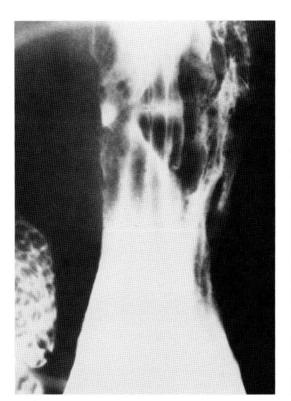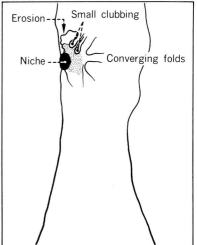

Fig. 245 Upright compression film demonstrating the small niche and the surrounding erosion. Two large folds reveal slight clubbing.

Chapter 7

Radiographic Diagnosis of Peptic Ulcer

Single Ulcer

General considerations

Many investigators have studied the development of peptic ulcer of the stomach from its onset to its chronic state. Peptic ulcer may show spontaneous healing, but it is an extremely uncontrollable disease that exacerbates and recurs repeatedly. Being difficult to follow clinically, it is not well understood. Radiographic diagnosis can identify the presence or absence of ulcer, and the number of ulcers, thereby aiding clinically in its medical management.

There are two ways to diagnose peptic ulcer. One is to detect a single round ulcer and make a definitive diagnosis. This method is the hallmark radiographic diagnosis and was instituted by Reiche (1909) and Haudek (1910). The other is to deduce the existence or absence of an ulcer, its location and its morphology by the deformity of the stomach in cases when a niche is not easily found. Among the deformities of the stomach "Beutelmagen" (Riedel 1909) and "schnecken-förmige Einrollung" (Schmieden and Härtel 1909), for example, are terms used for decades. Murakami et al. (1959) and Shirakabe et al. (1959a, b) later proved the relationship between these deformities and linear ulcer. Kumakura (1960) made a great contribution to radiographic diagnosis of multiple ulcers which cause specific deformities of the stomach. Their studies will be discussed later.

Shirakabe et al. (1956a, b, 1957, 1958, 1959a, b) studied peptic ulcer in their early investigations of the radiographic diagnosis of the stomach. According to Kumakura, the texts by Eschbach (1949a, b) and Bücker (1950) were suggested to him when he began his research. Kumakura made a detailed analysis of the nature of gastric ulcer, both acute and chronic using a single radiographic examination but without follow-up. Kumakura noticed that Eschbach analyzed the radiographic findings of ulcer and its surrounding region based upon histopathological findings contained in Hauser's textbook (1926) and Bücker (1950) did similarly with Konjetzny's textbook (1926). He began his own research on the radiographic diagnosis of gastric ulcer based upon operated cases. His method was to make as many microscopic preparations as possible of the operated specimen and to compare them with radiographic findings. This is a time-consuming process but is the best means of making a reliable diagnosis, and it was this method that made radiographic diagnosis of peptic ulcer applicable to early gastric cancer.

Shortly after he began his study, Kumakura (1960) noticed a wide discrepancy between radiographic diagnosis and histologic diagnosis if he followed Eschbach's and Bücker's textbooks exactly. One of the causes of this discrepancy, Kumakura presumed, was the abstract description by Eschbach and Bücker. But the main difficulty was the absence of a comparative study between radiographic findings and histo-pathologic ones, even though Eschbach and Bücker analyzed the radiographic findings according to Hauser's and Konjetzny's histological descriptions. This realization forced Kumakura (1960) to reexamine the radiographic diagnosis of gastric ulcer, and was a major turning point in Japan's history of the radiographic diagnosis of the stomach. Radiographic diagnosis departed from traditional methodology, which relied on textual facts, and evolved the topological idea of a one-to-one correspondence between resected specimens and radiographic findings. Shirakabe et al. (1956, a, b, 1957, 1958, 1959, a, b, 1961, 1967), Kumakura (1960, 1965, 1967) investigated the best method of radiographic examination. They compared pre-operative radiographic films with the corresponding films of resected specimens filled with barium, and discovered that precise macroscopic findings were obtainable. They made as many histological preparations of a lesion as possible in order to compare the radiographic findings with the histological findings in minute detail. Shirakabe's and Kumakura's theories were based on the premise that precise macroscopic findings can be demonstrated by high-quality, well-performed radiography. In Japan, radiographic studies of the digestive tract have since been performed with this in mind.

Histologic classification of ulcer

The depth of an ulcer can be described radiographically or surgically. Hauser (1926) used the term penetrating ulcer to mean an ulcer which has broken through a large area of the entire thickness of the gastric wall. On the other hand, surgeons mean by that term an ulcer that has penetrated the neighboring organs such as the pancreas or the spleen. Since it was hardly possible to describe the depth of ulcer objectively, Murakami and his co-workers (Murakami et al. 1959, Murakami 1961, Koide 1961) classified the depth of ulcer histologically, as shown in Figure 246. Murakami's classification, which presently is in wide use in Japan, is not only adequate to describe the depth of an ulcer his-

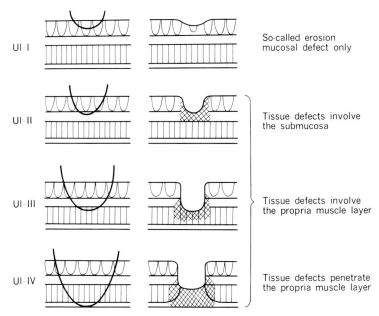

Fig. 246   Murakami's classification of peptic ulcer according to its depth (Murakami et al. 1959).

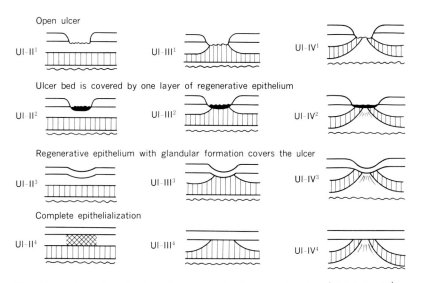

Fig. 247   Murakami's classification of healing peptic ulcer (Koide 1961).

tologically but also valuable in clinically evaluating its healing process. This classification also has enabled us to discuss ulcer-cancer sequence for all ulcers without considering the specific conditions of Hauser's criteria for ulcer-cancer sequence. This matter will be discussed later (Chapter 12).

Murakami's classification is simplified as follows: UI-I means a tissue defect limited to the mucosa. In general, this tissue defect of UI-I is called an erosion, not an ulcer. UI-II is a tissue defect breaking through the muscularis mucosae into the submucosal layer. UI-III is a tissue defect reaching the propria muscle without penetrating it. In UI-IV the tissue defect penetrates the entire thickness of the gastric wall.

Accordingly, the tissue defect from UI-II to UI-IV is the so-called ulcer, UI-II being the shallowest and UI-IV the deepest.

Figure 247 shows the formation of ulcer scar according to the depth of the ulcer. Four stages are present for each degree of ulceration. This classification according to the degree of healing is not so widely used as the classification of ulcer itself. In generally accepted usage, the letter S (scar) is employed and a scar is expressed as UI-IIS, UI-IIIS or UI-IVS. For example, UI-IIS means a shallow ulcer with tissue defect remaining within the submucosal layer and healing with scar. This method to express the degree of ulcer and ulcer scar is employed in this book to deal with the histological diagnoses when discussing the depth of an ulcer coexisting with early cancer, or when discussing the degree of healing.

Converging folds or mucosal convergence

The term *converging folds* is applied to folds which converge more or less toward a niche as visualized radiographically. Eisler and Lenk (1921) were the first to report converging folds. This had long been thought to be the sign of scar contracture (Rendich 1923, Chaul 1929, 1931). Chaul pointed out that converging folds were clearer in vivo than in the operated stomach and resulted from the contraction of the muscularis mucosae. Little change has been made in the interpretation of converging folds, which was considered to be the result of contraction of the muscularis mucosae or of scar formation in the vicinity of the ulcer. It was a general understanding that converging folds were formed by "Autoplastik" (autoplasty) according to Forssell's (1927) terms, together with scar contracture of the ulcer (Berg 1930, Assmann 1949, 1950, Tamiya 1958, Katsch and Pickert 1953).

Attempts were made to utilize converging folds as an indicator of the age of an ulcer. Baensch (1926) considered converging folds as an early sign of ulcer. They were considered to be the sign of ulcus callosum by Porcher et al. (1959) and Teschendorf (1949); a reliable evidence of ulcer scar or healed ulcer by Stoerk (1925) and Bayer (1936). Schinz et al. (1952) felt that the absence of a niche at the center of converging folds was evidence that an ulcer was healed. Eschbach (1949) stated that converging folds can be seen at a comparatively early stage, at an advanced stage, and also at a healing stage. According to Eschbach, coexistence of the rod-like converging folds as a result of marked thickening, plus an irregular niche situated in the center, are the characteristic signs of ulcus callosum.

The presence or absence of the converging folds and their stage of development are discussed from the standpoint of radiographic diagnosis. For example, the appearance of the converging folds is greatly influenced by the degree of distension of the resected specimen or by the degree of fixation. The same is true for the radiographic findings. The radiographic method used, and the distension of the gastric wall affect the appearance of the converging folds.

A comparison of the histologic findings of converging folds and their surrounding region with the macroscopic findings follows: When the converging folds surround the ulcer, there is a marked fusion of muscularis propria and muscularis mucosae almost entirely around the ulcer. And when the converging folds are either absent or present but not very distinguishable, either no fusion or only a very slight fusion occurs. These findings are evaluated on the freshly operated stomach, which is unfixed, incised along the greater curvature and laid out on a flat surface.

Although converging folds of a benign ulcer usually reach the ulcer edge without interruption, in some cases they are interrupted and do not reach the ulcer edge (Eschbach 1949, Kumakura 1960, Gonoi 1965).

Kumakura (1960) classified the various forms of converging folds macroscopically: (1) interrupted converging folds, (2) uninterrupted converging folds, (3) special type of converging folds (Fig. 248).

In the interrupted converging folds there is an elevated edge (ulcer mound) interrupting them (Figs. 249, 250). The mucosal convergence is not remarkable or absent in such a case. Histologically, thickening of the entire layer of the gastric wall is observed at the elevated portion of the ulcer edge,

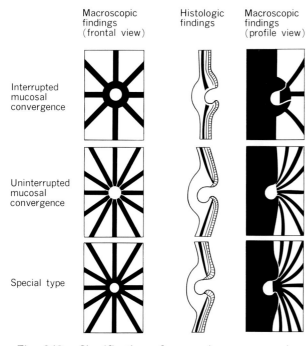

Fig. 248 Classification of mucosal convergence in peptic ulcer (From Kumakura 1960).

and is especially marked in the submucosal layer. The fusion of the muscularis propria and muscularis mucosae is wholly absent or slight if present. The elevated portion is radiographically observed as a radiolucent band (Figs. 249, 250, 252, 254) around which the slight converging folds are present. This radiolucent band corresponds to the so-called ulcer collar in the English literature and to the Schwellungshof in the German literature. These findings will be referred to in "ulcer mound" below.

The uninterrupted converging folds reach the ulcer edge without interruption, as macroscopic and histological findings disclose (Fig. 253). Histologically, fusion is observed almost entirely around the ulcer, and no localized thickening of the submucosal layer is found. This type of converging folds is encountered most frequently.

When mucosal thickening presents elevation at the ulcer edge and fusion is clearly observable, the converging folds belong to the special type. A feature shared by this type and the interrupted converging folds is the failure of the converging

---

Case 62   Peptic Ulcer with Interrupted Converging Folds.
A 43-year-old man (CIH). (Figs. 249-251)

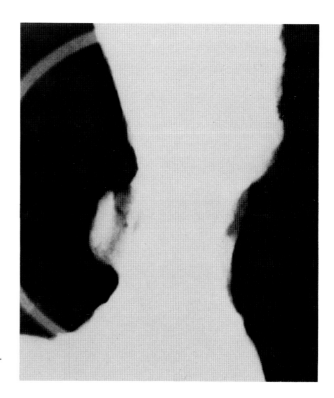

Fig. 249 Upright compression film demonstrates an ulcer collar.

131

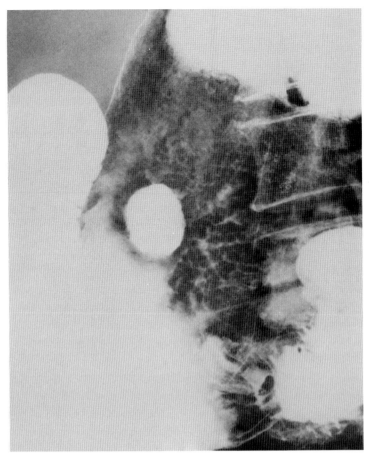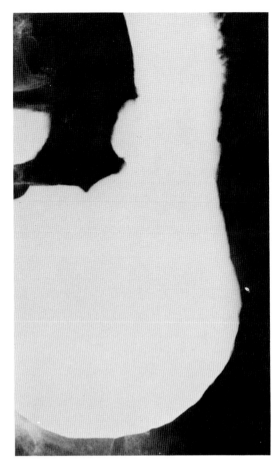

Fig. 250   Fig. 251

Fig. 250 Double contrast film in the left anterior oblique position demonstrates a frontal view of the niche seen in Figure 249. Slight mucosal convergence is interrupted by a large radiolucency.

Fig. 251 Barium-filled film demonstrates depression of the margin above and below the niche (arrow).

folds to reach the ulcer edge. The mucosal folds of the special type, however, are often gathered together radiographically. Kumakura claims that differentiation between the special type of the converging folds and the interrupted converging folds is possible radiographically.

In summary, when the uninterrupted converging folds form a complete circle around the ulcer, fusion can be observed circularly in almost all of the cases; when the converging folds are partially interrupted, fusion is observed at the corresponding uninterrupted portion and fusion is absent or very slight in the interrupted converging folds.

It is known from clinical observations that definite uninterrupted converging folds appear when a large and deep ulcer, i.e. Ul-IV, becomes smaller. It is also known that marked interrupted converging folds appear with scar formation in an

ulcer classified Ul-III or Ul-IV and larger than 10 mm in diameter (Hauser 1926).

Clinical significance of converging folds

Clinically, both fusion and uninterrupted converging folds indicate a healing process at the edge of an Ul-III or Ul-IV. A fusion would not exist if healing were incomplete at the ulcer edge or if the ulcer were still active. In an ulcer with partial uninterrupted converging folds, there are some portions where fusion is clearly observable and others where it is not. This means that healing does not occur uniformly in the same ulcer. On the basis of his experience, Kumakura (1960) concluded that uninterrupted converging folds are a sign of healing (Fig. 254). With a complete circle of

Case 63   Peptic Ulcer with Interrupted Converging Folds.
A 42-year-old man (CIH). (Fig. 252)

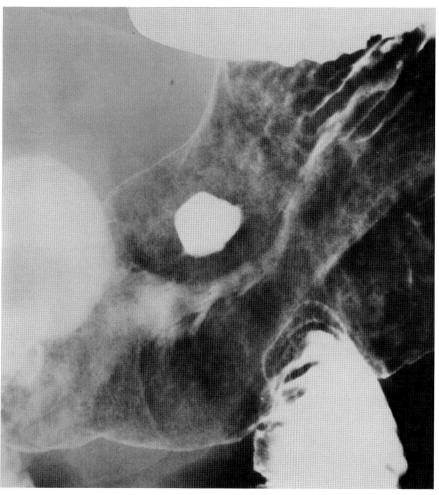

Fig. 252   Double contrast film in the right anterior oblique position demonstrates a frontal view of a niche with surrounding radiolucency. Coverging folds are barely visible.

uninterrupted converging folds an ulcer has markedly shrunk and no further shrinkage is expected. In such a case the ulcer depth is Ul-IV or at least Ul-III and it is comparatively old (Fig. 255). On the other hand, an ulcer with interrupted converging folds is comparatively acute and healings is minimal. Recent recurrence or exacerbation of an ulcer is suspected when uninterrupted converging folds are found in only a limited portion of the ulcer (Kumakura 1960). This situation, however, needs further study, because in some of these cases the ulcer clinically appears inactive.

Interrupted converging folds are found in an acute ulcer. Shrinkage of the ulcer occurs with adequate therapy. The special type of the converging folds are found in relatively chronic ulcers, whose depth is of Ul-IV or at least Ul-III. Clinically, the same interpretation of uninterrupted converging folds applies to this type because of the marked fusion mentioned above. The exact depth of the ulcer cannot be estimated by the converging folds only.

Case 64   Peptic Ulcer with Uninterrupted Converging Folds.
A 68-year-old man (JU). (Fig. 253)

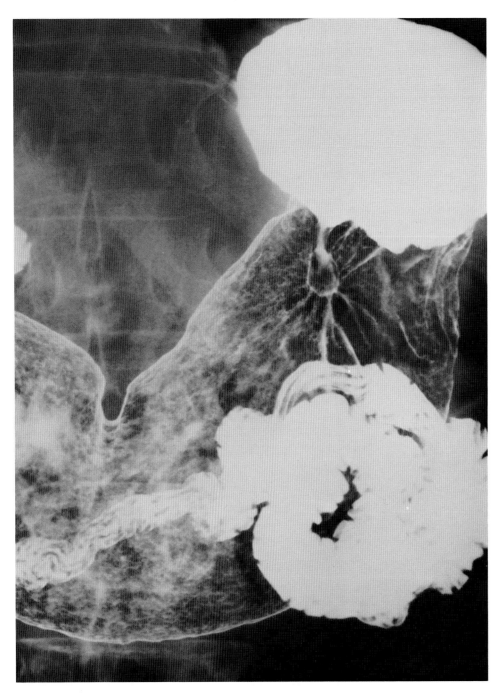

Fig. 253   Double contrast film in the supine frontal position demonstrates a niche with uninterrupted mucosal folds.

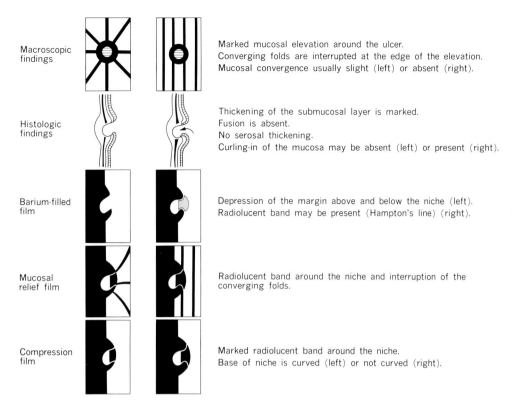

Macroscopic findings

Marked mucosal elevation around the ulcer.
Converging folds are interrupted at the edge of the elevation.
Mucosal convergence usually slight (left) or absent (right).

Histologic findings

Thickening of the submucosal layer is marked.
Fusion is absent.
No serosal thickening.
Curling-in of the mucosa may be absent (left) or present (right).

Barium-filled film

Depression of the margin above and below the niche (left).
Radiolucent band may be present (Hampton's line) (right).

Mucosal relief film

Radiolucent band around the niche and interruption of the converging folds.

Compression film

Marked radiolucent band around the niche.
Base of niche is curved (left) or not curved (right).

Fig. 254   Characteristics of acute peptic ulcer, which heals easily (From Kumakura 1960).

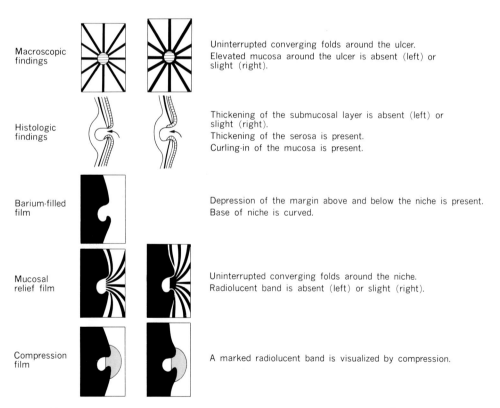

Macroscopic findings

Uninterrupted converging folds around the ulcer.
Elevated mucosa around the ulcer is absent (left) or slight (right).

Histologic findings

Thickening of the submucosal layer is absent (left) or slight (right).
Thickening of the serosa is present.
Curling-in of the mucosa is present.

Barium-filled film

Depression of the margin above and below the niche is present.
Base of niche is curved.

Mucosal relief film

Uninterrupted converging folds around the niche.
Radiolucent band is absent (left) or slight (right).

Compression film

A marked radiolucent band is visualized by compression.

Fig. 255   Characteristics of chronic peptic ulcer, which heals with difficulty (From Kumakura 1960).

Ulcer mound

The region surrounding a niche depicted on a radiograph has been called various names. "Randwall" and "Schutzwall" (Forssell 1927); "Ringwall" and "Schwellungshof" (Berg 1930); Schwellungsring (Kuhlmann 1950); Ulkuswall (Shinz 1952); ulcer mound (Wolf and Marshak 1957), etc. The depth of the niche radiographically is always deeper than the true depth of the ulcer. Subsequently, the elevation surrounding a niche (ulcer mound) was utilized to define the ulcer's nature. The cause of an ulcer mound has been ascribed to inflammatory swelling of the sub-mucosa (Gutmann 1956, Berg 1930, Chaul and Adam 1931, Prévôt and Lasrich 1959) or the autoplasty of the surrounding mucosa (Forssell 1927, Kurokawa 1956).

On a radiograph it appears as a depression above and below a niche in the profile view on the barium-filled film, as disappearance of the folds in the mucosal relief film and as a ring-like radiolucency around the niche in the compression film. These findings are called Schwellungshof or ulcer mound and are associated with an acute ulcer.

The cause of the ulcer mound in a chronic ulcer, however, has been considered to be proliferation of connective tissue in the submucosa and subserosa at the ulcer edge (Gutzeit 1929, Teschendorf 1949, Schinz et al. 1952, Prévôt and Lasrich 1959). Teschendorf in particular regards the proliferation of connective tissue as the cause of the depression above and below a niche in the profile view and of the radiolucency around the niche in the compression film. He attributes these two findings to the features of ulcus callosum.

Eschbach disagrees, claiming that the ulcer mound can occasionally be seen in ulcus callosum near the pylorus, but usually the ulcer edge in ulcus callosum is basically flat without a mound. He sees little importance in the recognition of an elevation at the ulcer edge. Generally speaking, a majority opinion in Europe and in the United States has been that one cannot distinguish radiographically whether the ulcer mound is an inflammatory swelling or a proliferation of connective tissue (Katsch and Pickert 1953, Schinz et al. 1952, Carman 1921).

Among the varied and puzzling descriptions of the ulcer mound, the term, Schwellungshof evokes the clearest image. The ulcer mound generally appears in the barium-filled film, the mucosal relief picture and the compression film. However occasional cases occur in which radiographic findings identical to Schwellungshof are absent in the barium-filled films and the mucosal relief film, while in the compression film a radiolucency is present around a niche (Kumakura 1960). In such a case, the mucosa surrounding the ulcer is rather flat and the gastric wall is markedly thickened as a result of thickening of the serosa side (Kumakura 1960). Forssell (1927), Gutzeit (1929) and Schinz (1952) took notice of this fact but a review of their work demonstrates a divergence of opinion between Schinz and the others (Fig. 256). Schinz states that the findings of the thickening on the serosa side can be obtained radiologically only by the compression method. Based on this fact and the special converging folds of mucosal thickening (mentioned previously), Kumakura (1965) classified ulcers into the three types: (1) thickening of the submucosal layer, (2) thickening on the serosa side only and (3) thickening of both the mucosa and the serosa side.

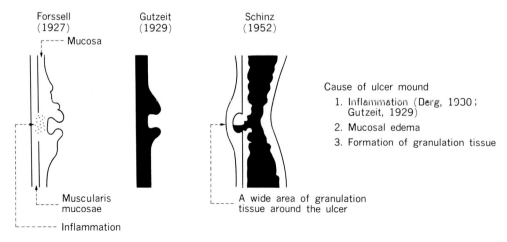

Fig. 256 Cause of ulcer mound.

Thickening of the submucosa

The ulcer mound can be observed in the barium-filled film, the mucosal relief film and the compression film. The compression film produces the clearest image, equivalent to the Schwellungshof or ulcer collar (Fig. 249). The depression above and below the niche is seen in the profile view of the barium-filled film (Fig. 251). A radiolucency between the niche and the stomach is sometimes observable. This is the so-called Hampton's line (Fig. 257) when the radiolucency has a linear appearance (Hampton 1937). This is considered to be a reliable sign of benign ulcer but occurs in early cancer. In the mucosal relief picture, the mucosal folds are interrupted near the niche. In the compression picture it is observed as a well-defined radiolucent band. Occasionally, however, no depression above or below a niche and/or no Hampton's line is observable in the barium-filled film when the ulcer mound is minimally elevated.

Thickening on the serosa side only

The image of the ulcer mound can be obtained only in the compression film. In the barium-filled film, there is flatness above and below a niche, and sometimes distorsion of the gastric wall is present where it is markedly thickened. In the compression picture, a radiolucency is seen around the niche, but it is not as well defined as Schwellungshof or ulcer collar. A radiolucency is absent when the thickening on the serosa side is not marked. In the mucosal relief picture and the double contrast

---

Case 65   Peptic Ulcer with Hampton's Line.
A 36-year-old man (CIH). (Fig. 257)

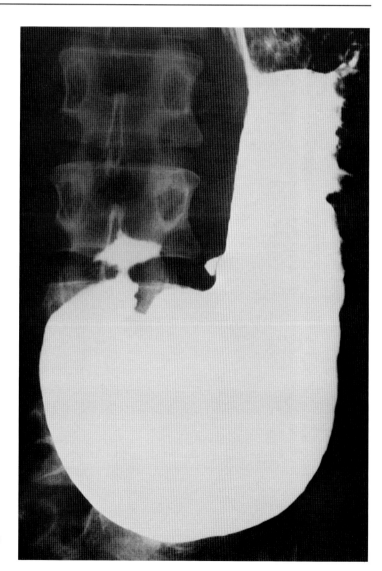

Fig. 257 Barium-filled film demonstrates Hampton's line.

picture, the ulcer mound is not delineated unless pressure is applied. Ulcer mound of this type depends on compression for identification.

Thickening on both the mucosa and the serosa side

This is a special type of ulcer mound. In the mucosal relief picture or double contrast image (Fig. 258) a radiolucency is observed at the site of the corresponding mucosal thickening, around which are the special converging folds described above. In the compression picture, the radiolucency is located at the site of the corresponding thickening on the serosa side (Fig. 259). An ulcer mound of this type takes the form of a small ulcer mound in the mucosal relief film and double contrast image, a large ulcer mound in the compression picture and a kind of mixture of "depression" above and below the niche and "distortion of the gastric wall" in the barium-filled film. Clinically, the findings of so-called Schwellungshof and ulcer collar strongly suggest the possibility of inflammatory swelling and are a sign of comparatively acute ulcer. The ulcer is expected to get smaller. On the other hand, an ulcer mound which is only revealed by the compression method is usually due to proliferation of connective tissue and an ulcer mound of this type can be regarded as a sign of a chronic ulcer.

Case 66   Peptic Ulcer with a Special Type of Ulcer Mound.
A 50-year-old man (CIH). (Figs. 258 and 259)

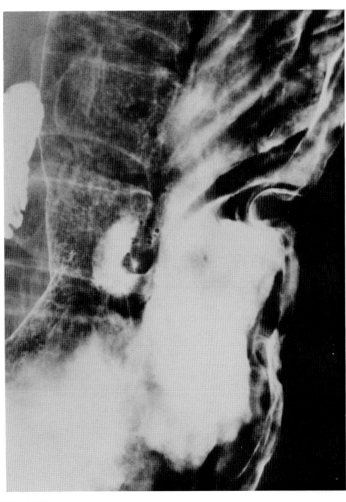
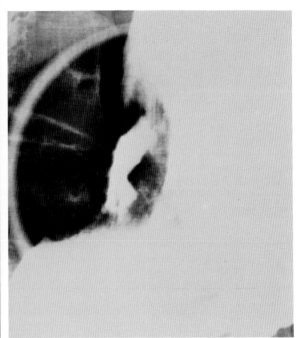

Fig. 258   Fig. 259

Fig. 258   Double contrast film in the left anterior oblique position demonstrates submucosal thickening.
Fig. 259   Upright compression film demonstrates thickening of the submocosa and serosa.

The shape and depth of the niche

As mentioned in the section on **Converging folds** the Western world has not made a precise one-to-one comparison between the radiographic diagnosis of ulcer niche and the histologic findings of gastric ulcer. Niche refers to its profile view and shape to the border between the niche and the gastric wall. It seems that in the United States the terms niche, ulcer and ulcer crater are used in the literature indiscriminately. For decades it has been argued that the radiographic niche is always deeper than the true ulcer depth. The terms true ulcer depth and depth of niche should be distinct from each other. If the term ulcer crater is used interchangeably with niche, the radiographic diagnosis is noncontributory.

The determining factors of the shape and the depth of the ulcer are curling-in of the mucosa and undermining (Kumakura 1960), the former causing a curve at the base of the niche, making it deeper, the latter causing a constriction at the border between the niche and the gastric wall, causing the margin of the niche to protrude. Coexistence of the two makes the niche deeper and the constriction marked. Figure 260 illustrates this principle according to Kumakura (1960). As illustrated in this figure, there are two different niches, i.e. niche(a) and niche(b). Niche(a) is the depth from the apex of the niche to the gastric wall, in other words the false depth. Niche(b) is the depth of the mucosal defect, the true depth of the ulcer. Various factors affect niche(a), but niche(b) is generally constant. The niche vs. true ulcer depth argument continuing since the days of Reiche and Haudek will be resolved by closely examining the histology of the ulcer and referring to the combination of factors of curling-in and undermining. In the same way Prévôt's assertion that the depth of a niche becomes deeper than the true depth of an ulcer by the presence of an edematous ulcer mound, autoplasty of the mucosa, non-opacifying substance in the niche or gastric motility and secretion, etc. will be refuted.

A well-defined film of the profile niche taken of the barium-filled stomach or double contrast film (Figs. 261, 262) is indispensible for depicting the shape or depth of a niche. The principle of curling-in and undermining is applicable to a very

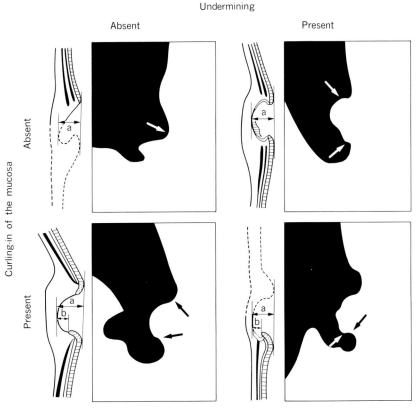

a : The depth from the apex of the niche to the gastric wall.
b : The depth of the mucosal defect.

Fig. 260 Schematic representation showing the difference in depth between niche and ulcer (Modified from Kumakura 1965).

Case 67   Peptic Ulcer with Uninterrupted Converging Folds.
A 60-year-old woman (JU). (Figs. 261 and 262)

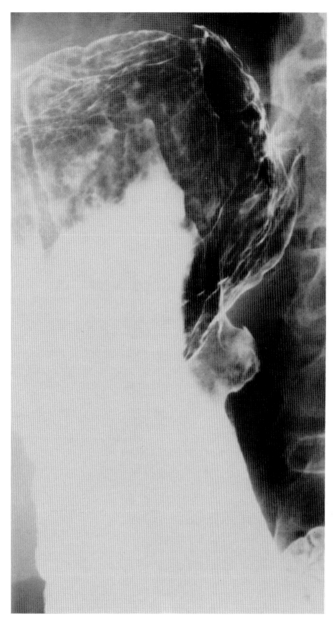

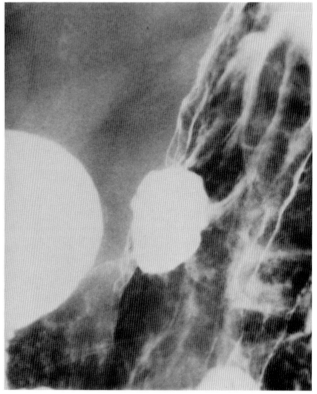

Fig. 261   Fig. 262

Fig. 261   Prone double contrast film demonstrates undermining and curling-in of the profile niche.
Fig. 262   Double contrast film in the left anterior oblique position (of Figure 261) demonstrates uninterrupted converging folds.

small ulcer provided a good profile niche is demonstrated. On occasion, however, it is not applicable when barium filling is incomplete, compression is added or peristalsis is present. In some cases the depth of the tissue defect can be estimated while the depth of niche cannot. It is difficult to recognize the shape and/or the depth of

the niche when there is a marked gastric deformity such as hourglass stomach or pyloric stenosis. However, these deformities have diagnostic significance overshadowing the shape and depth of niche.

The goal in measuring the true depth of the ulcer by the depth of niche is to distinguish simple

Case 68　　Peptic Ulcer with Double Layer Formation.
A 43-year-old man (JU). (Figs. 263 and 264)

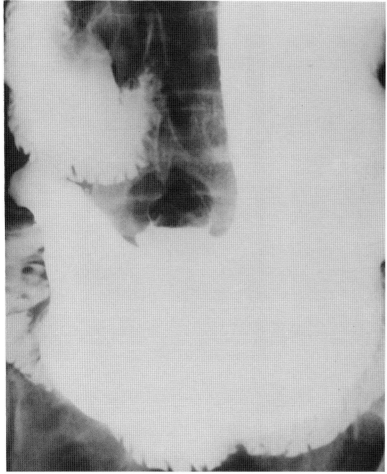

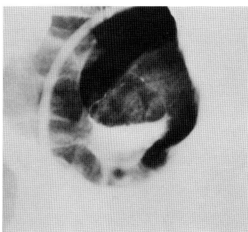

Fig. 263

Fig. 264

Fig. 263　Barium-filled film demonstrates three layers in the niche at the incisura (penetrating ulcer).

Fig. 264　Upright compression film demonstrates an ulcer collar.

non-penetrating ulcers from persistent penetrating ulcers. Emphasis has been put on such radiographic findings of penetrating ulcer as double layer (Figs. 263, 264) or triple layer formation (Assmann 1949, 1950, Haenisch 1951, Schinz 1952). Eschbach disagrees, asserting that the above findings are exceptional cases and that penetrating ulcer has no specific characteristics. He simply mentions that penetrating ulcer is suspected in cases of a deep niche. Kumakura (1960) states that the diagnosis of a deep ulcer (Ul-IV) is possible when the above-mentioned niche(b), not niche(a), is deep, and that, in addition, suspicious findings of Ul-IV are irregular ulcer beds and immobility of the niche by palpation.

Generally speaking, however, differentiation is impossible in the strictest sense, since Ul-II ulcers sometimes have deep niches and penetrating ulcers occasionally present with shallow niches. Use of the ulcer depth to distinguish Ul-II and Ul-III and Ul-IV is the next topic of discussion.

141

Linear Ulcer

History

Schmieden and Härtel (1909) reported the presence of *schneckenförmige Einrollung* or *Tabaksbeutelform* of the stomach in their investigation of gastric deformities. Uemura (1919) described linear ulcer and linear ulcer scar in autopsy findings of the stomach. Tamiya (1923), referring to the relationship between shortening of the lesser curvature and ulcer, stated that such shortening may be caused by a linear ulcer which gradually extends and results in subsequent scar formation. Hauser (1926) stated that linear scars measuring 20 to 30 mm or more were not infrequently observed pathologically and that a long linear ulcer nearly encircling the stomach perpendicular to its longitudinal axis is sometimes observed. In 1929 Eisler and Lenk suggested that linear scars do not show marked radiographic findings and that double ulcers without recognizable niches radiographically may reveal shortening of the lesser curvature, which is often observed in linear scar. In 1910 Haudek described a so-called "snail-like spiral" of the stomach and attributed it to shortening of the lesser curvature. In the English literature Ivy et al. (1950) suggested that a large saddle ulcer of the lesser curvature might cause marked deformity of the stomach, but he did not show an example.

Murakami et al. (1954) are the first to have proven that the radiographic findings of "snail-like spiral" and "pouch-like stomach" are caused by linear ulcer. This conclusion was based on detailed pathologic investigations of the relationship between deformity and symmetrical ulcers. Two years later, Shirakabe et al. (1956) successfully demonstrated a linear ulcer radiographically and they called it "linear groove" or "linear niche."

Stein (1963) cited the descriptions of linear ulcer by Murakami and Shirakabe in "Gastroenterology" by Bockus and showed a radiograph of a typical example. Frik (1965) also described the radiographic diagnosis of linear ulcer and discussed in general the typical deformities of the stomach caused by gastric ulcer.

Incidence of linear ulcer

The incidence of linear ulcer varies according to the author. Its incidence was high in the 1950s and decreased slightly in the 1960s. Nishizawa et al. (1970) stated that long linear ulcers were not recently observed, especially in large cities, and that relatively short linear ulcers are often visualized by endoscopy.

Morphogenesis of linear ulcer and pouch-like stomach

A linear ulcer is defined as a linear ulceration recognized in the resected specimen of the stomach. Sometimes a round ulcer or kissing ulcer is associated with linear ulcer. A typical linear ulcer develops in the region of the incisura, and is located perpendicular to the lesser curvature and nearly equidistant between the anterior and posterior wall. The morphogenesis of the linear ulcer as proposed by Murakami et al. (1954) is shown in Figure 265. Murakami thought that a short linear ulcer became longer as it repeatedly recurred and healed. As a consequence of this, the pylorus-to-ulcer distance becomes so shortened that the pyloric ring cannot be distinguished from the incisura. And the pouch-like stomach results.

Radiographic aspects of linear ulcer

The typical pouch-like stomach is usually observed in the upright barium-filled film (Figs. 266, 267, 270) and the shortening of the lesser curvature is observed in a double contrast film (Figs. 269, 272).

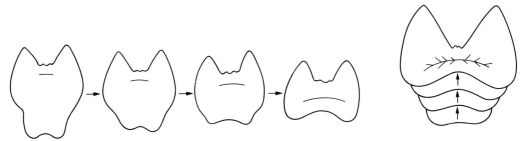

Fig. 265 Development of linear ulcer and the process of central atrophy (From Murakami et al. 1954).

Shirakabe et al. (1961) reported that there is a close relationship between the length of the linear ulcer and the degree of shortening of the lesser curvature (Fig. 274). Generally, a long linear ulcer (Figs. 275, 276) may result in marked deformity (+++ to ++++) and be called "pouch-like deformity" or "snail-like spiral." A medium-sized linear ulcer may cause "right-angled stomach" or shortening of the lesser curvature to a moderate degree (++, Fig. 277). A short linear ulcer may cause only slight deformity of the incisura (+, Figs. 278, 279).

When a linear ulcer has kissing ulcers at its end, an incisura deformity is observed at the greater curvature (Figs. 266, 267, 269). The narrowing of the antrum is caused by another ulcer which is usually located in or near the greater curvature of the antrum (Fig. 275). Marked contraction or

---

Case 69   Linear Ulcer.
A 64-year-old man (CIH). (Figs. 266-273)

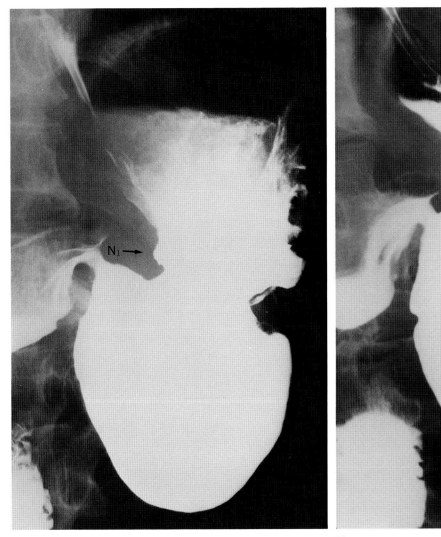
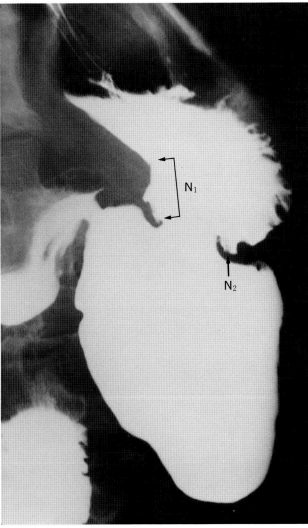

Fig. 266

Fig. 267

Fig. 266   Upright frontal barium-filled film demonstrates a niche (arrow N_1) at the incisura and incisura deformity of the greater curvature with shortening of the lesser curvature. Deformity of the stomach may be (+++) according to Shirakabe.

Fig. 267   Upright barium-filled film in the right anterior oblique position demonstrates a niche at the lesser curvature (arrow line N_1) and a niche on the posterior wall near the greater curvature (arrow N_2). The latter appears in the incisura deformity upon rotation of the patient.

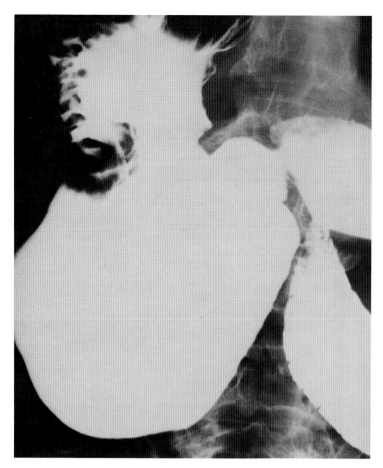

Fig. 268   Prone barium-filled film demonstrates typical snail-like spiral.

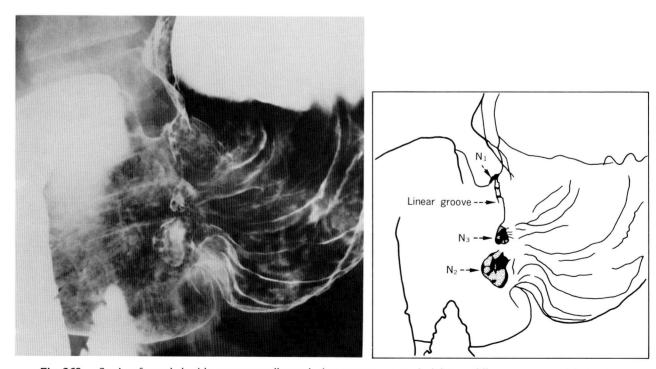

Fig. 269   Supine frontal double contrast radiograph demonstrates round niches and linear grooves with shortening of the lesser curvature.

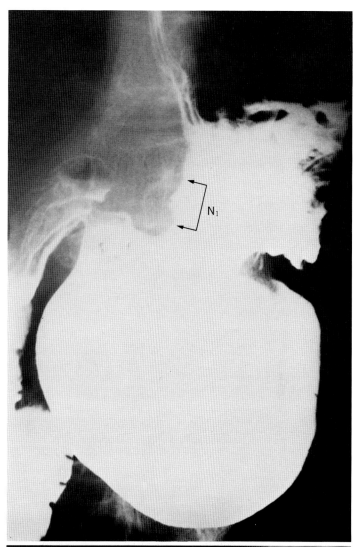

Fig. 270 Barium-filled film taken 2 weeks after the first examination demonstrates niche (N_1) and incisura deformity of the greater curvature.

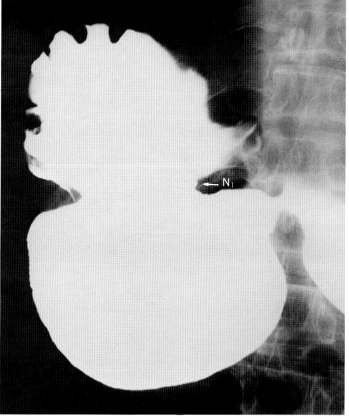

Fig. 271 Prone barium-filled film demonstrates marked snail-like spiral.

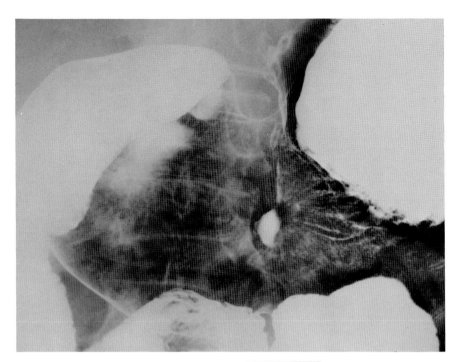

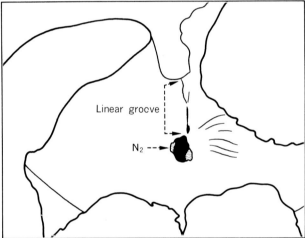

Fig. 272 Supine double contrast film demonstrates the niche (arrow N_2) and the linear groove. The ulcer is still open on the posterior wall.

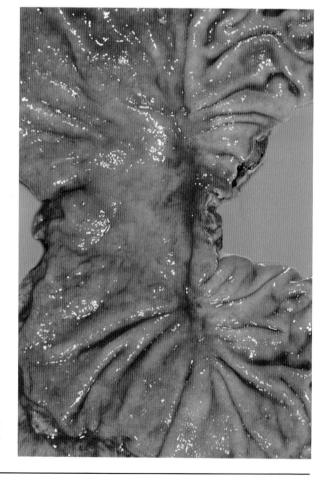

Fig. 273 Resected specimen showing the linear groove measuring 80 mm.

shortening of the lesser curvature may reveal out-pouching of the lower portions of the body (Frik 1965) termed "teapot-like" deformity of the stomach (Meuwissen, 1955)

Typical pouch-like stomach or snail-like spiral in a barium-filled film may be sufficient to make the definite diagnosis of linear ulcer. But it is necessary to differentiate short to medium-sized linear ulcers from other conditions such as kissing ulcer, multiple ulcers of the antrum or chronic single ulcer, when there is slight to moderate shortening of the lesser curvature (Nishizawa et al. 1970). For ulcers of these sizes direct visualization of linear niche by double contrast radiography is required.

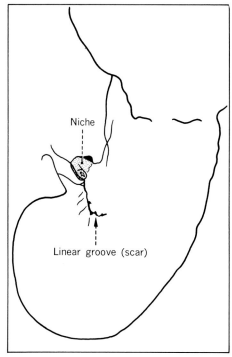

Degree of deformity		
Slight	+	
Moderate	+ +	
Marked	+ + +	
	+ + + +	

Fig. 274   Deformity of the stomach resulting from a linear ulcer (From Shirakabe et al. 1961).

Case 70   Linear Ulcer.
A 58-year-old man (JU). (Fig. 275)

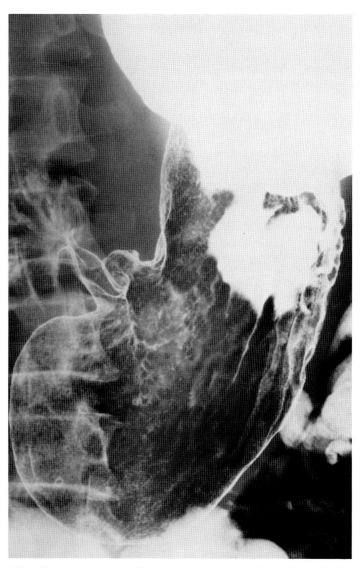

Niche

Linear groove (scar)

Fig. 275   Double contrast film demonstrates a niche at the incisura and a linear groove extending to the posterior wall. Deformity of the stomach may be (++++) according to Shirakabe.

Case 71 Linear Ulcer.
A 58-year-old man (JU). (Fig. 276)

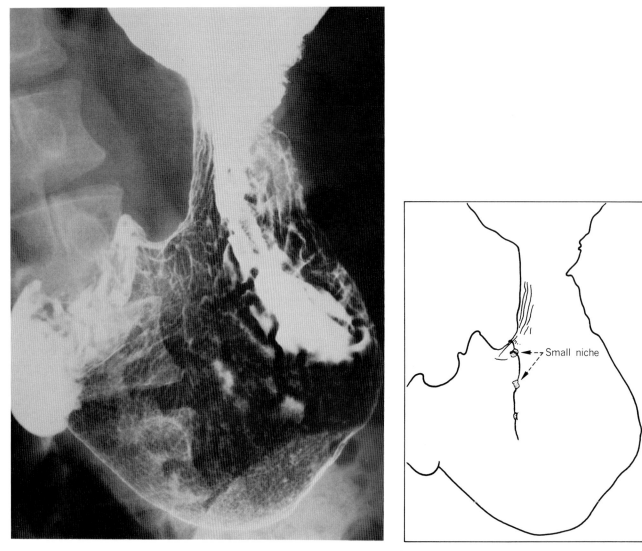

Fig. 276 Double contrast film in the supine right anterior oblique position demonstrates a long linear groove. Deformity of the stomach may be (+++) according to Shirakabe.

Case 72   Linear Ulcer.

A 36-year-old man (JU). (Fig. 277)

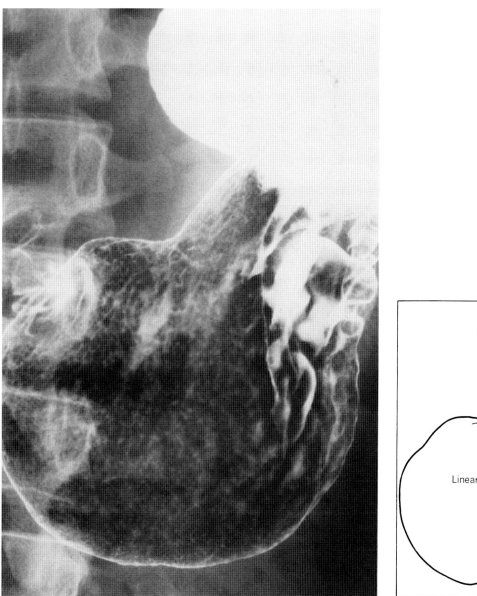

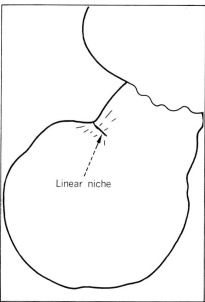

Linear niche

Fig. 277   Double contrast film demonstrates a short linear groove with shortening of the lesser curvature. Deformity of the stomach may be (++) according to Shirakabe.

Case 73 Linear Ulcer.
A 61-year-old man (CIH). (Figs. 278 and 279)

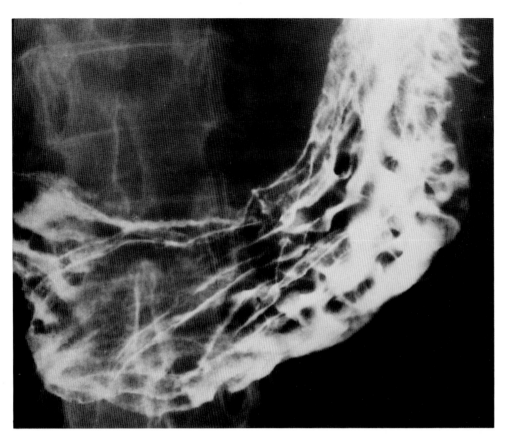

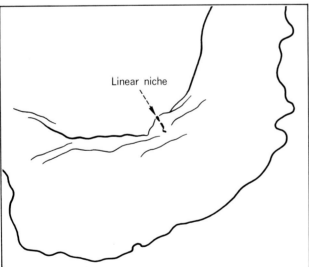

Fig. 278 Mucosal relief film demonstrates a short linear groove with slight shortening (+) of the lesser curvature.

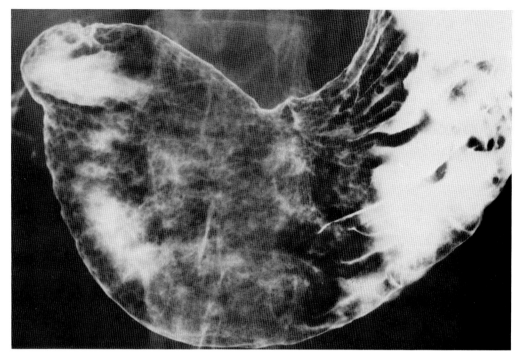

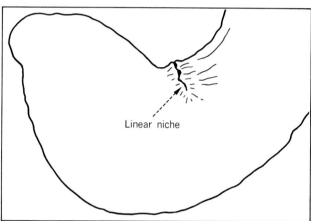

Linear niche

Fig. 279   Double contrast film demonstrates the linear groove.

Multiple Ulcers

General considerations

It was well known that more than 30 per cent of stomachs operated on for peptic ulcer disease had multiple ulcers (Nishizawa et al. 1970) and most of these were associated with ulcer scars. Very few cases were discovered in which multiple active ulcers were present. This was given as the reason for the apparent low incidence of multiple ulcers in the routine radiographic examination. However, recent developments in radiographic examination, especially the advent of double contrast radiography, has made it possible to detect ulcer scars, thus improving diagnostic accuracy. In the last several years, however, the exact incidence of multiple ulcers has not been determined, because the gradual decrease in operated cases has made it difficult to compare radiographic findings with macroscopic diagnoses.

At the present time multiple ulcers are considered to be curable because of the frequent co-existence of ulcer scar. Follow-up examinations, however, are needed to assess healing.

151

Location and orientation

The most frequent site for multiple ulcers is the gastric body. They usually occur in one segment of the stomach, but sometimes they appear in two or three segments, i.e. upper, middle and lower third. They occur in any portion of the stomach (Fig. 280). This contrasts with single ulcer which occurs frequently in the incisura. Ulcer scars are characteristically associated with multiple ulcers.

Multiple ulcers are oriented as follows: per-

Table 22 Orientation of multiple ulcers of the stomach in operated cases (From Nishizawa et al. 1970).

Number of ulcers	Orientation of multiple gastric ulcers		
	Oriented mainly perpendicular to the lesser curvature	Oriented parallel to the lesser curvature	Oriented irregularly
2	○—○	○—○	○—○
	○—○		○—○
	○—○		○—○
	○—○		○—○
	○—○		○—○
	○—○		○—○
	○—○		
	○—○		
	○—○		
	○—△	○—△	○—△
	○—△	○—△	
	○—△	○—△	
	○—△		
	○—△		
	○—△		
	○—△		
	△—△	△—△	△—△
	△—△	△—△	△—△
	△—△		△—△
	△—△		△—△
	△—△		
	△—△		
3	○—○—○	○—○—○	○—○—○
	○—○—○		
	○—○—○		
	○—○—△	○—○—△	○—○—△
	○—○—△		
	○—○—△		
	○—○—△		
	○—○—△		
	○—△—△		○—△—△
	○—△—△		○—△—△
	○—△—△		
	△—△—△		△—△—△
4	○—○—○—△		
	○—○—△—△		○—○—△—△
			○—△—△—△
			○—△—△—△
			△—△—△—△
			△—△—△—△
5			○—○—○—△—△—△

○ Ulcer   △ Ulcer scar

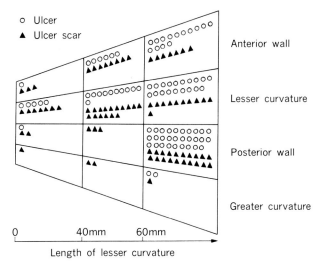

○ Ulcer
▲ Ulcer scar

Anterior wall

Lesser curvature

Posterior wall

Greater curvature

0   40mm   60mm

Length of lesser curvature

Fig. 280   Distribution of multiple ulcers of the stomach in operated cases (From Nishizawa, Ito and Kariya 1970).

Table 23 Number of operated gastric and gastroduodenal ulcers, 1960–1965, First Department of Internal Medicine, Faculty of Medicine, Chiba University (From Nishizawa, Ito & Kariya, 1970)

	Gastric ulcer	Gastroduodenal ulcer
Single	86	17
Multiple	66(9)*	4
Linear	31	8
Total	183	29 Cases

*: Including 9 cases of kissing ulcer

Diagnosed by direct and indirect signs	Diagnosed by direct signs only	Diagnosed as a single ulcer
32 cases (58.2%)	10 cases (18.2%)	13 cases (23.6%)

Fig. 281   Radiographic diagnosis of multiple ulcers of the stomach in 55 operated cases (From Nishizawa, Ito and Kariya 1970).

pendicular to the lesser curvature, parallel to the lesser curvature and irregularly oriented. Of these, the most frequent orientation is perpendicular to the lesser curvature (Table 22). The incidence of so-called kissing ulcer is relatively lower than expected (Table 23). In most cases of multiple ulcers with ulcer scars the number of ulcerations may be two or three.

Direct visualization of niche and scar in multiple ulcers

In considering the location of ulcers and ulcer scars, it may be difficult to demonstrate every lesion by the routine radiographic examination. Nishizawa et al. (1970) described that about 25 per cent of the niches could not be visualized in the lesser curvature and the posterior wall. In Nishizawa's series (Fig. 281), 58.2 per cent of multiple ulcers and ulcer scars were diagnosed by the direct signs of demonstration of a niche and converging folds, and another 18.2 per cent were diagnosed by a combination of direct signs and the indirect sign of gastric deformities. The remaining 23.6 per cent were diagnosed as single ulcer. Thus, the identification of gastic deformities improves the radiographic diagnosis of multiple ulcers.

Gastric deformities as an indirect sign

The hourglass stomach may be the most famous deformity characteristic of kissing ulcers (Fig. 282). Incisura deformity of the greater curvature may therefore lead to the diagnosis of kissing ulcers, when niches cannot be demonstrated. Kumakura, analyzed the relationship between the orientation of ulcerations on the resected stomach and deformities on the radiographs and proposed a formula for easily estimating the orientation of multiple ulcers by means of these basic deformities

153

Case 74 Multiple Ulcers.
A 50-year-old woman (JU). (Figs. 282 and 283)

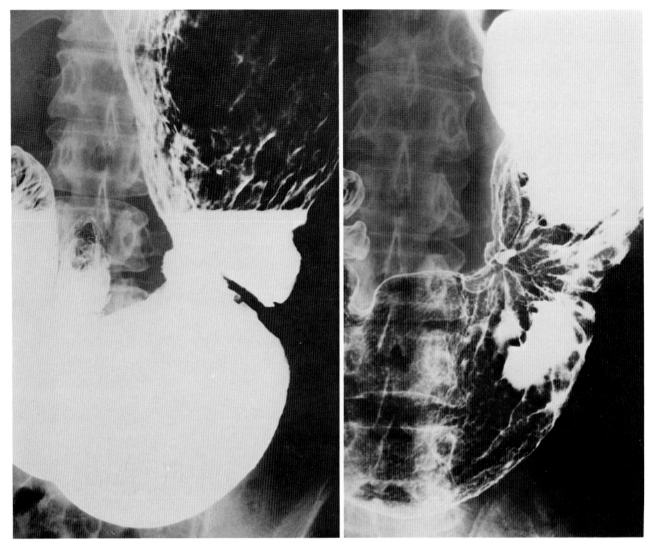

Fig. 282   Fig. 283

Fig. 282   Barium filled film showing a niche on the lesser curvature and marked incisura formation of the greater curvature opposite the niche ("hourglass" stomach). Although only one ulcer is visualized in this film, the diagnosis of multiple ulcers should be made, because of the marked incisura formation of the greater curvature.

Fig. 283   Double contrast radiograph of multiple ulcers showing one niche on the lesser curvature just above the incisura and another niche on the posterior wall near the lesser curvature. These two ulcers are very close together. The lesser curvature around the niches became twisted and slight incisura formation is visualized in the greater curvature.

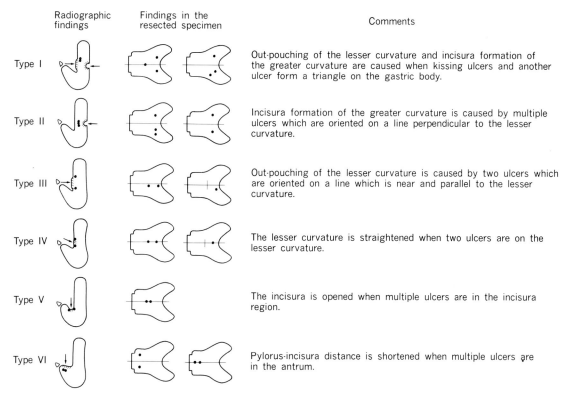

Radiographic findings	Findings in the resected specimen	Comments

Fig. 284   Relationship between the orientation of multiple ulcers and resultant radiographic deformaties (From Kumakura 1965).

(Fig. 284). Following this formula, the incisura deformity of the greater curvature is observed in kissing ulcers as well as in multiple ulcers which are perpendicular to the lesser curvature (Figs. 285, 286).

When a third ulcer is present on the lesser curvature together with the kissing ulcers, an out-pouching of the lesser curvature appears opposite the incisura deformity of the greater curvature (type I). When two ulcers are oriented parallel to the lesser curvature, an out-pouching of the lesser curvature appears. When two ulcers are situated on the lesser curvature, a straightening occurs between them (type IV, V). When multiple ulcers are present in the antrum, the distance between the pylorus and incisura becomes shortened, regardless of the orientation of the ulcers (type VI).

As Nishizawa has stated, however, Kumakura's formula is only a guideline in estimating the orientation of multiple ulcers. The signs of deformity appear to be mixed in many cases. The distance between ulcers may be more important in the formation of these deformities. When multiple ulcers are widely separated, they do not cause a specific deformity. On the other hand, when they are close together, the resultant deformity is that of single ulcer (Fig. 283). The average distance

between multiple ulcers causing specific deformities is 10 to 30 mm (Nishizawa et al. 1970). Kissing ulcers are an exception.

In some cases of multiple ulcers no deformity or only slight deformity is observed (Fig. 287). In such cases demonstration of a direct sign is necessary. In the fornix of the stomach, however, the theory of deformity cannot be applied (Fig. 288). Generally, a niche or center of converging folds is located in the vicinity of an incisura formation or indentation. This finding may be applied to any part of the stomach.

Kissing ulcers in the gastric antrum

The gastric antrum is the most frequent site of acute mucosal lesions, including kissing ulcers. Kissing ulcers are also called symmetrical ulcers. These lesions often present with the acute onset of epigastric pain, frequently followed by hematemesis and melena. The ulcers have an irregular shape but are sharply demarcated and lack a marked surrounding ulcer mound (Figs. 289, 290). They are usually large at their onset. The depth of the ulcer is almost always UI-II in its deepest portion. In its peripheral portion it may

155

Case 75 Multiple Ulcers.
A 55-year-old woman (JU). (Figs. 285 and 286)

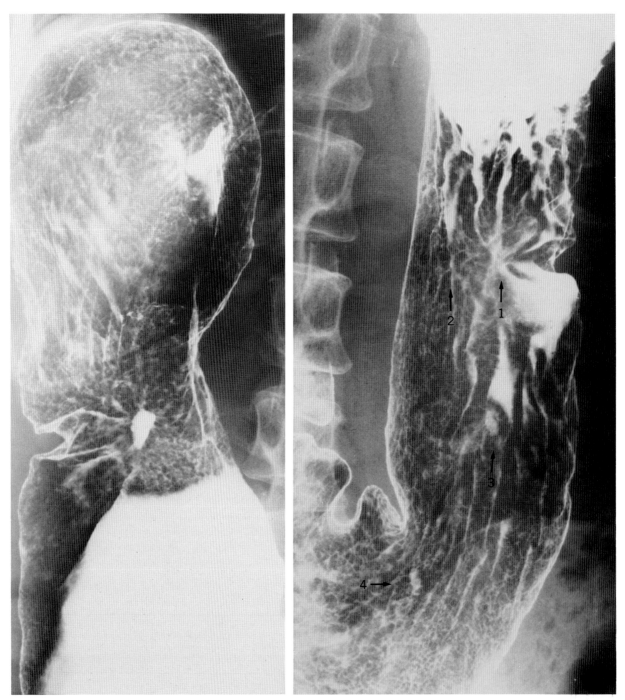

Fig. 285   Fig. 286

Fig. 285 Phone double contrast radiograph demonstrates a niche on the anterior wall. The niche on the posterior wall (arrow 1) and the one in this film are oriented as kissing ulcers.

Fig. 286 Supine double contrast radiograph of multiple ulcers. Two mucosal convergences in the mid-gastric body are oriented perpendicular to the lesser curvature. A niche is visualized in the center of the larger mucosal convergence (arrow 1). The smaller one is an ulcer scar (arrow 2). Other small niches without mucosal convergence are visualized in the lower gastric body (arrow 3) and near the incisura (arrow 4).

Case 76   Multiple Ulcers.
A 50-year-old man (JU). (Fig. 287)

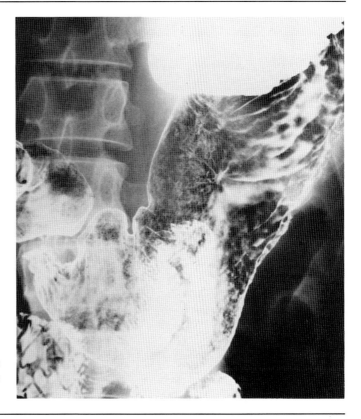

Fig. 287 Double contrast radiograph of multiple ulcers on the posterior wall without deformity of the gastric body.

Case 77   Multiple Ulcers.
A 65-year-old man (CIH). (Fig. 288)

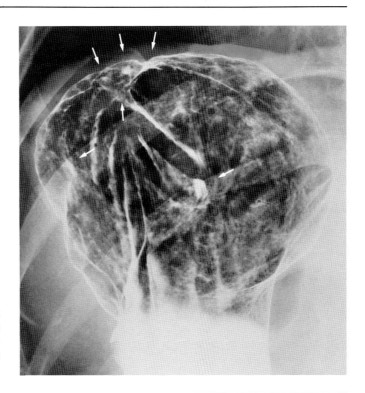

Fig. 288 Double contrast radiograph in the upright prone position shows multiple ulcers in the gastric fundus. Direct signs of niche and mucsal convergence indicate the presence of multiple ulcers (arrows).

Case 78   Multiple Ulcers (Kissing) of the Antrum.
A 25-year-old man (Courtesy of Dr. N. Komatsubara, Kosei Hospital, Tokyo). (Figs. 289-294)

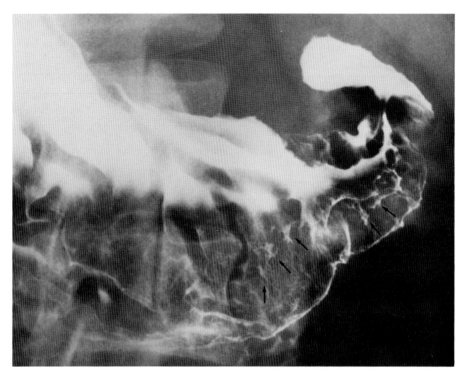

Fig. 289   Kissing ulcers of the antrum. Double contrast radiograph in the prone position shows a large niche on the anterior wall and small erosions scattered around the niche (arrows).

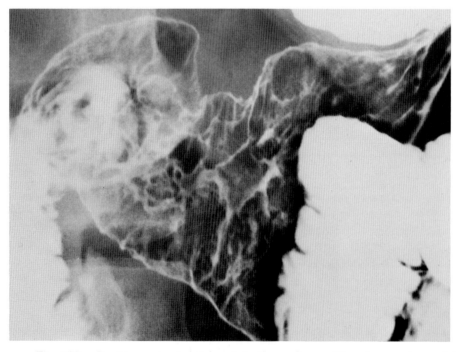

Fig. 290   Double contrast radiograph in the supine position shows a large niche on the posterior wall. In this film the niches on the anterior and posterior wall are superimposed. Small erosions are also scattered around the niche on the posterior wall.

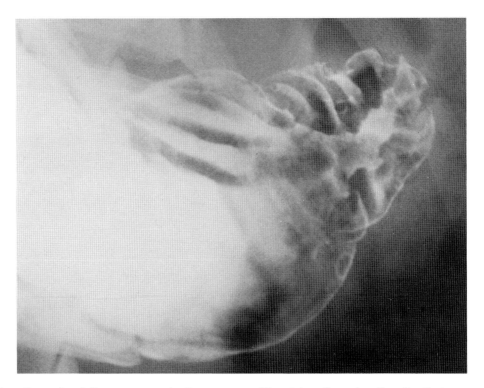

Fig. 291 Double contrast radiograph of the same case in the prone position taken 2 weeks after the first radiographic examination. The large niche on the anterior wall persists. Marked mucosal convergence appeared, but the erosions around the niche disappeared.

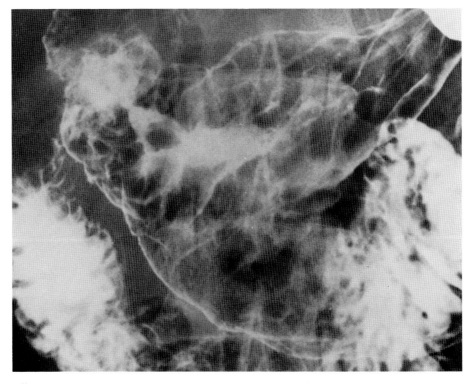

Fig. 292 Double contrast radiograph in the supine position. The large niche on the posterior wall persists without marked mucosal convergence.

159

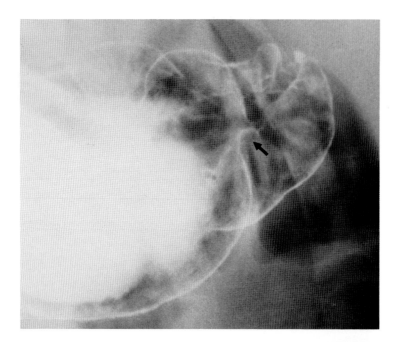

Fig. 293 Double contrast radiograph of the same case in the prone position taken 4 weeks after the first examination. The niche on the anterior wall disappeared almost completely with persistance of mucosal convergence (arrow).

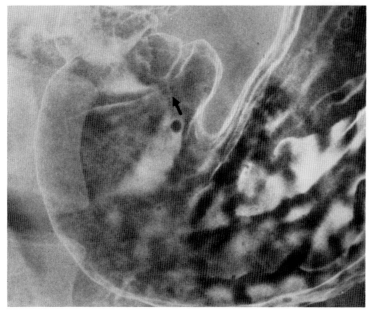

Fig. 294 Double contrast radiograph in the supine position. The niche on the posterior wall disappeared completely (arrow).

show an erosion (Ul-I). Sometimes small erosions are scattered around the ulcers (Figs. 289, 290). Mucosal convergence is not marked at their onset but becomes pronounced in time (Figs. 291, 292). Kissing ulcers of the antrum heal in a few weeks, leaving only mucosal convergence (Figs. 293, 294). They never recur.

Ulcer Scar

General considerations

European and American literature dealing with the radiographic diagnosis of ulcer scar is extremely rare. This suggests that those countries do not regard ulcer scar as very important but simply as one of the radiographic findings encountered in follow-up studies of ulcers. The radiographic diagnosis of ulcer scar, however, should be precise, since meticulous analysis can improve radiographic diagnosis. The presence of ulcer scar is essential in judging ulcer healing and in estimating the ulcer's size and shape in case of future recurrence. In Japan, the diagnosis of ulcer scar utilizes double contrast radiography and this method has aided in the diagnosis of type IIc early gastric cancer. However, it still remains difficult to make the differential diagnosis between ulcer scar and type IIc early cancer (Fig. 295). The presence of ulcer scar is also important in studying deformities of the stomach associated with gastric ulcer and cancer. The incidence of ulcer scar varies according to the author (Table 24). It is most frequent in UI-III, except for Yokoyama's report. Ulcer scar of

UI-IV comprises not more than 10 per cent in the report of any authors.

Macroscopic and histologic features of ulcer scar

A delicate mucosal convergence to a single point is radiographically considered a feature of ulcer scar. But macroscopically, a scar is not a point but an area on the surface which histologically shows a defect in the muscularis mucosae. This area was named "scarring zone" by Gonoi et al. (1975), who have long studied the radiographic diagnosis of ulcer scar. They classified this scarring zone into three basic types: round, linear and girdle-like. For round ulcer, the width of muscularis mucosae

---

Case 79   Type IIc Early Cancer.
A 41-year-old man (JU). (Fig. 295)

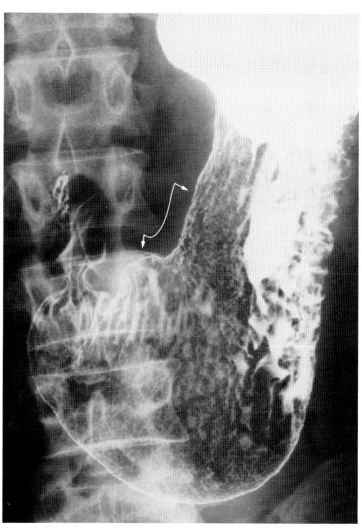

Fig. 295   Double contrast radiograph of early cancer, type IIc simulating ulcer scar (cf Case 83).

Table 24 Incidence of ulcer scar for each ulcer depth according to different authors.

Author	UI-II	UI-III	UI-IV
Koide, 1961 and Suzuki, et al., 1967 (combined data)	37.1%	61.7%	9.8%
	105 foci	107 foci	367 foci
Murakami, 1961 (excluding linear ulcer)	37.3%	66.7%	7.0%
	102 foci	90 foci	285 foci
Yokoyama, 1961	41.9%	31.2%	5.0%
	308 foci	176 foci	896 foci
Shirakabe, 1967	75%	56.8%	3.6%
	4 foci	37 foci	247 foci

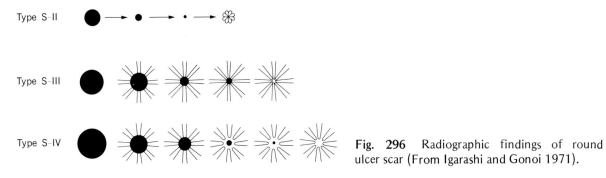

Fig. 296 Radiographic findings of round ulcer scar (From Igarashi and Gonoi 1971).

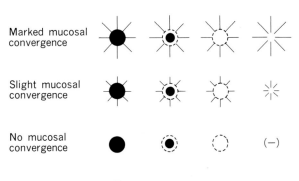

Fig. 297 Macroscopic findings of ulcer scar (From Ito 1969).

defect is 1 to 2 mm in diameter for UI-IIS, 1 to 3 mm for UI-IIIS, 2 to 6 mm for UI-IVS; i.e. the deeper the ulcer, the wider the muscularis mucosae defect.

The fundamental macroscopic findings of ulcer scar are mucosal convergence, minute depression and alteration of "areae gastricae" pattern (Figs. 296, 297).

Mucosal convergenece

Mucosal convergence of ulcer scar is similar to that of an ulcer, but is more minute and frequently appears in a dappled pattern. There are two types of mucosal convergence. One converges uninterrupted to a point and the other is interrupted, leaving a small area in the center similar to that of an ulcer. When there is uninterrupted convergence, the muscularis mucosa is unaffected. When there is interrupted convergence, the area surrounded by the interrupted folds lacks muscularis mucosae and is called the "scarring zone" (Gonoi et al. 1975).

Minute depression

Minute depression applies to a depression remaining in the course of an ulcer's healing, but excludes a benign erosion or an erosion in a type IIc early cancer. The depression is closely related to the depth of the ulcer. UI-IVS is accompanied by a definite depression, while UI-IIS and UI-IIIS have none or only a slight depression (Gonoi et al. 1975). Ito (1969) reported that minute depression which was shallower than 1 mm was seen in 25 per cent of ulcer scars (Table 25). He also reported that even active ulcer revealed flat or slightly irregular surface at the ulcerated portion in about 18 per cent (Table 25).

Alteration of areae gastricae pattern

Different patterns of areae gastricae may be found on the mucosal surface and in the region of the scarring zone. One type of areae gastricae pattern is identical with that of the surrounding mucosa. Another type has a larger pattern and therefore can be distinguished from it. Other scars lack an areae gastricae pattern, but present fine granularity of the mucosal surface, a velvety surface or a flat surface. In any case, an ulcer scar with macroscopically recognizable scarring zone presents mucosal convergence of interrupted type, in which the mucosa of the scarring zone consists of regenerative mucosa (Gonoi et al. 1975). On the other hand, the border of the scarring zone of the non-interrupted type is unrecognizable. In this case there usually is no distinct difference

Table 25 Macroscopic findings of ulcer scar and ulcer in operated cases. (From Shirakabe et al., 1967).

Depth			Ulcer scar	Open ulcer smaller than 5mm
I	Depression deeper than 1mm	⎇	0	21 (62%)
II	Depression not deeper than 1mm	⎇	7 (25%)	7 (21%)
III	Slight uneveness	∿	7 (25%)	5 (15%)
IV	Flat surface	-----	11 (39%)	1 (3%)
V	Slight elevation	⎍	3 (11%)	0
	Total		28 foci	34 foci

between areae gastricae pattern of the scarring zone and the surrounding mucosa. A difference is noticeable however, when some areae gastricae exist in the area surrounding the center of mucosal convergence. The epithelium however is not regenerative epithelium.

A "spatial type" of ulcer scar has no mucosal convergence. Areae gastricae of this type show a peculiar arrangement. The areae gastricae are not a regenerative epithelium but the so-called mucosal convergence is a formation of surrounding mucosa retracted to the ulcer scar.

Radiographic findings of ulcer scar

Radiographically, ulcer scar is classified in the same manner as the macroscopic findings (Gonoi et al. 1975). Ulcer scar consisting of uninterrupted type converging folds is characterized by a stellate mucosal convergence. Occasionally, some areae gastricae pattern is present in the center of convergence (Fig. 296). This areae gastricae pattern is called figure pattern of ulcer scar (Gonoi et al.). Radiographic evidence for ulcer scar consisting of interrupted type mucosal convergence is visualized as a faint collection of barium in a slight depression in the central area (Fig. 299). Areae gastricae pattern, so-called figure pattern of ulcer scar, is often found in the central area (Fig. 300). In the radiographic findings of ulcer scar formed solely of "spatially arranged" areae gastricae pattern the mucosal convergence is unclear. Spatially arranged areae gastricae pattern appears as petals of a

Case 80   Ulcer Scar, Uninterrupted Type.
A 66-year-old man (CPCC). (Fig. 298)

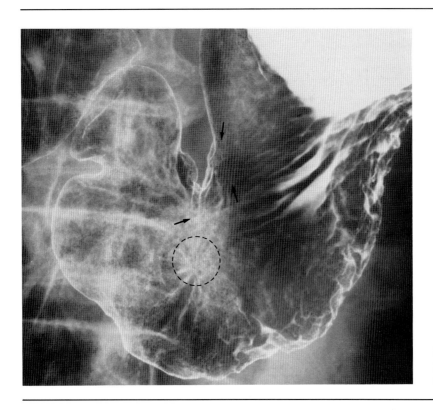

Fig. 298   Double contrast radiograph of ulcer scar, non-interrupted type. Three other ulcer scars are present (arrows).

Case 81   Ulcer Scar, Interrupted Type.
A 60-year-old man (CPCC). (Fig. 299)

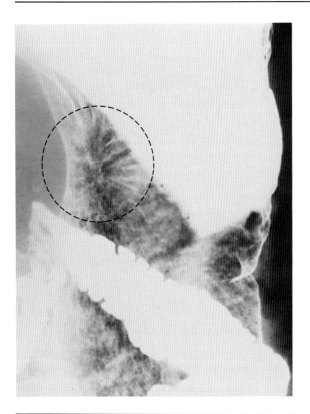

Fig. 299   Double contrast radiograph of ulcer scar, interrupted type.

Case 82 **Kissing Ulcer Scars of Figure Pattern with Interrupted Mucosal Convergence.** A 42-year-old man (CPCC). (Fig. 300)

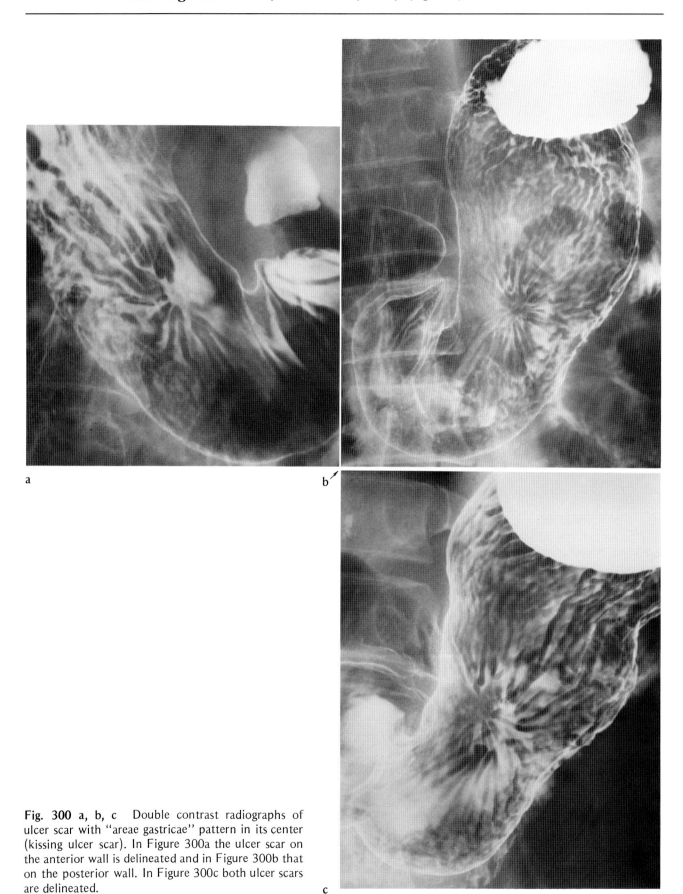

a

b

c

Fig. 300 a, b, c Double contrast radiographs of ulcer scar with "areae gastricae" pattern in its center (kissing ulcer scar). In Figure 300a the ulcer scar on the anterior wall is delineated and in Figure 300b that on the posterior wall. In Figure 300c both ulcer scars are delineated.

chrysanthemum or plum flower, as shown in Figures 301 and 302. This is one of the net patterns of ulcer scar. The "figure pattern" (Gonoi et al. 1975) appears in the follow-up of the ulcer scar when the niche completely disappears. There are two histologic kinds of figure pattern of the ulcer scar. One is that of ulcer scar presenting interrupted type mucosal convergence, formed of regenerative epithelium (Figs. 300, 301). The other is that of the ulcer scar presenting uninterrupting type mucosal convergence with the ulcer scar formed by the spatial arrangement of areae gastricae (Fig. 302), which retracts to the center of the scar. In each case, if the figure pattern of the ulcer scar is demonstrated the ulcer is cicatrized. Therefore, regardless of mucosal convergence or areae gastricae pattern, the figure pattern is most important in defining whether or not the lesion is

ulcer scar. When the figure pattern of ulcer scar is absent, as happens occasionally, ulcer scar is defined by a pair of mucosal converging folds directed toward the center as if they are touching each other (Figs. 303, 304).

Double contrast radiography is the only means that can delineate the ulcer scar. A good delineation, however, is not expected in the routine examination in which a fairly large volume of air is used. The double contrast radiograph must be taken with a proper volume of air, depending upon the shape of the stomach and location of the ulcer. A large to medium volume of air produces a good film of mucosal convergence of the interrupted type ulcer scar en face, while small volumes of air do not. Conversely, a large volume of air distends the gastric wall, resulting in the disappearance of mucosal convergence of noninter-

---

Case 83　Ulcer Scar of Figure Pattern with Interrupted Mucosal Convergence.
A 40-year-old man (JU). (Fig. 301)

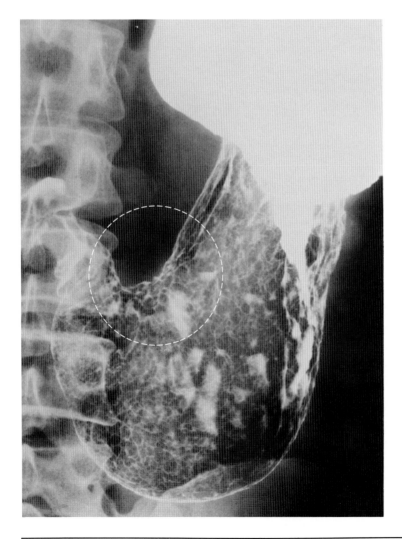

Fig. 301　Double contrast radiograph of ulcer scar, with interrupted type of mucosal convergence and regenerative epithelium.

rupted type ulcer scar, so that a fairly small volume of air is preferred.

The figure pattern of ulcer scar of any type can be well delineated with fairly large volume, of air which efface the mucosal folds. That volume of air will also delineate ulcer scar arranged as "spatial areae gastricae."

A complete profile view of the ulcer scar is necessary to demonstrate the distensibility of the gastric wall (Figs. 301, 302, 304), since the gastric margin is only visible in profile. When the ulcer scar is not radiographed in a complete profile view, areas of poor distensibility are not well seen. The further from the margin the less the ability to evaluate distensibility (Fig. 299).

Among ulcer scars situated in the lesser curvature of the gastric body, only UI-IVS presents a well-defined depression, but UI-IIIS and UI-IIS have better distensibility than UI-IVS because of the small extent of scarred areas. A strong retraction of UI-IVS gives rise to twisting at the gastric margin (Fig. 307) and the retraction may be recognized above and below the ulcer scar. Ulcer scar at the incisura presents angular deformity and rigidity (Fig. 304), which is always histologically ascribed to linear ulcer scar, according to Gonoi et al. Linear scar will be discussed in another section. Ulcer scar at the lesser curvature of the antrum is usually UI-IIS or UI-IIIS. Distortion of the antrum and poor distensibility of the margin are radiographically demonstrated. Benign ulcers at the greater curvature are exclusively UI-IIS (Gonoi et al. 1975). Its radiographic feature is depression at the margin.

Case 84   Ulcer Scar of Spatially Arranged "Areae Gastricae"
A 52-year-old man (CPCC). (Fig. 302)

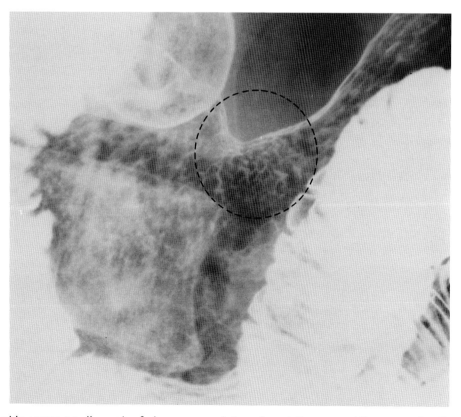

Fig. 302 Double contrast radiograph of ulcer scar consisting of spatially arranged "areae gastricae".

Case 85 Peptic Ulcer and Its Scar Formation.
A 60-year-old man (CIH). (Figs. 303 and 304)

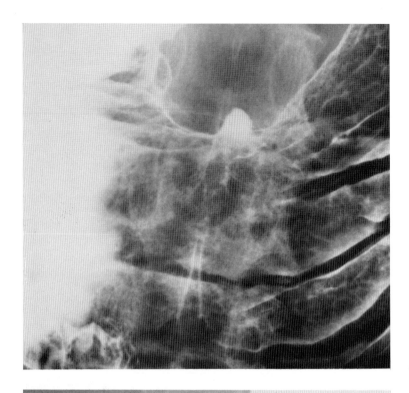

Fig. 303 Double contrast radiograph of an open ulcer at the incisura.

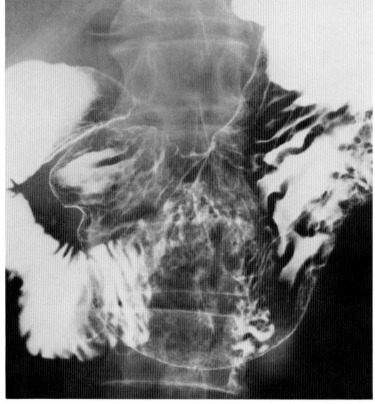

Fig. 304 Double contrast radiograph of ulcer scar shown in Figure 303. Two converging folds are touching.

Case 86   Multiple Ulcers and Their Scar Formations.
A 60-year-old woman (JU). (Figs. 305-307)

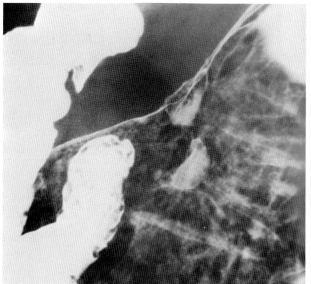

Fig. 305

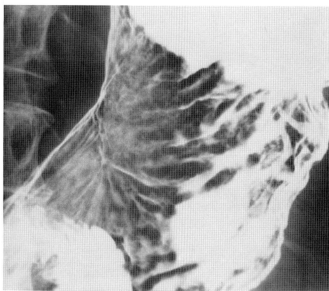

Fig. 306

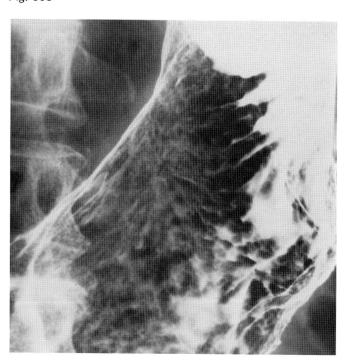

Fig. 307

Fig. 305   Double contrast radiograph of multiple ulcers.
Fig. 306   Double contrast radiograph of an almost completely healed ulcer, four weeks after Figure 305. There is retraction above and below the ulcer scar.
Fig. 307   Double contrast radiograph of a completely healed ulcer, two months after Figure 305. The margin is twisted.

Chapter 8

Radiographic Diagnosis of Gastric Erosions

General Considerations

Gastric erosion is histologically defined as a defect of the mucosa without involvement of the muscularis mucosae. On the other hand, a gastric ulcer is defined as a defect in the gastric wall, extending to the submucosal layer. In radiographic findings the distinction between mucosal and submucosal is made by the depth of the defect. And careful evaluation should be made, especially on a double contrast radiograph.

In Japan, since 1959 Murakami's classification concerning depth and reparative state of gastric ulcer (see Fig. 246, Chapter 7) has played an important role in the investigation of peptic ulcer and early gastric cancer. The concept of gastric erosions may be better understood if we follow Murakami's classification of gastric ulcer: An erosion corresponds to Ul-I, Ul-II is a shallow ulcer involving only the submucosal layer and Ul-IV is a deep ulcer penetrating the propria muscle layer.

In long-standing erosions, the muscularis mucosae is elevated and sometimes slight fibrosis of the submucosal layer is observed. But the fibrosis is not as marked as that of a Ul-II ulcer. Consequently, erosions never produce mucosal convergence, even when present in the stomach for a long time. In long-standing erosions surrounding mucosal elevations seem to be more prominent than mucosal depressions. This elevation, may change finally into a true polyp of the regenerative type (Nakamura T. 1962, Sano 1975).

Fresh erosions are not subject to radiographic diagnosis, since these cases are brought to urgent endoscopy with the diagnosis of acute mucosal lesions with hemorrhage. Incomplete or complete erosions (Table 26) are terms proposed by Kawai

Table 26   Classification of erosions according to endoscopic findings (From Kawai et al.: *Endoscopy*, 2: 168, 1970).

1. The flat hemorrhagic erosion
2. The incomplete or immature erosion
3. The complete or mature erosion

et al. (1970), based upon his endoscopic experience. He defined incomplete erosions as those which disappear in 2—8 days and complete erosions as those which remain for a long time. Hemorrhagic erosion reveals bleeding spots of various sizes, especially in the antrum (Table 26). When bleeding stops, the spots appear dark brown or black, because of the influence of the gastric juice. Sometimes, multiple ulcers are associated in the antrum and incisura, and Sano called this condition "ulcero-erosive gastritis" (1974). Incomplete erosion is the term used for lesions with the same morphology but without extensive bleeding. Accordingly, the erosions are not as numerous as in hemorrhagic gastritis. Sometimes, the erosion is solitary. The term complete erosion is used for lesions with marked surrounding elevation. This type has been called "Dellengastritis" (Berg 1953), gastritis veruccosa (Abel 1954) and gastritis valioliform (Walk 1955). This type is the most frequently discussed in the radiographic diagnosis.

Sano (1975), experienced in clinical pathology, classified those long-standing erosions into 4 types (Fig. 308) and called them gastritis veruccosa, because of their multiplicity and polypoid shape.

Radiographic Diagnosis

The diagnosis of gastric erosions has not attracted the interest of Western radiologists in recent years, despite early descriptions by Henning and Schatzki (1933), Abel (1954), Walk (1955) and Frik (1956). Bücker (1964) and Frik (1965) discussed the radiographic diagnosis of gastric erosions in detail. Descriptions of their radiographic diagnosis have appeared only sporadically in text books published in the United States, Such scarce descriptions may be partly ascribed to the advent of endoscopy, which has made it possible to observe subtle detail of the gastric mucosa.

In Japan, Aoyama (1964), Hirokado and Okabe (1964) and Yoshida et al. (1967) reported the radiographic diagnosis of gastric erosions. Those erosions are the so-called "gastritis erosiva" or "varioliform" erosions, which are characterized by multiple small flecks of the contrast medium

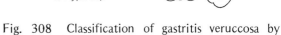

1. Varioli form

2. Polypoid form

3. Serpiginous form

4. Hypertrophied form

Fig. 308 Classification of gastritis veruccosa by Sano (1975).

surrounded by a radiolucent halo. As Kumakura (1967) stated, these erosions are morphologically different from the erosions which should be differentiated from depressed type early cancer (type IIc or type IIc + IIa). Macroscopically, these

---

Case 87   **Single Large Erosion.**
A 53-year-old man (JU). (Figs. 309 and 310)

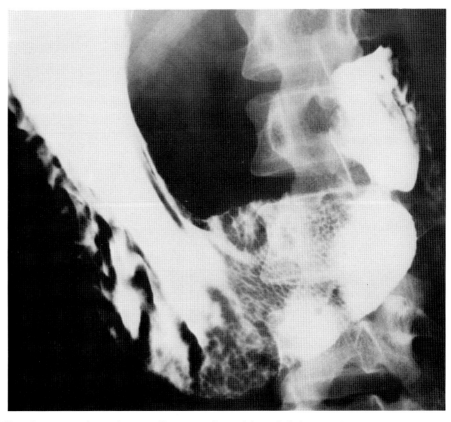

Fig. 309   Prone mucosal relief film demonstrating a large, solitary erosion with a slightly raised margin on the anterior wall of the antrum near the incisura. The raised margin has a slightly enlarged pattern of "areae gastricae".

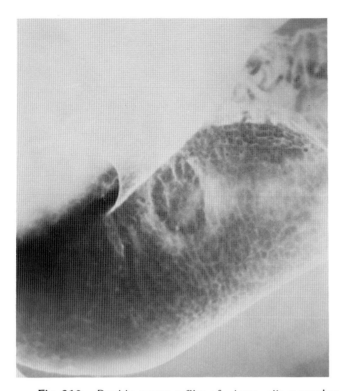
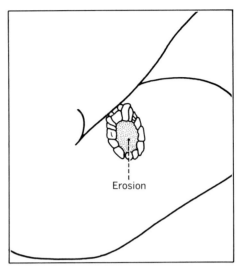

Erosion

Fig. 310   Double contrast film of a large solitary erosion. Compare the surface pattern of the raised margin with that of "areae gastricae" in the gastric antrum.

erosions appear as relatively large, flat depressions of the mucosal surface. Figures 309 and 310 show a single large erosion, which can be confused with cancer. This type of erosion occurs infrequently.

Only recently have gastric erosions been discussed radiographically in Western countries in such a way as to re-evaluate the usefulness of the Japanese style double contrast radiography of the stomach (Gelfand 1975, Laufer and Trueman 1976).

Varioliform erosions are shown in Figure 311. Only a central depression points to an erosion histologically, although the surrounding halo is more pronounced than the depression itself. This type of erosion is identical to that reported by Henning and Schatzki (1933), who successfully demonstrated them by compression technique. Compression technique is an effective method for delineating typical varioliform erosions as long as they are located in the gastric antrum or in the lower portion of the stomach (Figs. 312, 313). Compared with a compression image (Fig. 312), a double contrast radiograph (Fig. 313) is able to demonstrate very small erosions in the proximal portion of the antrum. These are visualized as punctiform barium flecks without remarkable surrounding halo. This case also reveals several forms of erosion, new and old.

The morphology of the gastric erosions is varied, depending upon their age and their repaired stage (Fig. 314). In fresh erosions the depressed surface may be relatively large and the surrounding margin not be significantly raised. This type may disappear in a short time (disappearing type). The varioliform erosions may disappear or persist, depending upon the nature of their raised margin and depression. Long-standing erosions are rounded, oval or stick-shaped, as Sano (1975) described, and the central depression may appear or disappear during the period of observation (Sata 1974). Sometimes, they resemble type IIa early cancer.

When varioliform erosions are on the crest of the folds, they reveal a pearlstring arrangement which is very typical. However, changes of the folds in erosions vary, depending upon the intensity of involvement (Fig. 315). In fresh erosions the folds show only edematous swelling or change of caliber. In long-standing erosions the fold simulates a snake that has swallowed an egg.

172

Case 88 Varioliform Erosions.
A 32-year-old man (CPCC). (Fig. 311)

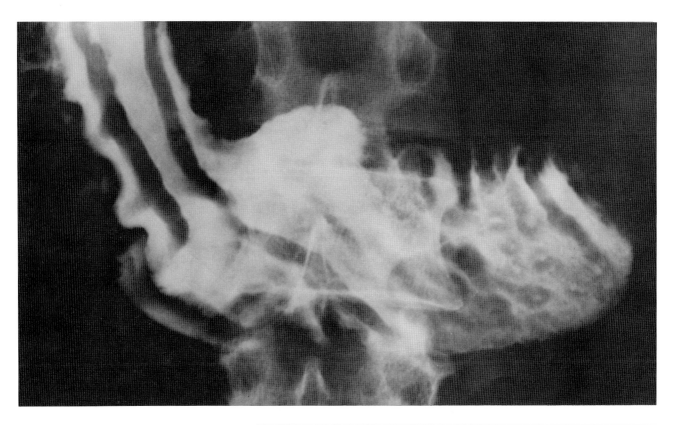

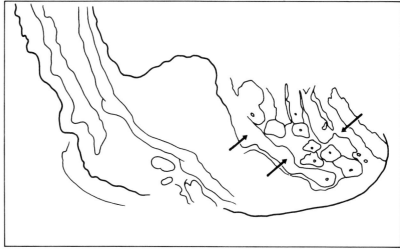

Fig. 311 Prone mucosal relief film demonstrates varioliform erosions and changes of caliber (arrows) of mucosal folds of the antrum.

Case 89   Varioliform Erosions.
A 39-year-old woman (JU). (Figs. 312 and 313)

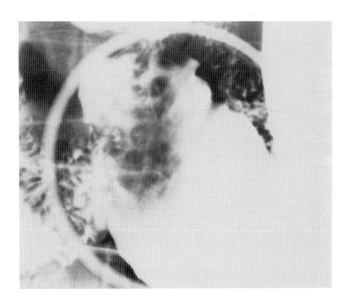

Fig. 312   Upright compression film demonstrates varioliform erosion of the antrum.

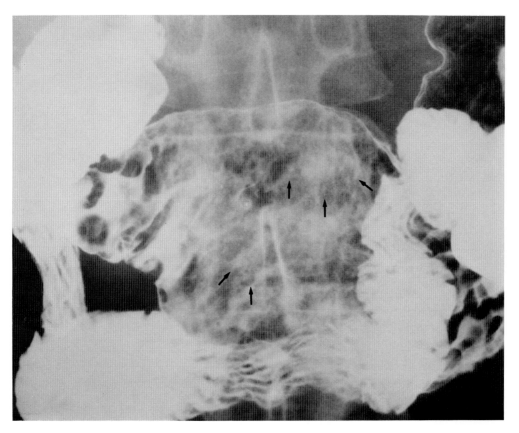

Fig. 313   Double contrast film demonstrates punctate erosions without remarkable surrounding halo (arrows).

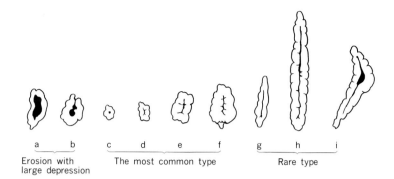

Fig. 314   Schema of macroscopic findings of gastric erosions (Aoyama 1964).

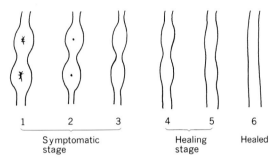

Fig. 315   Macroscopic findings of gastric erosions on the crest of mucosal folds (various changes of caliber, Aoyama 1964).

Erosions in Acute Phase

As was mentioned above, varioliform erosions of the stomach are encountered most frequently in radiographic diagnosis. However, our experience in endoscopic diagnosis demonstrates a wide spectrum of macroscopic appearance and age of gastric erosions. Fresh erosions, which always occur with the onset of acute hemorrhage or acute abdomen, are discovered during emergency endoscopy. They rarely are examined radiographically.

Usually, a patient with acute erosions complains of severe epigastric pain which appeared one or two days previously (Figs. 316–321).

Figure 317 may be a mucosal relief image or a double contrast image with a small volume of air which reveals only the edematous mucosal folds. There is a rapid passage of the contrast medium into the proximal jejunum despite the use of an antispasmodic agent (Coliopan). The enlarged shadow of the papilla of Vater (arrow) (Fig. 317), together with the compression of the descending duodenum, suggests associated pancreatitis. The patient was placed in the right anterior oblique position in order to shift air to the antrum (Fig. 318). Several barium flecks are observed in the

markedly enlarged mucosal folds. The greater curvature of the antrum is delineated as double contour, probably due to compression by the enlarged pancreas. The moderately distended air-filled stomach (Fig. 320) reveals only enlarged, edematous folds of the gastric body. By compression technique, the edematous, enlarged mucosal folds are demonstrated, and an erosion is visualized as small barium flecks (arrow) (Fig. 319). These compression images may be similar to those reported by Bücker in 1964. A barium-filled film (Fig. 316) reveals the irritable stomach with slight translucencies showing edematous mucosa. The enlarged papilla of Vater is also visualized.

In this patient, endoscopy was performed on the day following radiography. Figure 321 is the endoscopic picture of the antrum. Petechial bleeding spots are scattered on the fresh edematous antral mucosa.

There is another type of lesion which may also belong to an acute stage of gastric erosions (Figs. 322–332). In a mucosal relief image (Fig. 322), edematous, enlarged mucosal folds in the anterior wall are characteristic. In an upright barium-filled film (Fig. 323), the incisura is deformed and the lesser curvature above it seems to show a very rigid wall.

On a prone barium-filled film (Fig. 324),

175

Case 90   Erosions in Acute Phase.
A 45-year-old man (CIH). (Figs. 316-321)

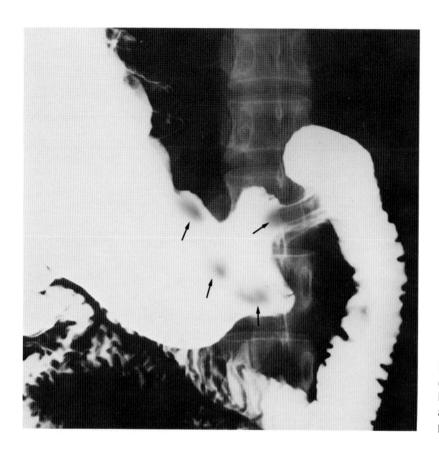

Fig. 316 Prone barium-filled film demonstrates faint radiolucency caused by edematous mucosal folds of the antrum (arrows) (erosions in acute phase).

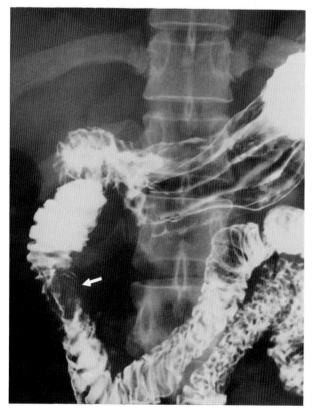

Fig. 317 Supine mucosal relief film demonstrates edematous mucosal folds and enlarged papilla of Vater (arrow). The descending portion of the duodenum is displaced laterally due to the enlarged pancreas.

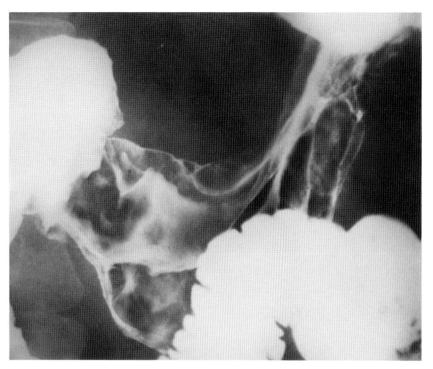

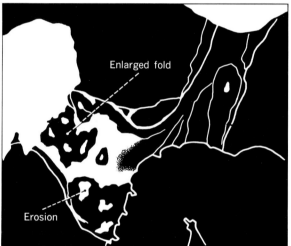

Fig. 318 Supine right anterior oblique double contrast film with a very small volume of air demonstrates barium flecks on the markedly enlarged mucosal folds.

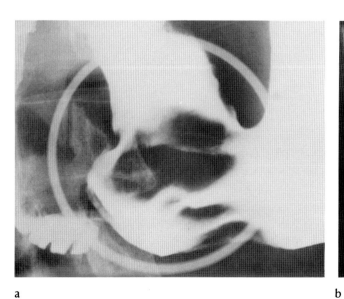

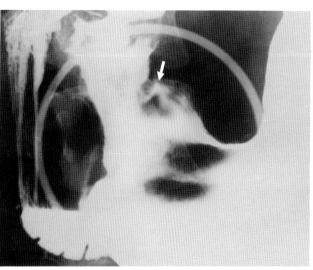

a   b

Fig. 319 a and b Upright compression films demonstrate large edematous folds of the antrum. An arrow points to an erosion.

177

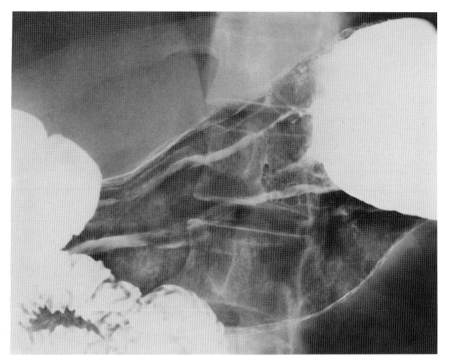

Fig. 320 Supine left anterior oblique double contrast film with a large volume of air demonstrates the marked edematous folds of the gastric body.

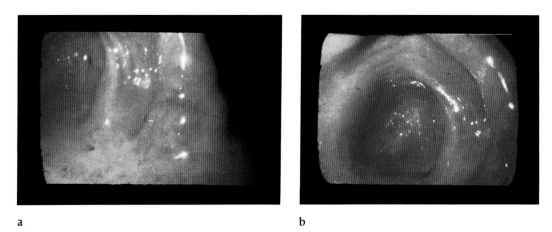

a   b

Fig. 321 a and b Endoscopic findings demonstrate petechial bleeding spots on the edematous antral mucosa.

distensibility of the gastric body seems to be so poor that one inevitably has to think of linitis plastica type cancer. A double contrast radiograph in the supine, right anterior oblique position (Fig. 325) reveals faint, irregular collections of barium in the posterior wall of the proximal antrum which extends to the incisura in a pseudopod-like fashion. These radiographic findings are interpreted as those of multiple erosions. A supine frontal double contrast radiograph (Fig. 326) clearly reveals tiny multiple erosions which are located in the posterior wall along the lesser curvature (arrow).

A double contrast radiograph in the left anterior oblique position reveals fairly large, irregular erosions in the lesser curvature of the lower gastric body, and a double contrast radiograph in the right decubitus position (Fig. 327) reveals erosions of the same form which are located in the middle part of the gastric body. Compression radiographs (Fig. 328a, b) demonstrate an irregular but sharply defined mucosal depression in the proximal antrum which is delineated in the first double contrast radiograph.

Just one month after the medical treatment,

Case 91 Erosions in Acute Phase.
A 42-year-old woman (ClH). (Figs. 322-332)

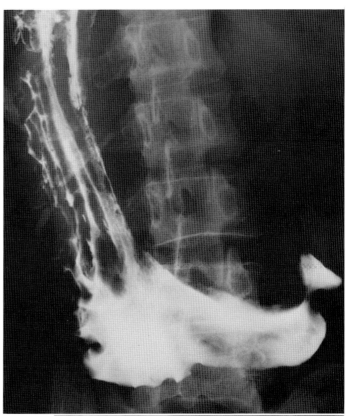

Fig. 322 Prone mucosal relief film demonstrates the edematous mucosal folds from the antrum to the body.

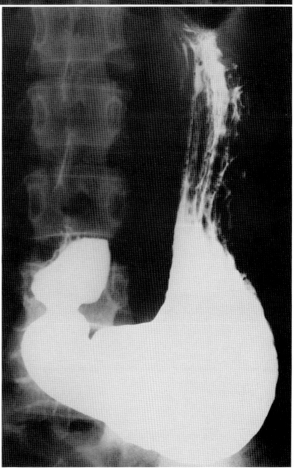

Fig. 323 Upright barium-filled film demonstrates deformity of the incisura and rigid appearance of the lesser curvature of the lower body.

179

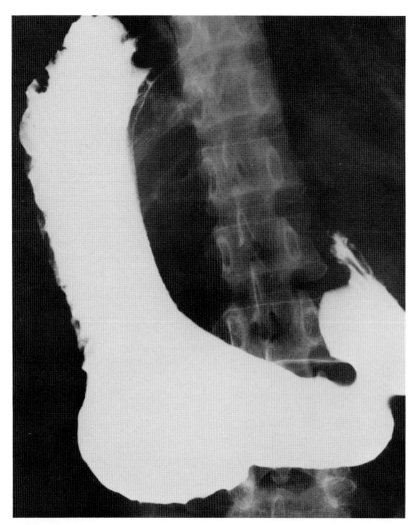

Fig. 324 Prone barium-filled film demonstrates poor distensibility of the gastric body, which gives an impression of linitis plastica type cancer.

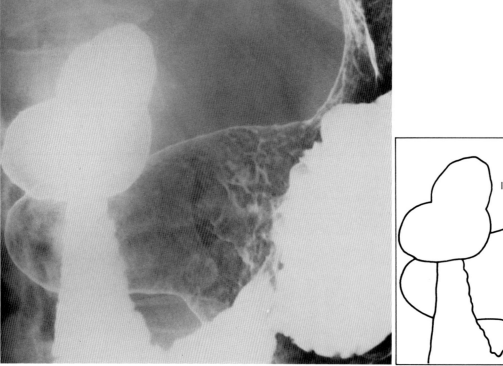

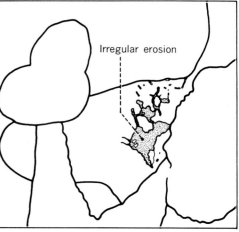

Irregular erosion

Fig. 325 Supine right anterior oblique double contrast film demonstrates faint, irregular collections of barium in the proximal antrum, simulating pseudopods. The small barium collections extend to the incisura.

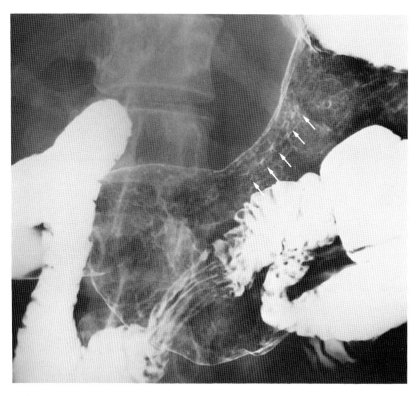

Fig. 326 Supine frontal double contrast film demonstrates large erosions of the proximal antrum and tiny erosions on the posterior wall of the gastric body along the lesser curvature (arrow).

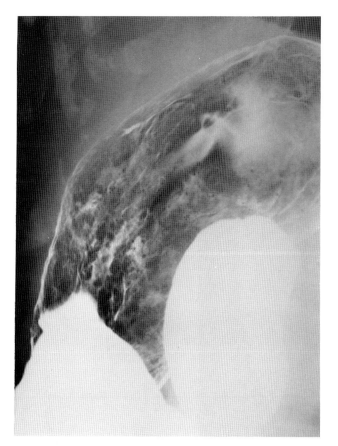
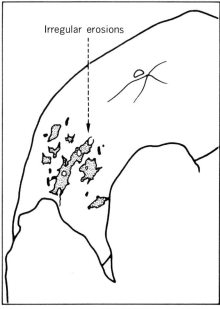

Fig. 327 Supine double contrast film in the right lateral decubitus position demonstrates irregular erosions of the upper body of the lesser curvature.

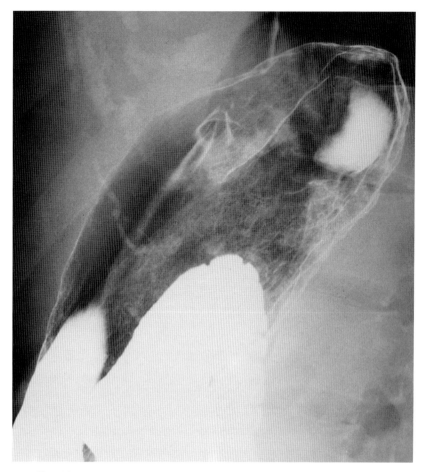

Fig. 332 Supine double contrast film in the right lateral decubitus position reveals normal mucosa of the upper body.

the deformity of the incisura still remains in the barium-filled stomach (Fig. 329), but the extensive erosions in the proximal antrum and middle gastric body seem to have disappeared almost completely (Figs. 331, 332), leaving only a small part of the slight mucosal depression (Fig. 330).

As mentioned, there is no mucosal convergence left in these two cases after healing, despite the extent of the erosions.

Another type of fresh gastric erosion is often observed in patients with symmetrical ulcers of the antrum, as shown in Figures 289—294 in Chapter 7. The main ulcers in the anterior and the posterior wall are almost always shallow. Histologically, they are Ul-II acute ulcers according to Murakami's classification, and small collections of barium scattered around the main ulcers are diagnosed as multiple erosions.

So-called Gastric Erosions

So-called gastric erosions are those lesions which reveal central depression with surrounding elevation of the mucosa. Clinically, they can be classified into two groups, namely, the disappearing type and the long-standing type. In most cases of disappearing type the lesions disappear within 3 months. In Sata's (1974) series the longest persistence was 45 months.

There is no marked seasonal difference in the occurrence of the long-standing type, but the highest incidence is in October, while the disappearing type reveals a bimodial curve in April and October (Sata 1974). The disappearing type is most frequently seen in the 4th decade and the long-standing type is most frequently seen in the 5th decade (Sata 1974). In the disappearing type the lesion is most frequently located from the antrum to the incisura in the 20—30-year age group. They appear in the gastric body in the thirties and become distributed in the entire gastric mucosa in the forties. In the long-standing type the entire gastric mucosa becomes affected in the fifties. Slight differences in the time of proximal spread of the lesions is observed between the disappearing and the long-standing type (Sata 1974).

Abel (1954) is the first in the radiographic literature to have observed that there are two types of gastric erosions, disappearing and long-standing. He presented two cases of gastric erosion which disappeared in 6 weeks and in 3 months, respectively. Abel called the disappearing type "gastritis erosiva" and the long-standing type "gastritis veruccosa." He emphasized the usefulness of the compression method for the differential diagnosis. In the disappearing type polypoid components are effaced by a relatively strong compression and in the long-standing erosion they remain visible despite the same amount of compression. Abel stated that the polypoid lesion is soft in the former and hard in the latter (warzige Schleimhauterhebungen). Sano et al. (1970), analyzing the findings of endoscopy and surgical specimens in so-called gastric erosions, classified them into two types in the same way as Abel. Sano et al. (1970) stated that the surrounding elevation of the mucosa is produced by hyperplasia of the foveolar epithelium associated with round cell infiltration and edema and suggested that this change may shift into atrophic-hyperplastic gastritis. In the long-standing type, proliferation of the pyloric glands simulating neoplasia may cause mucosal elevation in the antrum, and hyperplasia and cystic formation of the foveolar epithelium may be the components of the surrounding mucosal elevation in the fundic gland area.

Disappearing Type

In the radiographic diagnosis of the disappearing type the wider surface of the mucosal elevation is seen to be occupied by a shallow depression and the mucosal elevation itself reveals rather gradual sloping to the normal mucosa (Figs. 333–336). The depression may be shallow (Sata 1974). In Figure 334 marked erosions are located in the intermediate zone between the pyloric gland and fundic gland area, which is a frequent site of peptic ulcer. Some folds in the fundic gland area reveal changes in caliber and contain specks of barium.

Case 92   **Erosions in Acute Phase.**
A 39-year-old man (JU). (Fig. 333)

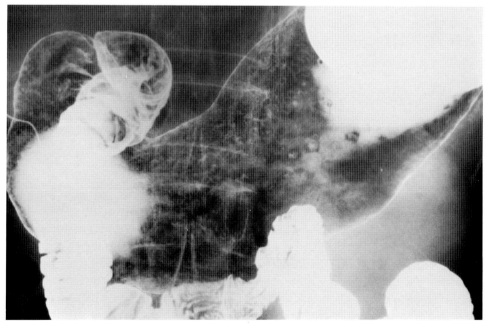

Fig. 333   Supine frontal double contrast film demonstrates disappearing erosions on the posterior wall of the gastric body.

Case 93   Erosions, Disappearing Type.
A 44-year-old man (CIH). (Fig. 334)

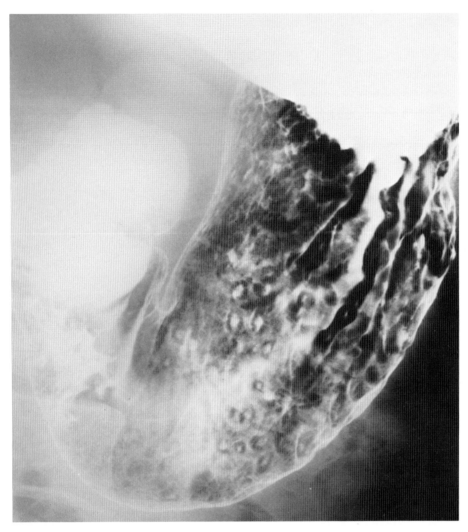

Fig. 334   Supine right anterior oblique double contrast film demonstrates disappearing erosions which are mainly localized in the intermediate zone. The mucosal folds of the fundic gland area show caliber changes.

The surrounding halos of the marked erosions are faintly demarcated, just as is seen in the mound surrounding a peptic ulcer which has a rapid healing tendency. In Figure 333 those erosions near the lesser curvature side show no definite surrounding halos. They may disappear rapidly. In Figure 336 those erosions in the anterior wall near the lesser curvature do not reveal the surrounding halos. In Figure 337 the two erosions (arrows) with large mucosal depression may be the disappearing type but the depression is not visualized in the compression image (Fig. 338). In this case a moderate degree of compression may have effaced

the central depression. It is characteristic of the disappearing type that the margin of the radiolucent halo is rather faintly delineated in the double contrast images. This contrasts with a long-standing erosion such as that shown in Figure 339 (arrow 1). Arrow 2 points to that type of erosion. In this case some erosions of the disappearing type (arrows) are scattered in the proximal antrum. The mucosal relief image (Fig. 341) reveals changes of caliber and a long-standing erosion at the incisura (arrow). A double contrast radiograph in this case was taken with too much air, which effaced the mucosal details (Fig. 342).

Case 94 Erosions, Disappearing Type.
A 60-year-old woman (JU). (Figs. 335 and 336)

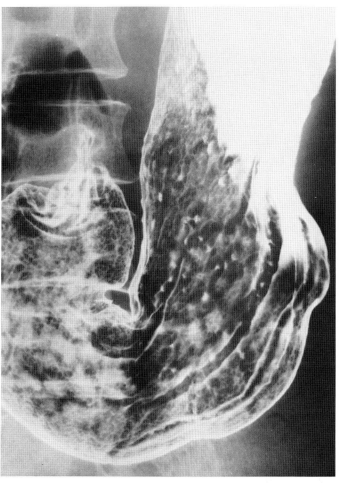

Fig. 335 Supine frontal double contrast film demonstrates disappearing erosions without remarkable surrounding halo in the gastric body.

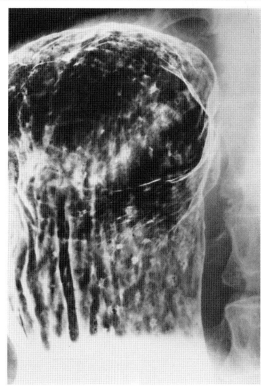

Fig. 336 Semi-upright prone double contrast film demonstrates disappearing erosions without remarkable surrounding halo in the gastric body and fundus.

Case 95 Erosions, Disappearing Type.
A 40-year-old man (JU). (Fig. 337 and 338)

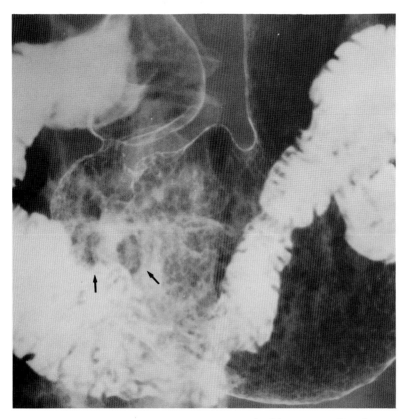

Fig. 337 Supine right anterior oblique double contrast film demonstrates two erosions of the disappearing type in the antrum (arrows).

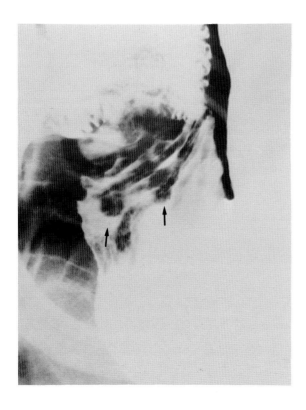

Fig. 338 Upright compression film demonstrates surrounding halos without marked depression (arrows).

188

Case 96   Erosions, Disappearing and Long-Standing Type.
A 58-year-old man (CIH). (Figs. 339-342)

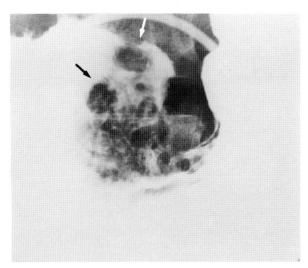 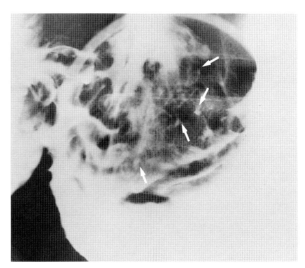

Fig. 339   Fig. 340

Fig. 339   Upright compression film demonstrates two erosions of the long-standing type in the antrum (arrows).

Fig. 340   Upright compression film demonstrates erosions of the disappearing type (arrows).

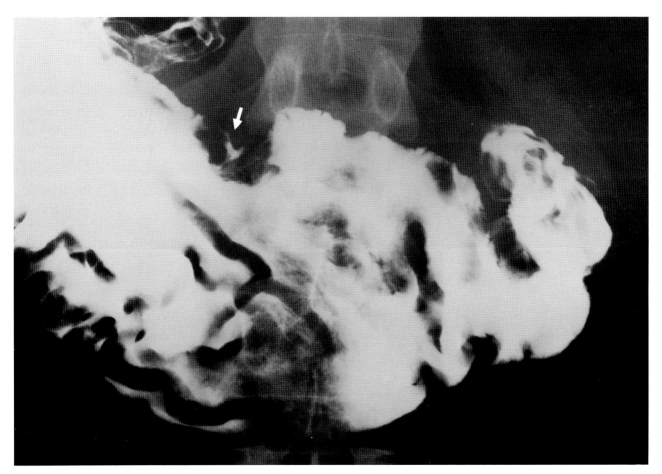

Fig. 341   Prone mucosal relief film demonstrates a long-standing erosion in the incisura (arrow) and changes in caliber of the mucosal folds of the antrum.

189

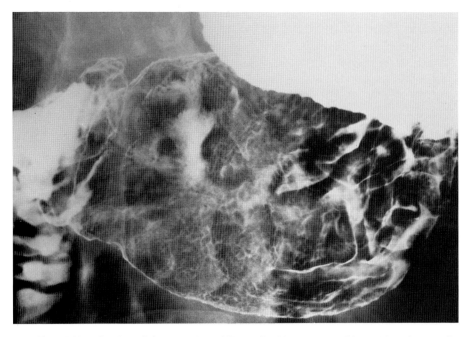

Fig. 342 Supine right anterior oblique double contrast film with a large volume of air does not demonstrate mucosal details.

Long-standing Type

Long-standing erosion may sometimes be solitary when discovered (Figs. 343–350). In such cases the lesion initially might have been multiple with only one persisting. The margins of the radiolucent halos are smooth and sharply outlined, compared with those of the disappearing type. Sometimes, the lesion has the same appearance as that seen in a hyperplastic polyp. However, in most cases of long-standing type, the lesions are multiple (Figs. 351 and 352). As mentioned above, surface depressions appear and disappear during the period of observation (Fig. 351). Sometimes, the gastric

Case 97 **Single Erosion, Long-Standing Type.**
A 45-year-old man (CIH). (Figs. 343-346)

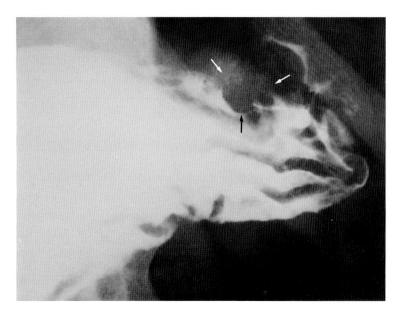

Fig. 343 Prone compression film with a small volume of air demonstrates a solitary long-standing erosion at the lesser curvature of the antrum (arrows). A central depression is not delineated.

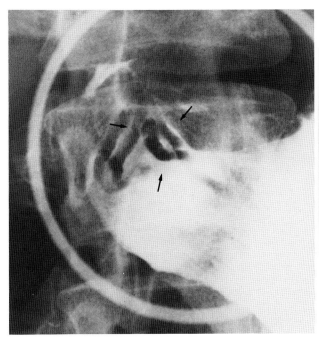

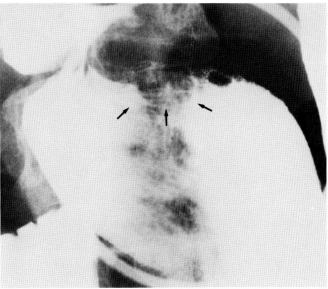

Fig. 344   Fig. 345

Fig. 344 Upright compression film with a small volume of air demonstrates the solitary long-standing erosion. The central depression is delineated (arrows).

Fig. 345 Upright compression film with a moderate volume of air faintly demonstrates the lesion (arrows).

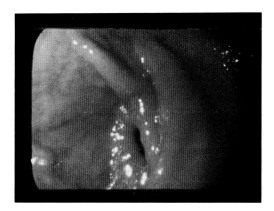

Fig. 346 Endoscopic picture of a solitary long-standing erosion.

mucosa is widely involved by erosions with various stages of development (Fig. 352–354). In such cases the long-standing erosions are usually observed in the antrum and the incisura (Fig. 352), and those of the disappearing type are observed in the lower gastric body (Fig. 353). In time, longstanding erosions with sharply outlined margins are observed (Fig. 354).

Case 98   Single Erosion, Long-Standing Type.
A 50-year-old woman (CIH). (Figs. 347 and 348)

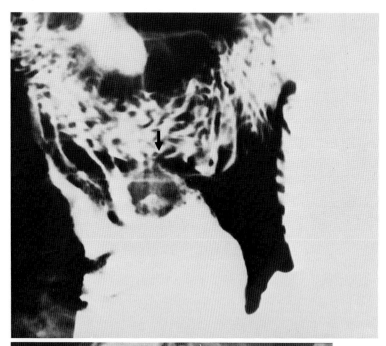

Fig. 347 Upright compression film demonstrates a relatively large solitary erosion of the long-standing type on the antrum near the lesser curvature (arrow).

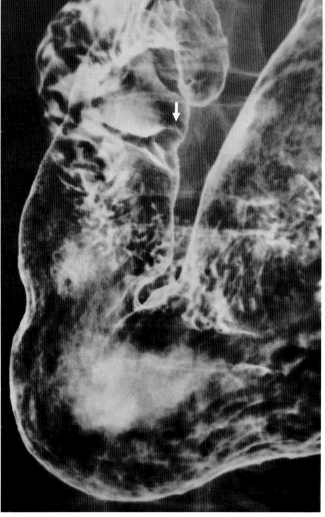

Fig. 348 Supine frontal double contrast film demonstrates a solitary long-standing erosion on a mucosal fold (arrow).

Case 99 Single Erosion, Long-Standing Type.
A 48-year-old man (CIH). (Figs. 349 and 350)

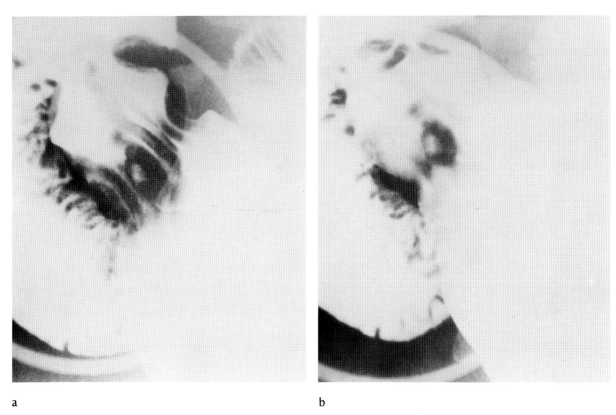

a   b

Fig. 349 a and b   Upright compression films demonstrate a solitary long-standing erosion on the antrum. The size of the surrounding elevation changes according to the intensity of the compression applied.

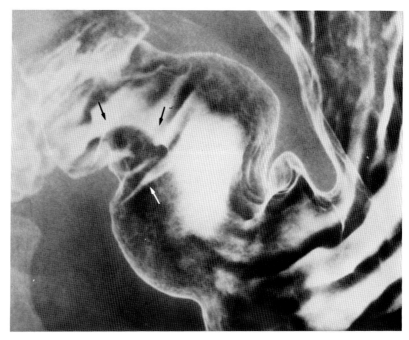

Fig. 350   Supine right anterior oblique double contrast film demonstrates a solitary long-standing erosion (arrows).

Case 100 Erosions, Long-Standing Type.
A 53-year-old man (ClH). (Fig. 351)

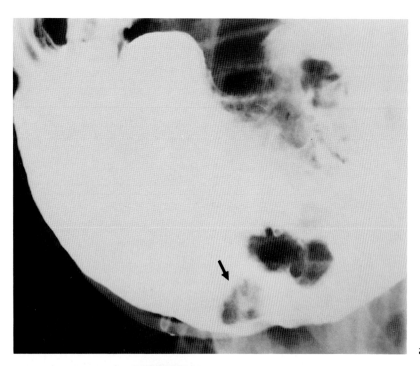

a

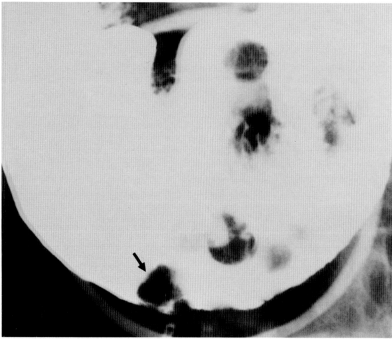

b

Fig. 351 a and b Upright compression films demonstrate appearance and disappearance of a surface depression in a long-standing erosion in an interval of 6 months (arrows).

Case 101   Erosions, Long-Standing Type.
A 45-year-old man (CIH). (Figs. 352-354)

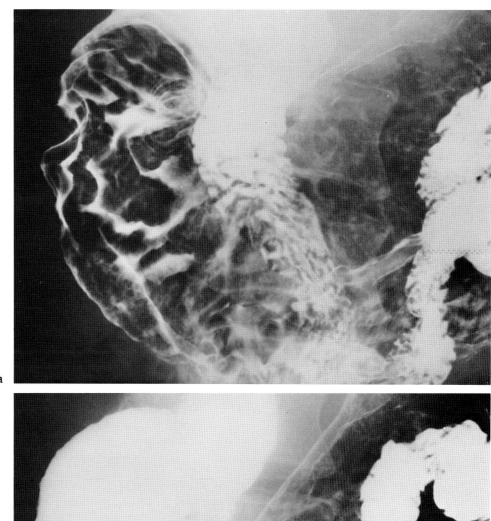

a

b

Fig. 352 a and b Supine frontal double contrast films demonstrate extensive erosions with a mixture of disappearing and long-standing types.

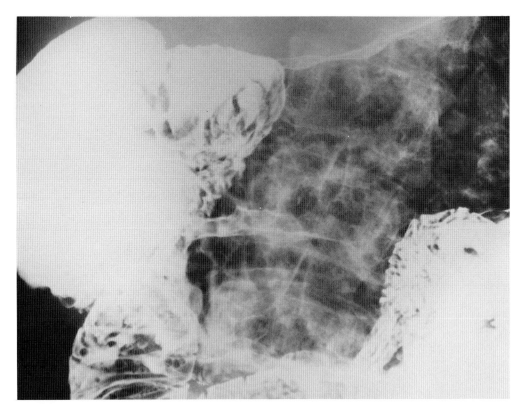

Fig. 353 Supine left anterior oblique double contrast film demonstrates erosions of the disappearing type in the lower gastric body which are faintly delineated due to a large volume of air.

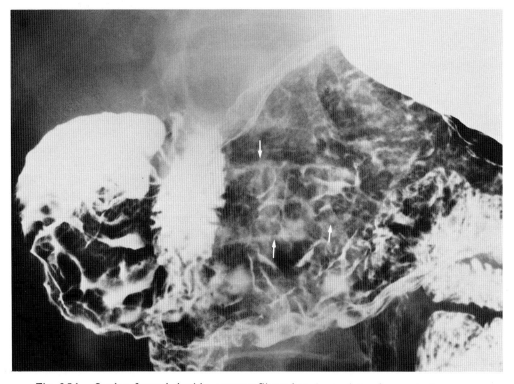

Fig. 354 Supine frontal double contrast film taken 1 year later demonstrates appearance of some long-standing erosions in the lower gastric body (arrows).

Differential Diagnosis

Solitary erosions should be differentiated from small type IIc lesions. In the type IIc lesion the depression is always irregular and sharply outlined (Figs. 576–583), though it is very small. Multiple erosions, regardless whether of disappearing or long-standing type, are usually not difficult to differentiate from malignancy, except in unusual case (Figs. 355–359).

Case 102   Type IIa Early Cancer Simulating Long-Standing Erosions.
A 62-year-old woman (CIH). (Figs. 355-359)

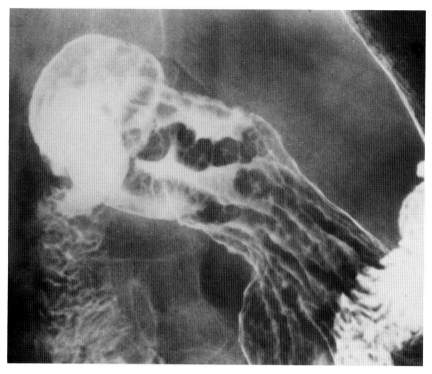

Fig. 355   Supine right anterior oblique double contrast film demonstrates a peculiar lesion of early cancer type IIa + (IIc), which may be confused with long-standing erosions.

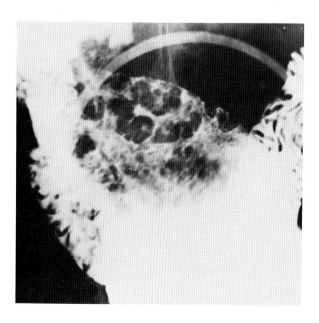

Fig. 356   Upright compression film demonstrates aggregation of radiolucencies with surface depression which appear to be long-standing erosions.

197

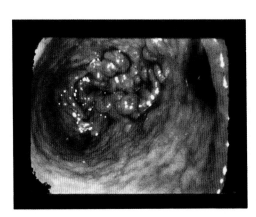

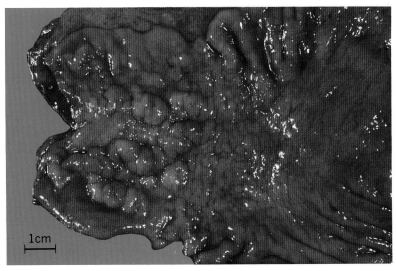

1cm

Fig. 357

Fig. 358

Fig. 357 Endoscopic picture of early cancer simulating long-standing erosions (dye-spraying method by Ingigocarmin).

Fig. 358 Resected specimen.

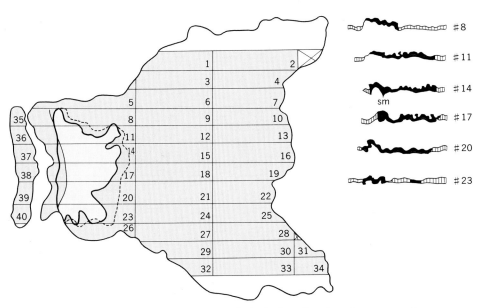

Fig. 359 Schematic representation of the lesion showing the extent of cancer spread. Histologic examination revealed a small type IIc lesion (adenocarcinoma papillotubulare) around the elevation. Cancer involved the submucosa (sm) only slightly (#14).

could be classified following Borrmann's classification of advanced cancer, based on the same principle as Kumakura. In Ninomiya's series, Borrmann type 3 was most frequent, comprising 65 per cent of all advanced malignant lymphoma (Table 30). Borrmann type 2 was second most frequent, comprising 25 per cent. There is some difference in the recognition of the macroscopic findings between Kumakura and Ninomiya. Kumakura's type II (Ulcerating Type) corresponds to Borrmann type 2, which was second most frequent in Ninomiya's classification.

Sugiyama (1974), considering the difficulty of using Kumakura's classification in early lesions, tried to classify the macroscopic form of malignant lesions into 4 types (Table 31). In his classification, superficial, depressed type is most frequently observed and must be differentiated from type IIc early cancer. Multiple ulcers in a depressed lesion are characteristic of this type. The polypoid type may reveal a smooth elevation of the mucosa with a bridging fold, or sharply demarcated multiple elevations of the mucosa suggesting submucosal origin. This type was not present in the operated cases, but was seen in the initial findings of radiography and endoscopy of two cases, observed over a period of time (Figs. 369–376). Akaike et al. (1972) reported a case of early malignant lymphoma belonging to the polypoid type. Multiple mucosal elevations with bridging folds were the characteristic findings in his case. The ulcero-polypoid type is a combination of multiple elevations simulating submucosal tumor and a shallow ulceration. Sometimes, an ulceration seems to be surrounded by multiple mucosal elevations instead of converging folds. The giant rugal type (Fig. 361) reveals a rather smooth pattern of the mucosal folds without narrowing of the gastric lumen. The presence of multiple ulcers is characteristic of this type. The giant rugal pattern is considered to be one of the characteris-

tics of advanced malignant lymphoma (Fig. 362). Rarely, however, it may be observed in early cases (Fig. 361). Ninomiya (1981) reported that most lesions of early malignant lymphoma were classified by the macroscopic classifications as early gastric cancer (Table 32). However, he found some lesions which revealed the macroscopic characteristics of the giant rugal type (Fig. 361) and a mixed variety of type IIc + Borrmann type 3 (Fig. 363). The ulcero-polypoid type in Sugiyama's classification corresponds to the type IIc + Borrmann type 3.

Radiographic findings of malignant lymphoma

Radiographic diagnosis of malignant lymphoma has been described mainly for large advanced lesions (Feldmann 1938, Rafsky et al. 1944, Marshall et al. 1950, Frank 1955, Franz 1962, Kumakura et al. 1970). Culver et al. (1955) described the radiographic diagnosis of early malignant lymphoma, but he did not refer to the definition of early malignant lymphoma. He doubted that one could detect early malignant lymphoma. In Japan, up to 1970, more than 20 cases of early malignant lymphoma were reported (a list of case reports is presented at the end of this atlas). Usually, malignant lymphoma of the stomach, including early and advanced lesions, is diagnosed radiographically with some difficulty. In the series of the Cancer Institute Hospital (Table 33) only 22 per cent (13/59) of all malignant lymphomas were diagnosed correctly. And 76 per cent (45/59) of them were initially diagnosed as cancer. Of the 15 early cases, 7 were diagnosed correctly and 7 were diagnosed as cancer. One case was diagnosed as multiple ulcers.

The radiographic findings of malignant lymphoma, whether early or advanced, consist of either mucosal elevation, suggesting submucosal origin, or multiple erosions or ulcerations (Figs. 364–368). In the early phase of malignant lymphoma a small polypoid lesion simulating a

Table 32 Macroscopic classification of early malignant lymphoma of the stomach (Ninomiya et al. 1981).

Macroscopic type	Cases
Type IIc	11 (58%)
Type IIa + IIc	3 (16%)
Giant folds type	3 (16%)
Type IIc + Borrmann 3 type	2 (10%)
Total	19 Lesions

1946–1980, Cancer Institute Hospital, Tokyo.

Table 33 Initial radiographic diagnosis of malignant lymphoma of the stomach (Ninomiya et al. 1981).

Initial diagnosis	Cases
Malignant lymphoma	13 (7) [22%]
Cancer	45 (7) [76%]
Multiple ulcers	1 (1) [2%]
Total	59 (15)

( ): Early malignant lymphoma
1946–1980, Cancer Institute Hospital, Tokyo.

submucosal tumor may be the only diagnostic sign (Fig. 369). This may develop rather rapidly into a large mass with multiple ulcerations (Fig. 370). Sometimes, localized thickening of the mucosal folds with a smooth surface configuration may be the initial sign (Figs. 376 and 377). In these cases the lesions develop into a large mass with giant rugae and ulcerations (Figs. 378–380). In early malignant lymphoma, the two above-mentioned features are visualized by careful examination of the compression and double contrast images. In the depressed type of malignant lymphoma simulating type IIc early cancer, a partially raised margin may suggest a submucosal origin (Figs. 386–392 and 393–400). This is unusual in early gastric cancer. Sometimes, multiple erosions are present when the depression is large (Figs. 401–405). In such cases it may be difficult to distinguish the border of a

Case 107   Advanced Malignant Lymphoma (Giant Rugal Type)
An 18-year-old girl (NCCH). (Figs. 364-368)

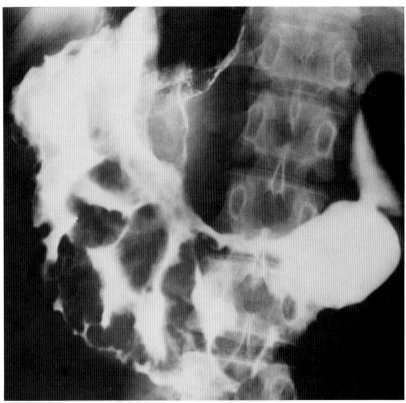

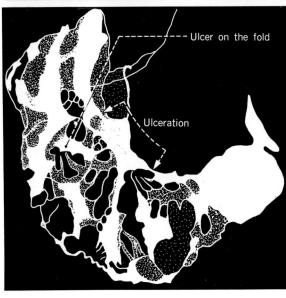

Ulcer on the fold

Ulceration

Fig. 364   Prone mucosal relief film demonstrates giant rugal folds with intervening depressions, from the upper gastric body to the proximal antrum.

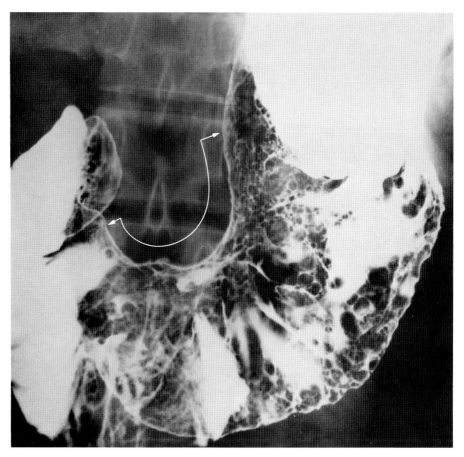

Fig. 365 Supine frontal double contrast film demonstrates multiple depressions (ulcer) and giant rugal folds. The lesser curvature is not well distended (arrow line).

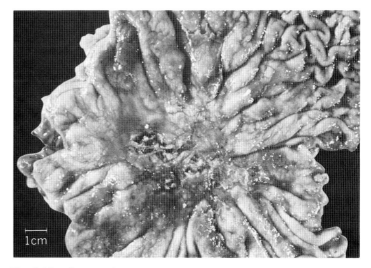

1cm

Fig. 366 Resected specimen.

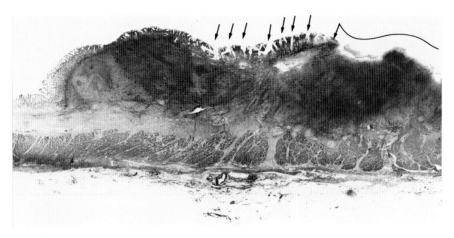

Fig. 367 Cross section of the lesion, showing marked submucosal proliferation of lymphatic tissue. Mucosal surface reveals multiple, tiny erosions (arrows) and ulceration (arrow line).

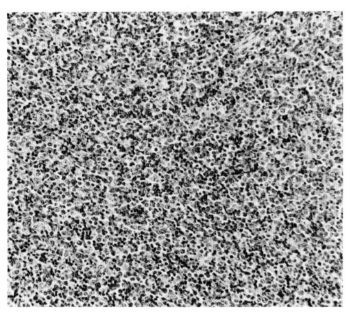

Fig. 368 Histologic findings show non-Hodgkin's malignant lymphoma.

depression from the normal surrounding mucosa. Sometimes, type IIc early cancer of the undifferentiated type is difficult to distinguish from the depressed type of malignant lymphoma. However, granularity in a depression is irregular and roughly distributed in the former, whereas in the latter it is regular and densely distributed. The presence of multiple ulcer scars may be a differentiating point. Also, converging folds show smooth enlargement or tapering, which is unusual in cancerous infiltration (Fig. 402).

Some cases of early malignant lymphoma are peculiar in that marked enlargement and reduction of the size of the tumor may occur in a short period of time (Ohashi et al. 1973, Takeuchi et al. 1971, Nakano et al. 1972). Takeuchi (1971) reported a case of early malignant lymphoma which decreased in size when it became ulcerated. In Nakano's case a part of the tumor became smaller with scar formation. In this case invasion of the malignant lymphoma was still limited to the submucosa even after reappearance of the tumor.

Case 108 Multiple Advanced Malignant Lymphomas (Borrmann Type 2).

A 46-year-old man (CIH). (Figs. 369-374)

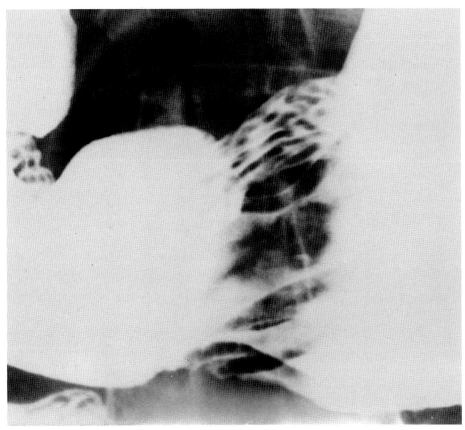

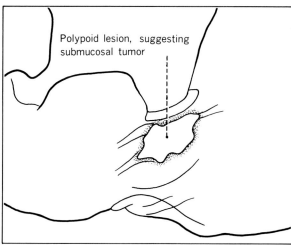

Polypoid lesion, suggesting submucosal tumor

Fig. 369   Initial compression film demonstrates an irregular radiolucency, suggesting a polypoid lesion of submucosal origin (arrow).

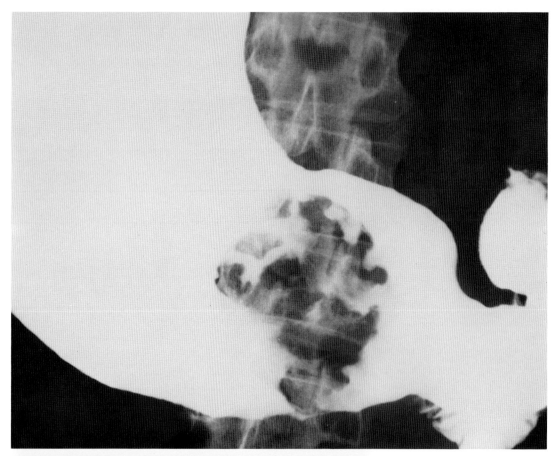

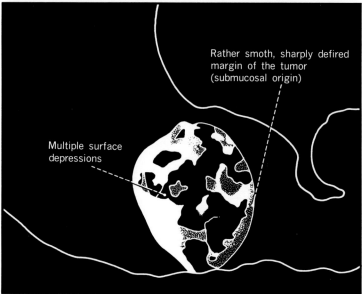

Fig. 370 Prone compresion film in the second examination about 3.5 months later demonstrates a large polypoid mass with multiple, irregular surface depressions in the antrum.

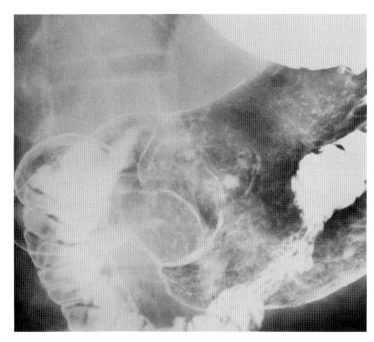
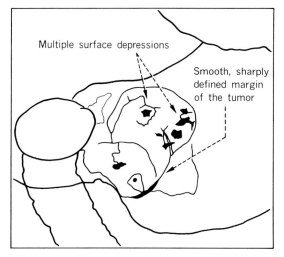

Multiple surface depressions

Smooth, sharply
defined margin
of the tumor

Fig. 371   Supine right anterior oblique film demonstrates large polypoid lesions suggesting submucosal tumors, with multiple irregular surface depressions.

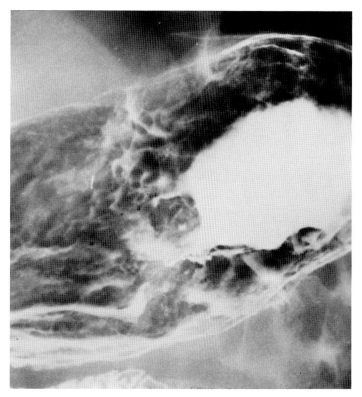

Fig. 372   Supine double contrast film in the left anterior oblique position. Another lesion in the upper gastric body near the cardia which was unchanged from the initial examination. This lesion also is an irregular polypoid mass with multiple surface depressions.

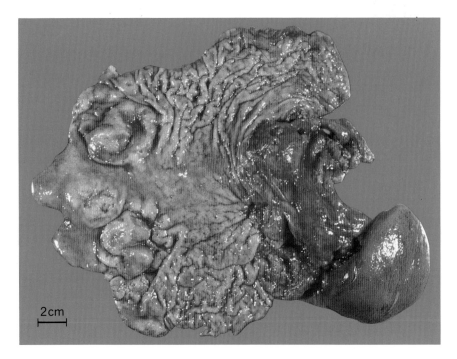

Fig. 373   Resected specimen.

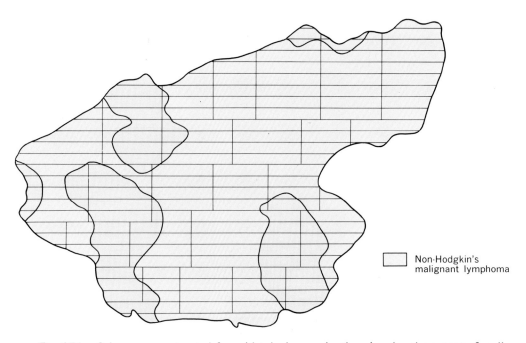

☐ Non-Hodgkin's
  malignant lymphoma

Fig. 374   Schema reconstructed from histologic examination showing the extent of malignant lymphoma in the resected specimen. The histologic examination revealed that both lesions were non-Hodgkin's malignant lymphoma, involving the serosa.

Case 109   Advanced Malignant Lymphoma (Borrmann Type 3).
A 51-year-old man (CIH). (Figs. 375-385)

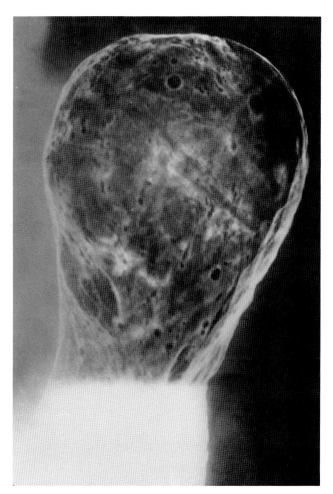 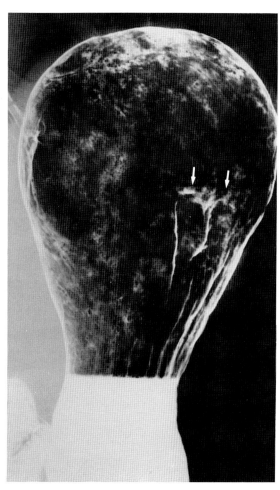

Fig. 375   Fig. 376

Fig. 375   Upright double contrast film from the initial examination reveals no abnormality.
Fig. 376   Upright double contrast film in the second examination about 7 months later reveals two enlarged folds in the upper gastric body (arrows.)

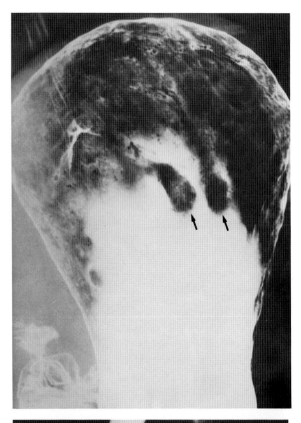

Fig. 377 Semi-upright prone double contrast film (on the same date) reveals localized enlargement of the two folds in the upper gastric body (arrows).

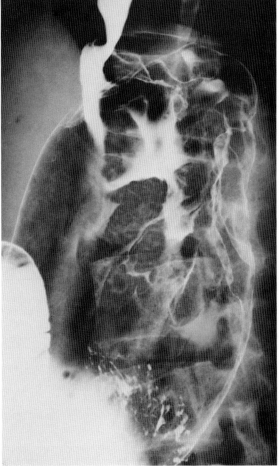

Fig. 378

Fig. 379

Fig. 378 and 379 Supine left anterior oblique double contrast film about 2 years and 2 months later demonstrates a large irregular collection of barium surrounded by a prominently raised margin consisting of enlarged mucosal folds. The lesion involves the upper gastric body and fundus.

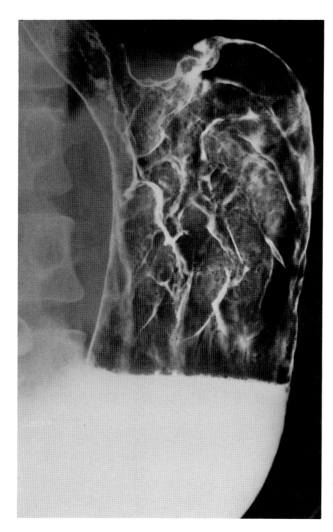

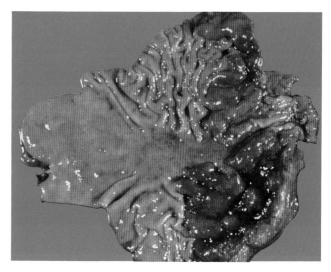

Fig. 381 Resected specimen.

Fig. 380 Upright double contrast film demonstrates the lesion, consisting mainly of prominently enlarged folds. It also involves the esophagus. The fundus and upper gastric body are poorly distended.

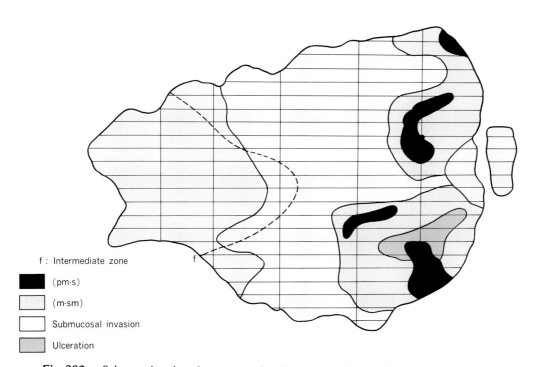

f : Intermediate zone

■ (pm-s)

▨ (m-sm)

□ Submucosal invasion

▨ Ulceration

Fig. 382 Schema showing the extent of malignant lymphoma. Histologic examination revealed non-Hodgkin's malignant lymphoma, involving the serosa.

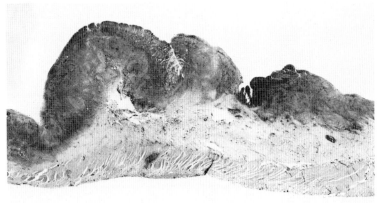

Fig. 383

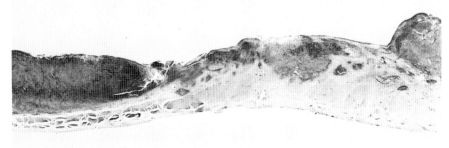

Fig. 384

Fig. 383 and 384   Cross sections of the lesion.

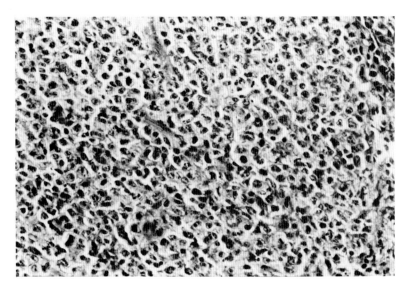

Fig. 385   Histologic findings show non-Hodgkin's malignant lymphoma.

Case 110 Early Malignant Lymphoma (Type IIc).

A 49-year-old woman (CIH). (Figs. 386–392)

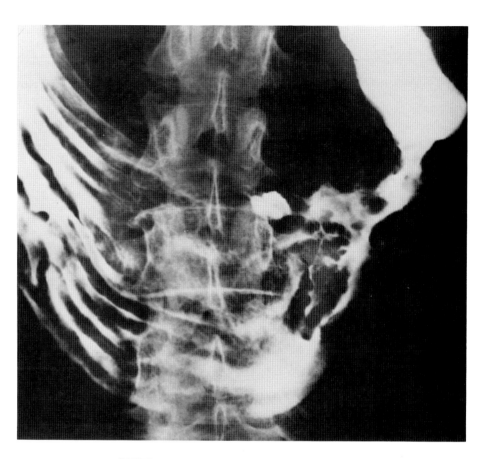

Fig. 386 Prone mucosal relief film.

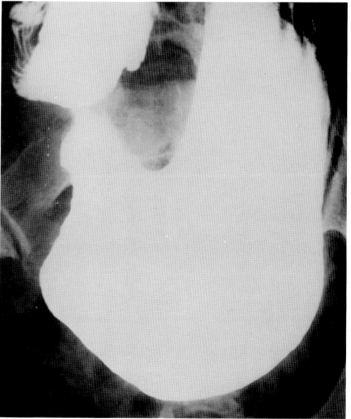

Fig. 387 Barium-filled film.

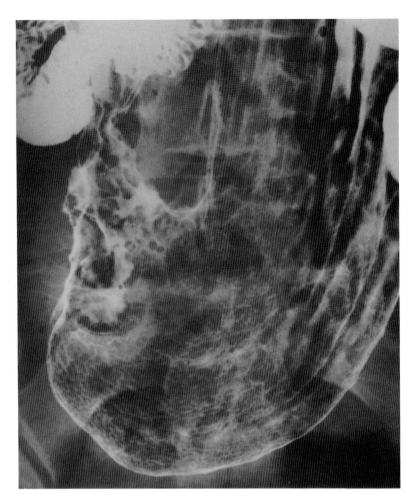
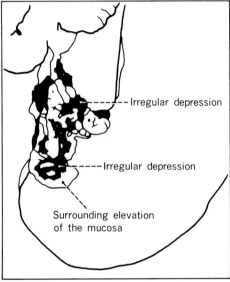

Irregular depression

Irregular depression

Surrounding elevation
of the mucosa

Fig. 388 Supine frontal double contrast film demonstrates multiple irregular collections of barium surrounded by radiolucencies in the poorly distended antrum.

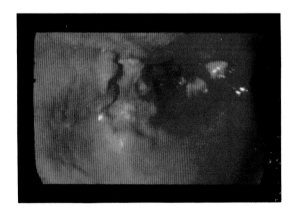

Fig. 389 Endoscropic findings.

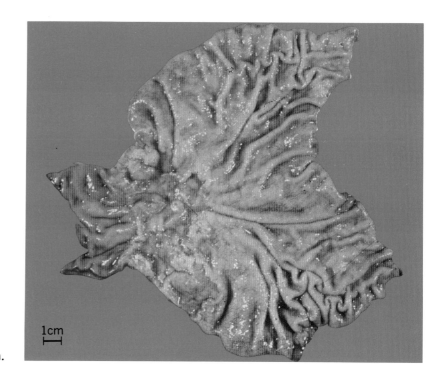

Fig. 390 Resected specimen.

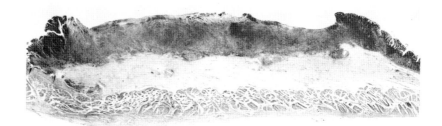

Fig. 391 Cross section of the lesion.

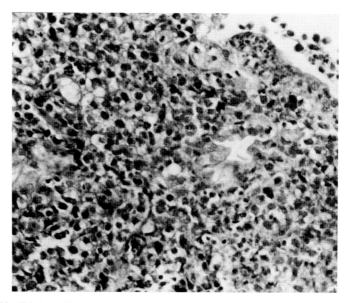

Fig. 392 Histologic examination revealed a non-Hodkin's malignant lymphoma, involving the submucosa.

Case 111 Early Malignant Lymphoma (Type IIc).
A 41-year-old man (CIH). (Figs. 393–400)

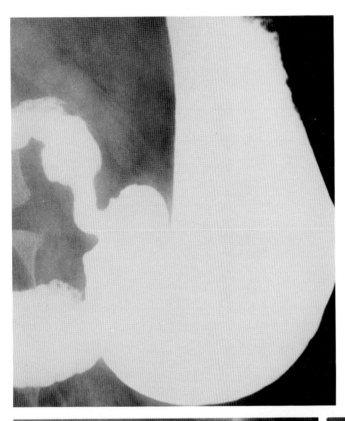

Fig. 393 Barium-filled film in the right anterior oblique position demonstrates marked narrowing of the distal antrum.

Fig. 394 Supine right anterior oblique double contrast film demonstrates radiolucencies of various sizes in the distended antrum. There is irregularity of the lesser and greater curvatures.

Fig. 395 Supine left anterior oblique double contrast film. The radiolucencies in profile appear as a slight mucosal elevation. The greater curvature of the antrum is well distended.

Fig. 393

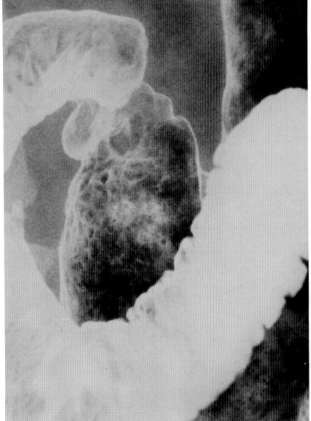

Fig. 394

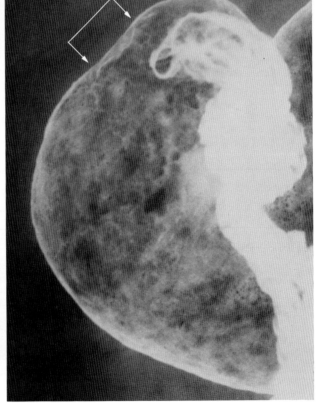

Fig. 395

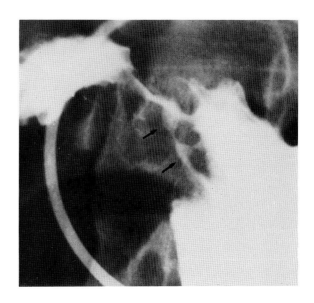

Fig. 396 Upright compression film of the distal antrum. Two niches with surrounding radiolucency are seen (arrows).

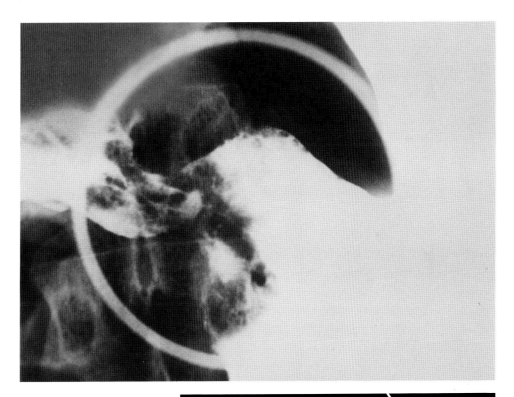

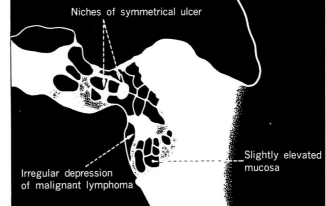

Fig. 397 Upright compression film of the proximal antrum. Irregular barium collection with surrounding radiolucency is seen in the proximal antrum near the greater curvature. The small niches in Figure 396 may correspond to the symmetrical ulcer scars in Figure 398, and the irregular depression in Figure 397 may correspond to the malignant lymphoma lesion itself.

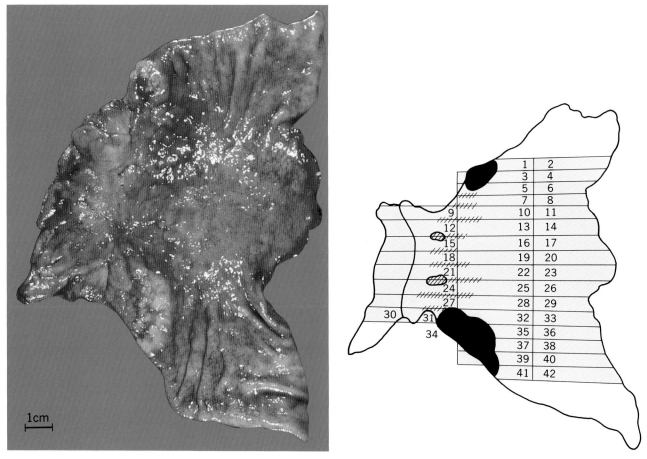

Fig. 398   Fig. 399

Fig. 398   Resected specimen. The malignant lymphoma appears as a yellowish mucosal elevation with irregular surface depressions and measures 35 x 30 mm. Symmetrical ulcer scars are present in the distal antrum.

Fig. 399   Schematic representation showing the extent of the malignant lymphoma as reconstructed from the histologic examination. Narrowing of the antrum is caused by fibrosis of the region surrounding the symmetrical ulcer scars.

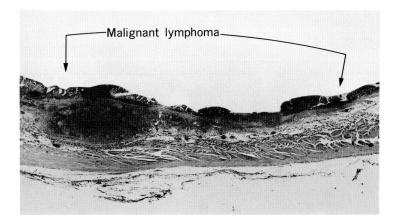

Fig. 400   Cross section of the lesion (Block number 35). The submucosa is involved by non-Hodgkin's malignant lymphoma.

Case 112   Early Malignant Lymphoma (Type IIc).

A 43-year-old woman (CIH). (Figs. 401-405)

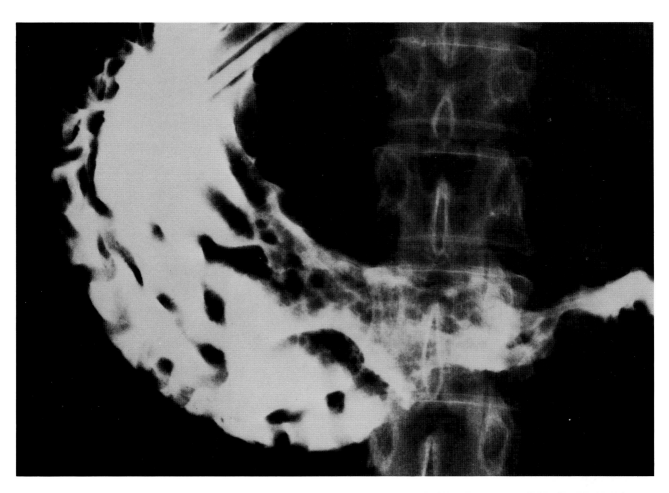

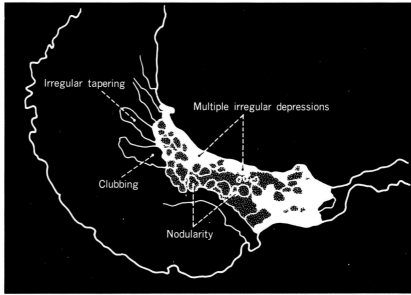

Fig. 401   Prone mucosal relief film demonstrates irregular collections of barium and intervening radiolucencies. Converging folds show irregular tapering and clubbing. The entire lesion is a large depression and contains multiple erosions with intervening nodularity.

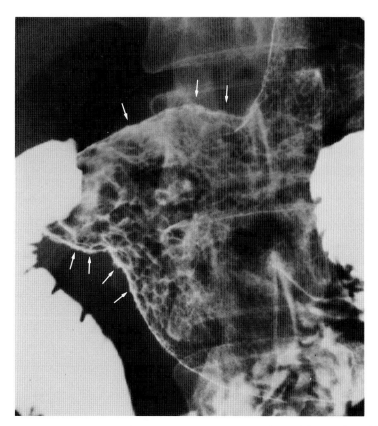

Fig. 402 Supine double contrast film in the right anterior oblique position with a moderate amount of air. Multiple erosions and nodularity are seen in the entire antrum. Irregular contours of the lesser and greater curvatures of the antrum result from multiple erosions in profile (arrows). The proximal border of the lesion is not clearly delineated as converging folds are effaced, probably due to overdistension of the stomach.

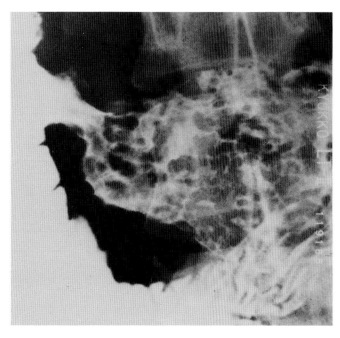

Fig. 403 Upright compression film clearly demonstrates the multiple erosions and nodularity.

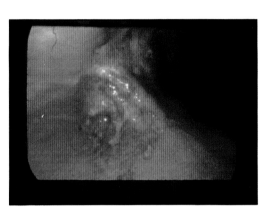

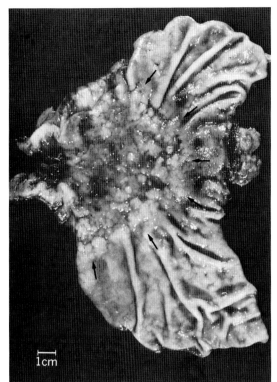

Fig. 404   Fig. 405

Fig. 404   Endoscopic findings. Multiple irregular depressions with surrounding raised mucosa are characteristic of early malignant lymphoma.

Fig. 405   Resected specimen. The entire lesion is depressed (arrows), and consists of multiple erosions and nodularity. The nodularity is most marked in the peripheral part of the lesion. Histologic examination disclosed, non-Hodgkin's malignant lymphoma, involving the submucosa. The duodenal bulb also was slightly involved.

Role of endoscopy and biopsy in the diagnosis of malignant lymphoma

The observations mentioned above are similarly applied to the endoscopic diagnosis of early malignant lymphoma. Multiple irregular depressions with surrounding raised mucosa are characteristic of early malignant lymphoma (Fig. 389). In this figure the surrounding raised mucosa in the greater curvature suggests that the lesion is of submucosal origin. On the other hand, the endoscopic findings shown in Figure 404 are not characteristic of early malignant lymphoma.

In the type IIa + IIc malignant lymphoma radiographic and endoscopic diagnosis is also difficult (Figs. 406–408). However, the endoscopic diagnosis may have an advantage, because submucosal origin of a lesion is strongly suspected in the endoscopic findings, as shown in Figure 408.

Result of biopsy in the diagnosis of malignant lymphoma

Biopsy is not always a reliable method for the diagnosis of malignant lymphoma, as shown in Table 34. In the cases of advanced malignant lymphoma, its positivity is 57 per cent and in those of early malignant lymphoma, it is 50 per cent. In four cases of early lesions in which biopsy was positive, the initial biopsy was positive in two cases. In one case malignant lymphoma was confirmed in the second biopsy. In the remaining case the initial biopsy diagnosis was scirrhous cancer and repeated hisologic examination finally confirmed malignant lymphoma.

In order to establish malignant lymphoma, biopsy fragments should be taken from the inner aspect of the surrounding raised mucosa. Otherwise, the histologic diagnosis may result in necrotic

223

mass or normal gastric mucosa. For this reason, it is very difficult to establish the diagnosis of malignant lymphoma without the surrounding raised mucosa by biopsy (Fig. 404).

Table 34 Result of biopsy for malignant lymphoma.

	Positivity
Advanced malignant lymphoma	57% (16/28)
Early malignant lymphoma	50% (4/ 8)

Case 113 Early Malignant Lymphoma (Type IIa+IIc, Non-Hodgkin).
A 30-year-old man (CIH). (Figs. 406 and 407)

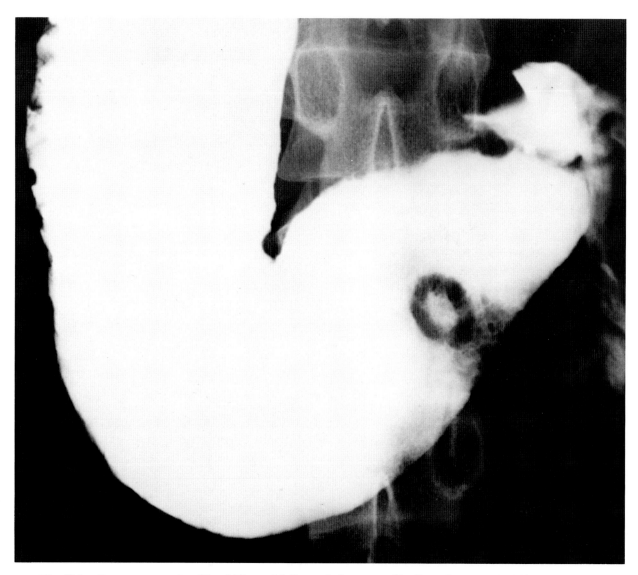

Fig. 406 Prone compression film. Differential diagnosis from type IIa+IIc early cancer is difficult.

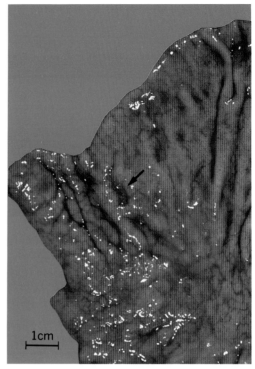

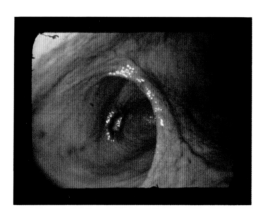

Fig. 407   Endoscopic findings.

Fig. 408   Resected specimen.

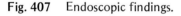

Reactive Lymphoreticular Hyperplasia (RLH)

Localized or diffuse proliferation of lymphoreticular tissue of the stomach is a non-epithelial lesion which is histologically visualized in the resected specimen. This lesion is recognized macroscopically as a mucosal change if the proliferation becomes marked. Konjetzny (1928) considered this lesion to be a type of chronic gastritis (lymphatisch-hyperplastischer Gastritis) and in 1938 reported three cases as "chronisch-lymphatischer Gastritis" which were often confused with cancer clinically and radiographically. Schindler (1937) described this lesion as "chronic atrophic lymphoblastomoid gastritis", a type of gastritis which is often diagnosed as cancer.

This lesion did not attract attention until 1958 when Smith and Helwig emphasized its importance in the differential diagnosis of malignant lymphoma. In their statistical investigation they noticed that malignant lymphoma of the stomach had a better prognosis than that of other organs, and they ascribed this to the fact that some benign lesions were difficult to differentiate histologically from malignancy and were included in the cases diagnosed as malignant lymphoma. They called these benign lesions "reactive lymphoid hyperplasia." Nakamura (1967) called the same lesions "reactive lymphoreticular hyperplasia" for the reason that not only lymphocytic hyperplasia but also reticulum cell hyperplasia is often visualized.

The lesion has not been accepted as a disease entity, but is referred to by name. The author uses the name, "reactive lymphoreticular hyperplasia" (RLH), following Nakamura (1967).

In Japan, it is considered important to differentiate RLH from early gastric cancer by radiography and endoscopy. Many cases of RLH have been reported which were difficult to diagnose.

Several authors pointed out that RLH reveals macroscopic characteristics that often are confused with malignancy. Generally, RLH is located in the intermediate zone between the pyloric and fundic glands and has a convolutional hypertrophy of the mucosa or hypertrophy of the mucosal folds (localized, hypertrophic form, by Nakamura 1967). In about 70 per cent to 80 per cent of cases with such macroscopic findings there are ulcerations in its center. This type of RLH is difficult to differentiate from type IIc + III. Sometimes it is confused with type IIa, if an ulcer is not present. Another type of RLH is characterized by an

225

extensive erosion in the antral portion of the stomach not extending beyond the intermediate zone (diffuse, flat form, by Nakamura 1967). This type is often confused with IIc type mucosal cancer (Y. Maruyama et al. 1969, Takeuchi et al. 1971, Doi et al. 1971).

Radiographically, RLH should be differentiated from cancer, malignant lymphoma, peptic ulcer and ulcer scar, erosions, benign polypoid lesions and giant rugae. The positive diagnosis of RLH is not difficult if the radiographic examination, including double contrast radiography and compression method, is performed effectively. RLH is first suggested by a hesitancy to make the diagnosis of early cancer because of inconsistency of radiographic findings, even after careful evaluation. RLH has poorly demarcated borders, compared with those of type IIa, and nodularity is not as densely distributed as in type IIa. When RLH simulates type IIc or type IIc + III, the margin of its depression is discontinuous, i.e.

its outline is interrupted in the macroscopic examination (Figs. 409–411). Abnormality of the converging folds such as clubbing and interruption is partially present around the depression (Figs. 409 and 410). Sometimes, the surrounding mucosa has fine granularity (Figs. 409 and 410). Changes in the radiographic findings are often observed in short periods of observation (Figs. 412 and 414). Follow-up study should be performed, even if biopsy reveals RLH, because it may sometimes be difficult to make a distinction between RLH and malignant lymphoma in the histologic examination of the biopsy fragments. In addition, there have been some reported cases in which malignant transformation of RLH is suggested (Konjetzny 1928, 1938, Castleman et al. 1956, Smith and Helwig 1958, Jacobs 1963, Faris and Salzstein 1964, Kay 1964, Schindler 1966, Takeuchi et al. 1973, Sannohe et al. 1976, Tsugane et al. 1978, Takasugi et al. 1978, Nakazawa et al. 1980, 1981, Katsumata et al. 1981).

Case 114   Reactive Lymphoreticular Hyperplasia (RLH).
A 50-year-old woman (JU). (Figs. 409-412)

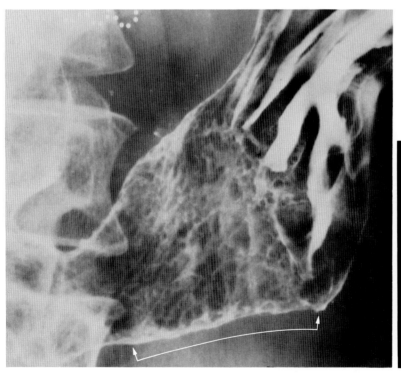
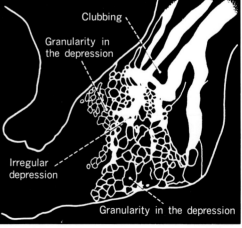

Fig. 409   Supine frontal double contrast film with a small volume of air. Faint irregular barium collections and granularity are seen in a wide area on the posterior wall, from the lower gastric body to the proximal antrum. The converging folds from the gastric body are interrupted and show clubbing. There is a slight indentation of the greater curvature (arrow line).

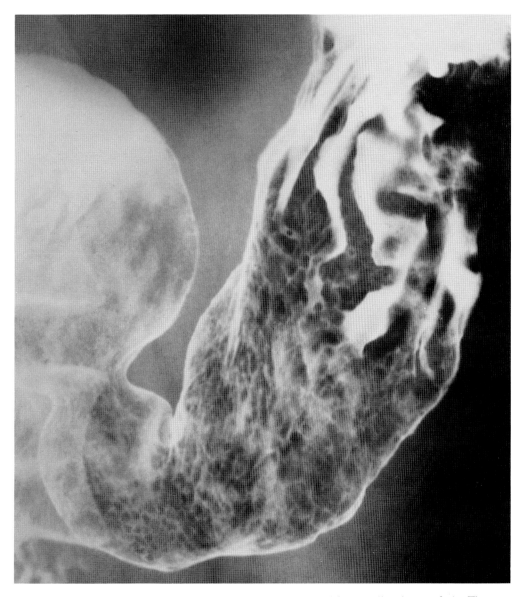

Fig. 410 Supine double contrast film in the right anterior oblique position, with a small volume of air. The wide area of mucosal abnormality with interrupted converging folds is suggestive but not diagnostic of early cancer (type IIc).

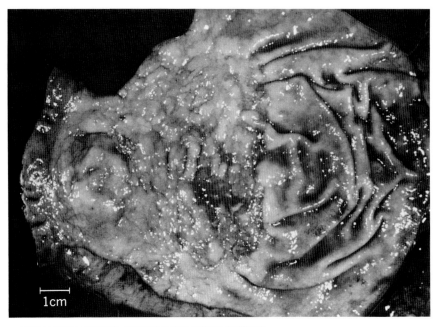

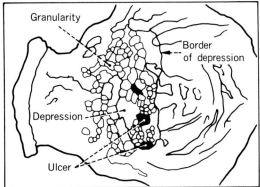

Fig. 411 Resected specimen, incised along the anterior wall aspect of the lesser curvature. There is a large irregular mucosal depression, located mainly on the posterior wall and involving the greater curvature. The granularity of the mucosa extends widely to the antrum and to the anterior wall. Interrupted folds frame the proximal border of the depression but the distal border is obscure. There are two small ulcerations in the depressed area.

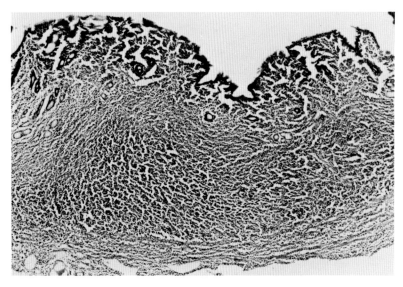

Fig. 412 Histologic findings of RLH.

Case 115 RLH.

A 43-year-old woman (CU). (Figs. 413 and 414)

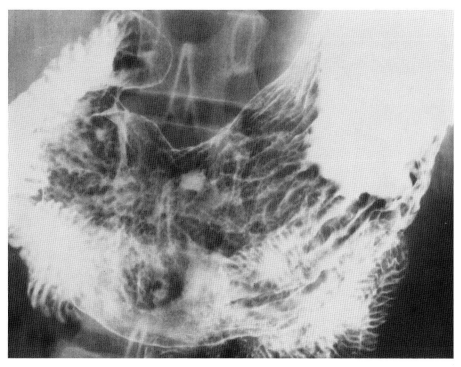

Fig. 413 Supine frontal double contrast film. A relatively irregular niche is seen on the posterior wall of the incisura region. The surrounding mucosa shows some irregular granularity. A converging fold from the antral side is interrupted far from the niche, and two folds reaching the niche show irregular tapering. The incisura is deformed, presumably as a result of fibrosis.

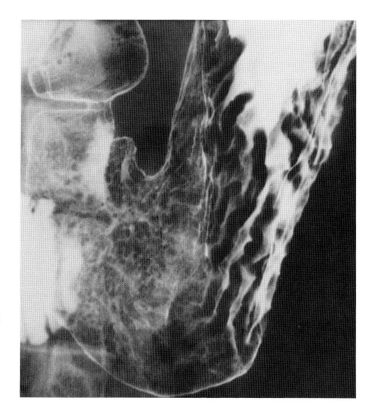

Fig. 414 Supine double contrast film in right anterior oblique position, taken 10 months later. The niche has disappeared, but there are irregular barium collections, suggesting multiple erosions in much wider region. The surrounding mucosa is roughly granulated.

Case 116 RLH.
A 53-year-old man (TMCDC). (Figs. 415-418)

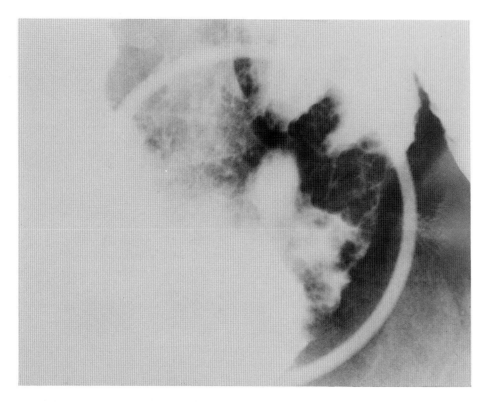

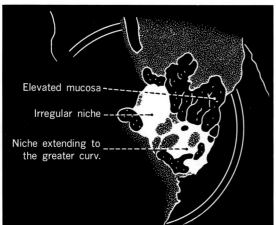

Elevated mucosa----

Irregular niche --

Niche extending to
the greater curv.

Fig. 415 Upright compression film. A large irregular niche extending to the greater curvature is seen in the lower gastric body. The surrounding mucosa is markedly elevated in the proximal region, which may explain the prominent clubbing of the converging folds. A normal, though elevated pattern of "areae gastricae" is seen.

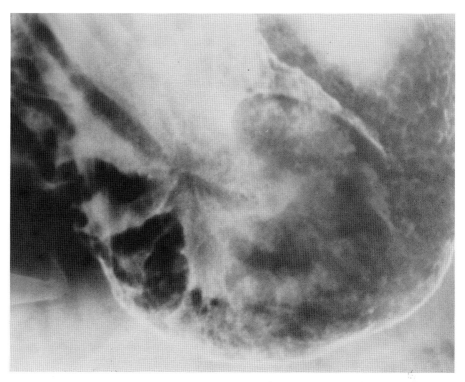

Fig. 416   Prone double contrast film taken 3 months later. The lesion is on the anterior wall. The irregular niche seems to have disappeared almost completely. The converging folds show smooth tapering.

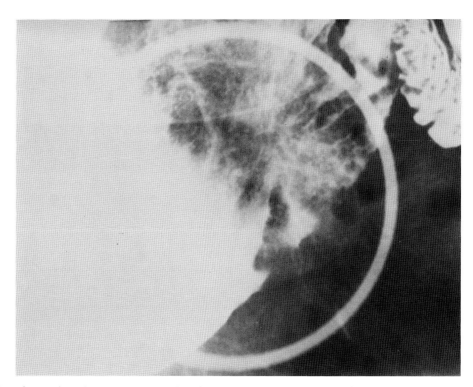

Fig. 417   Upright compression film taken 3 months later. The folds are converging toward the region of the deeper niche. The region between the point of the mucosal convergence and the greater curvature appears slightly granulated with multiple tiny erosions.

231

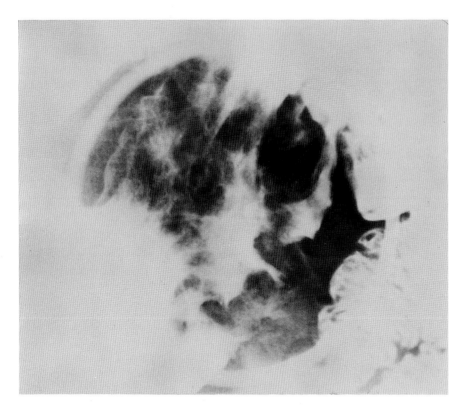

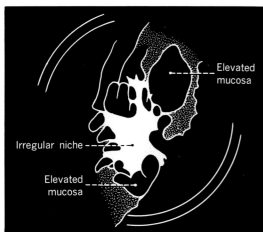

Fig. 418 Upright compression film taken about 4 months later than the second examination. A large, irregular niche reappeared. The surrounding mucosa is prominently raised, but appears smooth in outline and surface pattern, suggesting edematous mucosa.

Chapter 10

Radiographic Diagnosis of Depth of Invasion of Gastric Cancer

General Considerations

The aim of diagnosing the depth of invasion of gastric cancer is primarily to differentiate early from advanced cancer, since they have a considerably different prognosis. It is important for the surgeon to make an accurate differential diagnosis preperatively, as the type of operation and the extent of lymph node dissection may be changed if the depth of invasion is estimated.

In the routine radiographic diagnosis 21.1 per cent of early gastric cancers were diagnosed as advanced cancer or suspicious of advanced cancer (Fig. 419). In endoscopic examination 32.4 per cent were diagnosed as advanced cancer or suspicious of advanced cancer (Fig. 419). The X-ray examination was better in diagnosing the depth of invasion, which is a feature distinguishing early from advanced cancer. Advanced cancers occur most frequently of all gastric cancers. Most

of the Borrmann types are in the category of advanced cancer, as shown in Figure 421.

Among the lesions saddling the lesser curvature, as demonstrated in Figure 420, constant deformities such as severe rigidity of the wall (+++) and filling defects are found in 90 per cent of advanced cancers, and in 16 per cent of early cancers. Thus, the presence of severe rigidity of the wall (+++) or filling defects suggests that it is highly probable that the lesion is an advanced cancer.

Radiographic diagnosis can accurately differentiate early cancer from advanced cancer in nearly 90 per cent of all cases. Morphologic similarity of early cancer to an advanced cancer simulating an early lesion poses difficulty in the differential diagnosis, as illustrated in Figures 419 and 420.

The simpliest way to diagnose the depth of invasion is by the size of the lesion. As seen in Figure 421, the largest number of early cancers ranges from 10 to 40 mm, and advanced cancers

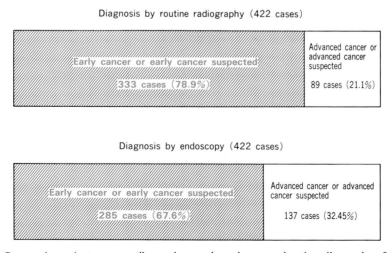

Diagnosis by routine radiography (422 cases)

Early cancer or early cancer suspected
333 cases (78.9%)

Advanced cancer or advanced cancer suspected

89 cases (21.1%)

Diagnosis by endoscopy (422 cases)

Early cancer or early cancer suspected
285 cases (67.6%)

Advanced cancer or advanced cancer suspected

137 cases (32.45%)

Fig. 419 Comparison between radiography and endoscopy in the diagnosis of depth of invasion of early gastric cancer.

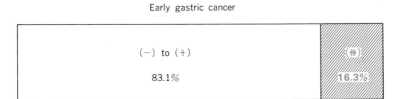

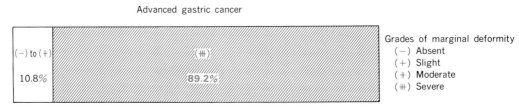

Grades of marginal deformity
(−) Absent
(+) Slight
(‡) Moderate
(‖) Severe

Fig. 420 Differential diagnosis of early and advanced gastric cancer by the radiographic sign of marginal deformity (lesser and greater curvature).

Size	<10mm	10-20mm	20-30mm	30-40mm	40-50mm	50-60mm	60-70mm	70-80mm	80-90mm	90-100mm	100-110mm	110-120mm	>120 mm
Early cancer 138 foci	10	23	33	24	14	14	8	5	3	3	1		
Advanced cancer 225 foci		4	11	20	40	47	39	30	12	9	4	5	4

Simulating early cancer

Borrmann type

Fig. 421 Comparison of size and depth of invasion of gastric cancer (363 foci) (I).

	Depth of invasion \ Size	<10mm	10-20mm	20-30mm	30-40mm	>40mm
Early cancer	Mucosa (m)					
	Submucosa (sm)					
Advanced cancer	Propria muscle (pm)					
	Serosa (s)					

Fig. 422 Comparison of size and depth of invasion of gastric cancer (363 foci) (II).

from 40 mm to 70 mm. Lesions less than 10 mm are all early cancers, and early cancers exceed advanced cancers in lesions ranging from 20 to 40 mm. With lesions larger than 40 mm advanced cancers predominate. If the lesion is less than 10 mm, the diagnosis of early cancer is made with certainty based upon size only. Lesions up to 20 mm can be diagnosed as early cancers with a fairly high degree of probability. Morphologic differences are necessary in order to differentiate between early and advanced cancers among lesions larger than 20 mm. Lesions belonging to the Borrmann types variety macroscopically can be diagnosed as advanced cancer based upon their morphology, but there are a large number of advanced cancers which simulate early cancer in macroscopic morphology and size. Under such circumstances the diagnosis of depth of invasion is actually required.

Diagnosis of depth of invasion would be more useful if it could correspond to the layer of the gastric wall involved. Usually, a lesion less than 10 mm is limited to the mucosa, but the depth of invasion of a lesion measuring more than 10 mm cannot be accurately determined (Fig. 422). Diagnosis of the depth of invasion of elevated and depressed cancers is studied separately, as they differ in their course of development and in their radiographic findings.

Elevated Cancer and Diagnosis of Depth of Invasion

Early cancers of the elevated type are classified as types I, IIa and IIa + IIc, and advanced cancers of elevated type correspond to Borrmann types 1 and 2. It is better to discuss early cancer and advanced cancer together because a number of advanced lesions simulate early lesions. This is because of the lack of a distinctive macroscopic transitional phase from early to advanced cancer.

For convenience, the elevated cancers are divided into two groups. One is polypoid cancer consisting of type I pedunculated lesions of considerable height and Borrmann type 1 lesions; the other consists of sessile cancers such as type IIa of flat elevation, type IIa + IIc with central depression, and Borrmann type 2. As shown in Figure 423 polypoid cancer may invade the propria muscle layer and the serosa, regardless of size. Among the sessile lesions, most of the type IIa cancers are limited to the mucosa. Type IIa + IIc frequently invades the submucosa, even in small lesions.

Depth of invasion of the polypoid lesions, as shown in Figure 424, is diagnosed by the form and

Appearance of elevated cancer		Depth of invasion \ Size	<10mm	10-20mm	20-30mm	30-40mm	40-50mm	50-60mm	60-70mm	>70mm
Polypoid	Type I or Borrmann type 1	Mucosa (m)	O	OO		OOOOO	OO			O
		Submucosa (sm)			⊗	⊗				
		Propria muscle (pm)			◉			◉		
		Serosa (s)				●	●			●
Flat elevation	Type IIa	Mucosa (m)	OOO	OOOOO	OOOOO OOOOO	OO	OOO	OOO		
		Submucosa (sm)		⊗						
		Propria muscle (pm)						◉		
		Serosa (s)								
	Type IIa + IIc or Borrmann type 2	Mucosa (m)		OOOO	OOO		O			
		Submucosa (sm)	⊗	⊗⊗⊗⊗⊗ ⊗⊗⊗⊗	⊗⊗	⊗⊗⊗	⊗		⊗	⊗⊗
		Propria muscle (pm)			◉◉◉◉◉	◉◉◉◉◉	◉◉	◉	◉	◉
		Serosa (s)			●●●	●●●●●	●●●●● ●●●●	●●	●●●●● ●	●●●●● ●●

Fig. 423 Comparison of size and depth of invasion of elevated cancer of the stomach (124 foci).

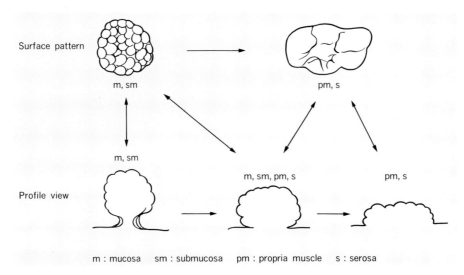

Surface pattern

m, sm   pm, s

m, sm

Profile view   m, sm, pm, s   pm, s

m : mucosa   sm : submucosa   pm : propria muscle   s : serosa

Fig. 424   Diagnosis of depth of invasion of polypoid gastric cancer (early cancer type I and Borrmann type 1).

Case 117   Type I Early Cancer.
A 75-year-old man (TMCDC). (Figs. 425-428)

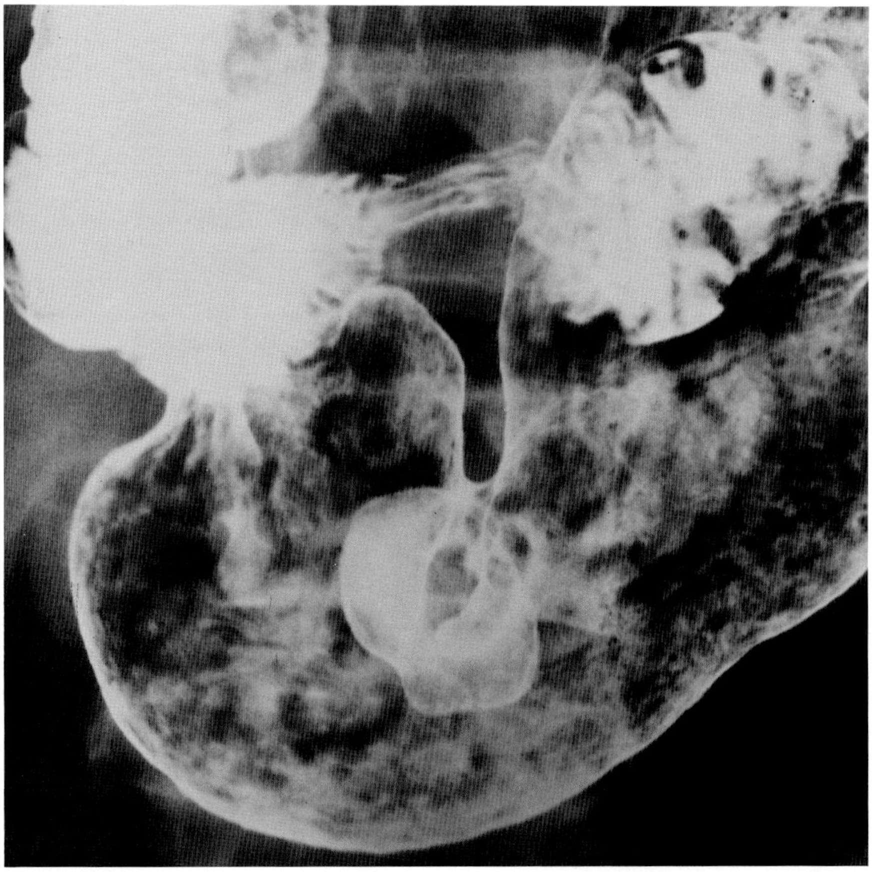

Fig. 425   Pedunculated lesion, early cancer, type I with submucosal invasion (sm). Supine double contrast film demonstrates an oval-shaped tumor mass at the incisura with a seemingly smooth outline. The central radiolucency extending to the incisura is the lesion's stalk, which suspends the head from the anterior wall.

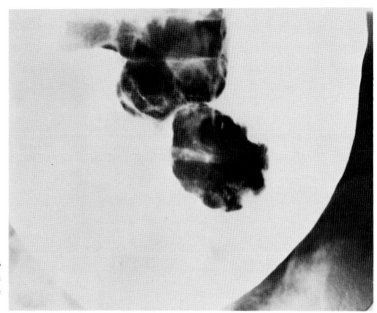

Fig. 426 Upright compression film demonstrates the notched outline of the lesion. Surface pattern is not delineated satisfactorily because severe compression was applied.

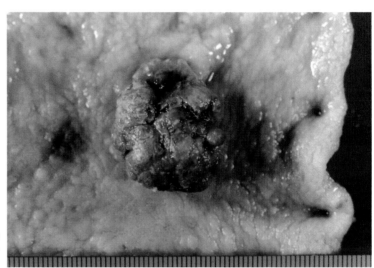

Fig. 427 Resected specimen demonstrates the lesion which measures 30 mm in the largest diameter, and has an irregular surface nodularity.

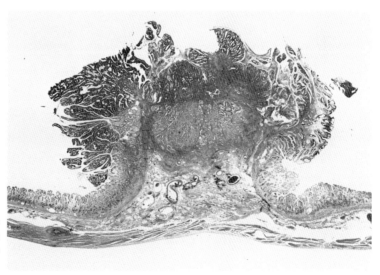

Fig. 428 Cross section of the lesion reveals the short stalk. The submucosa is involved (sm). It was histologically diagnosed as adenocarcinoma papillotubulare (well differentiated adenocarcinoma).

the nature of its surface (Nishizawa 1977). In pedunculated lesions, those with a granular or nodular surface are early cancers limited to the mucosa or submucosa (Figs. 425–428). Subpedunculated or narrow-base sessile cancers are most difficult to differentiate (Figs. 429–433). As the invasion becomes deeper, the surface pattern changes from fine regular granularity (Figs. 434–436) to rough, irregular nodularity (Figs. 437–439). Most sessile lesions presenting a smooth nodular surface may involve the propria muscle layer or the serosa.

Type IIa lesions with fine granularity are mostly limited to the mucosa and must be differentiated from atypical epithelium (ATP). Even a large lesion may present surface granularity which is similar to the pattern of areae gastricae (see Chapter 4).

A sessile lesion with central depression is early cancer type IIa + IIc or Borrmann type 2 advanced cancer. Although the lesions of this type measuring less than 20 mm are early cancers, as shown in Figure 423, many of them involve the submucosa. Figure 440 demonstrates that there are two ways in which this lesion develops. One starts from an elevated type early cancer (types I and IIa) developing into type IIa + IIc and finally into Borrmann type 2, and the other starts from a depressed type early cancer such as type IIc, developing into type IIa + IIc and finally into Borrmann type 2 (Nishizawa 1977). If two lesions with different developing processes are of the same size, the latter will disclose deeper invasion than the former. Hence it is important to judge whether a type IIa + IIc lesion has developed from an elevated lesion or a depressed one when diagnosing the depth of invasion of type IIa + IIc lesion.

Figure 441 demonstrates the morphological

Case 118   Borrmann Type 1 Advanced Cancer.
A 59-year-old man (TMCDC). (Figs. 429-433)

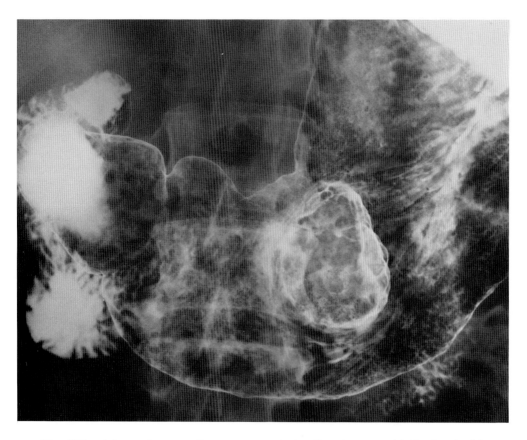

Fig. 429 Advanced cancer, Borrmann type 1, invading the serosa (s). Supine double contrast film demonstrates a large, narrow-base sessile tumor with irregular surface nodularity on the posterior wall of the incisura region. It measures about 55 mm in the largest diameter on the radiograph.

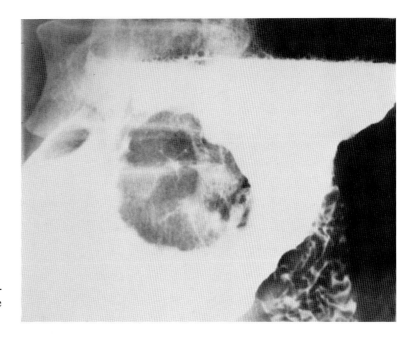

Fig. 430 Upright compression film demonstrates the irregular outline and surface nodularity.

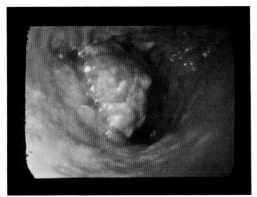

Fig. 431

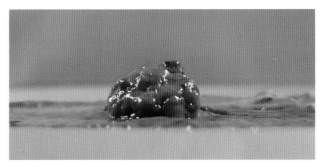

Fig. 432

Fig. 431 Endoscopic picture demonstrates the large polypoid mass with irregular surface nodularity. It appears to be a narrow-base sessile lesion.

Fig. 432 Picture of the lesion showing narrow-base sessile elevation. Cancer invades the serosa (s).

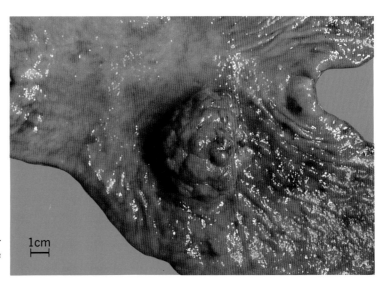

Fig. 433 Resected specimen. The lesion, measuring 50 x 50 mm, has an irregular surface nodularity.

1cm

Case 119 Type IIa Early Cancer.
A 55-year-old woman (CU). (Figs. 434-436)

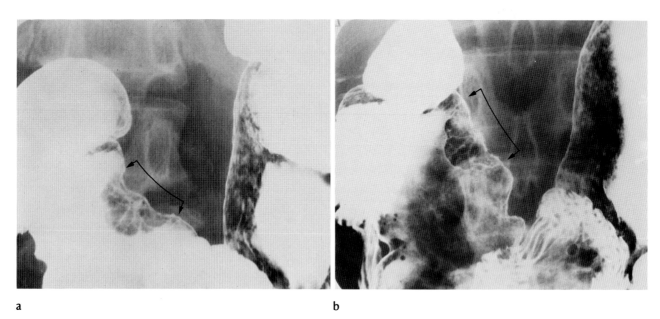

a   b

Fig. 434 Flat mucosal elevation. Early cancer, type IIa, limited to the mucosa (m). Supine frontal (a) and right anterior oblique (b) films demonstrate a flat mucosal elevation at the lesser curvature of the antrum (arrow line), measuring about 25 mm in the largest diameter. The surface pattern suggests a fine uniform granularity (intramucosal cancer??). Slight indentation or contour defect of the lesser curvature indicates that a part of the lesion is situated on the anterior wall (arrow line).

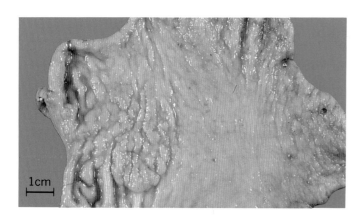

Fig. 435 Resected specimen. The lesion measures 35 × 25 mm. The uniform granularity of the surface may be typical of early cancer.

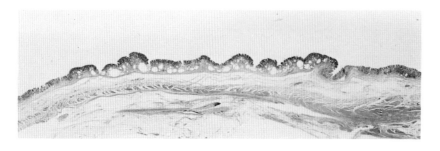

Fig. 436 Cross section of the lesion showing a flat mucosal elevation. Cancer is limited to the mucosa (m). Adenocarcinoma papillotubulare (well differentiated adenocarcinoma).

Case 120   Borrmann Type 1 Advanced Cancer.
A 55-year-old man (CU). (Figs. 437-439)

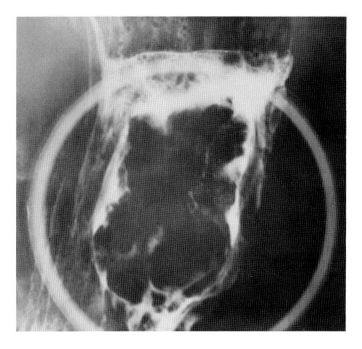

Fig. 437 Advanced cancer, Borrmann type 1, invading the serosa(s). Upright compression film demonstrates a large polypoid mass with marked surface nodularity of the upper gastic body measureing about 70 mm in the largest diameter. This picture is typical of advanced cancer Borrmann type 1.

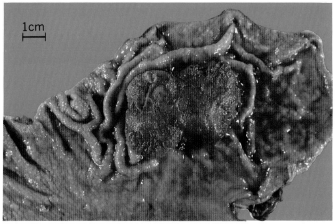

Fig. 438 Resected specimen. In this case the surface configuration has changed into a rough nodularity that makes diagnosis of advanced cancer is easy. The lesion measures 40 x 35 mm.

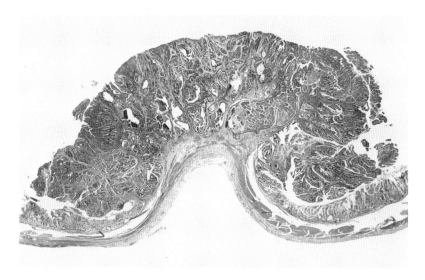

Fig. 439 Cross section of a lesion showing extensive involvement of the serosa (s).

difference between these two developing processes. Table 35 shows the differentiation method, intergrated from endoscopy and biopsy.

Cancers which have their origin in the elevated lesions (Figs. 442—445) are limited to the mucosa or submucosa if their size is less than 30 mm, with the former predominating. Lesions measuring more than 30 mm invade beyond the submucosa. The larger the size the more pronounced the raised margin, and the deeper and bigger the central depression the deeper is the depth of invasion.

Cancers which originate in depressed lesions (Figs. 446—449) may invade the submucosa, even if they are less than 20 mm, and those measuring more than 20 mm may invade the propria muscle layer or the serosa (Figs. 450—453). With lesions over 40 mm, serosal invasion is quite frequent.

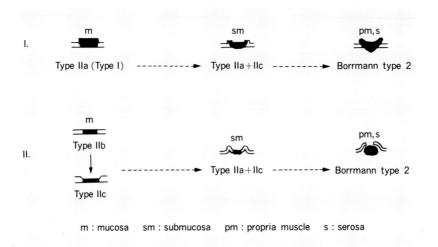

m : mucosa   sm : submucosa   pm : propria muscle   s : serosa

Fig. 440   Course of development of cancer into Borrmann type 2.

Table 35   Differential diagnosis of gastric cancer with central depression and peripheral elevation
(From Nishizawa, M.: *I to Cho*, 12: 1217, 1977).

	Radiography	Endoscopy	Biopsy	Depth of invasion and size		Note
Arising from depressed lesion	No mucosal convergence. Sharply defined radiolucency. Irregular outline. Granular or Nodular surface.	Wide base sessile. Totally discolored.	Positive at peripheral portion.	30mm _____ m, sm	30mm _____ sm, pm, s	Size being equal, the larger and deeper the depression, the deeper the depth of invasion. The more irregular a surface pattern, the deeper the depth of invasion.
Arising from elevated lesion	Mucosal convergence present or absent. If present, it simulates a bridging fold. Occasional clubbing and fusion. ───── Radiolucency. Smooth surface and outline.	Elevated lesion with gentle sloping. Smooth margin. No difference in color from the normal surrounding mucosa.	Normal mucosa at peripheral portion.	20mm _____ sm	20mm _____ pm, s	Size being equal, the higher the raised margin, and the larger and deeper the depression, the deeper the depth of invasion.

m: mucosa   sm: submucosa   pm: propria muscle   s: serosa

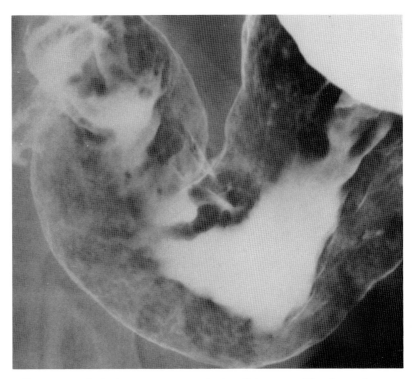

Fig. 460 Double contrast film with a small amount of air demonstrates marked radiolucency. The depression appears less marked than the surrounding elevation.

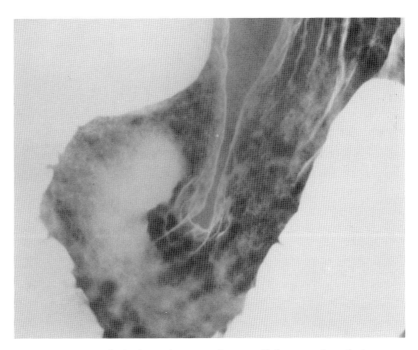

Fig. 461 Double contrast film with a moderate amount of air shows less prominent radiolucency than that in Figure 460. The radiolucency has also shifted to the distal side of the incisura. Due to positional change barium was not retained in the depression.

251

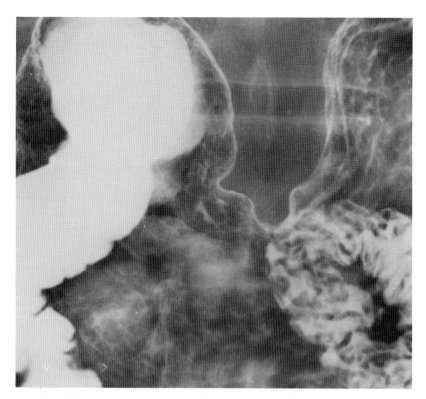

Fig. 462 Double contrast radiograph with a large volume of air demonstrates less prominent radiolucency than in the previous films. By changing the volume of air one can demonstrate that the lesion shifts distally to the incisura. This may be a sign that cancer has not invaded deeper than the serosa (Igarashi et al. 1977).

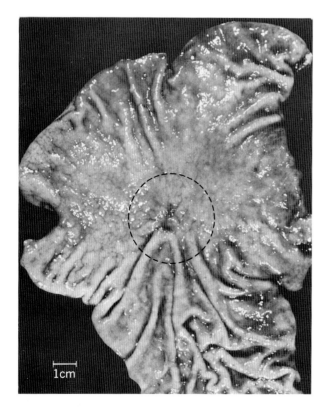

Fig. 463 Resected specimen. The lesion measures 18 x 15 mm and is located on the posterior wall of the incisura. The surrounding elevation is not as conspicuous as expected from the radiographic findings.

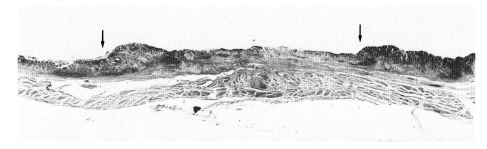

Fig. 464 Cross section of the lesion showing marked involvement of the submucosa and moderate involvement of the propria muscle layer (pm). Histologically, it is diagnosed as adenocarcinoma tubulare (well-differentiated adenocarcinoma).

advanced cancer, the latter revealing filling defect, surrounding raised margin and shrinkage of the affected portion of the entire thickness of the stomach (Figs. 474–480). An intramucosal cancer or a cancer with slight submucosal involvement does not reveal a tumor shadow on a double contrast radiograph, even with a small volume of air.

Case 126   Advanced Cancer Simulating Type IIc (pm).
A 63-year-old man (CIH). (Figs. 465-470)

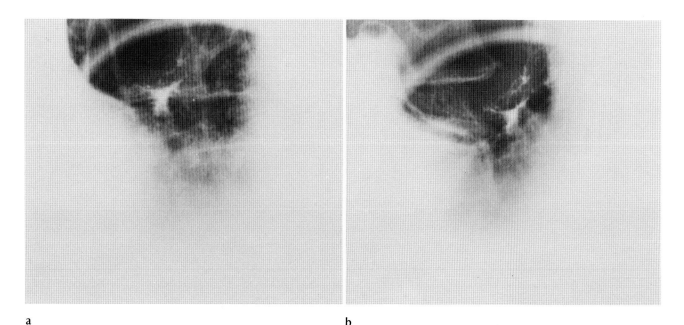

a   b

Fig. 465 a and b   Advanced cancer simulating type IIc, with marked involvement of the submucosa and slight involvement of the propria muscle layer. Compression films demonstrate only slight surrounding radiolucency. The incisura has an irregular and rigid appearance.

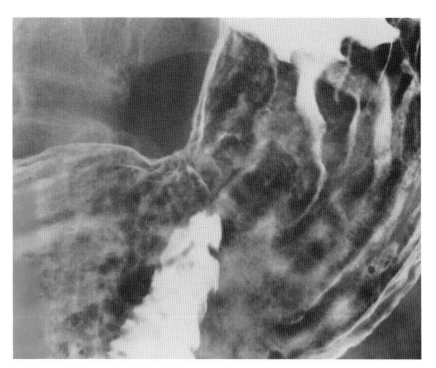

Fig. 466   Double contrast film with a small amount of air.

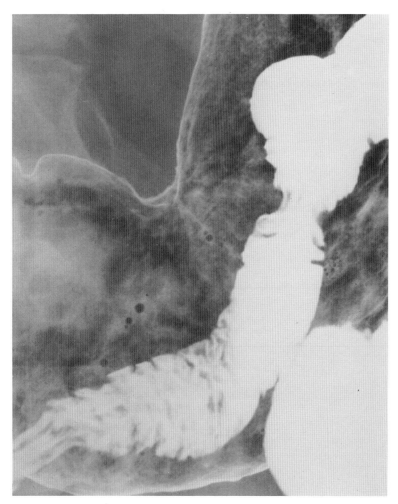

Fig. 467   Double contrast film with a moderate amount of air.

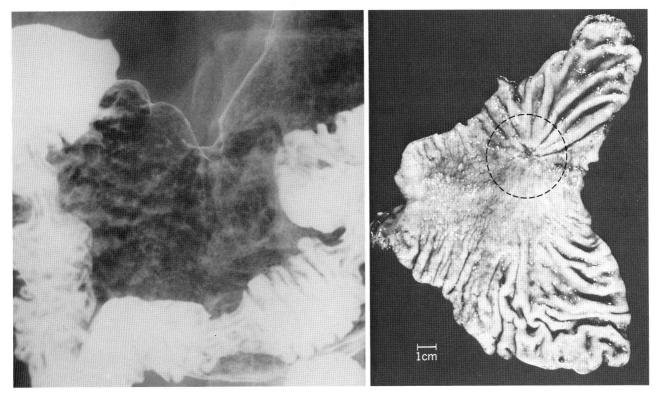

Fig. 468   Fig. 469

Fig. 468   Double contrast radiograph with a large volume of air. The constant deformity of the incisura is observed by changing the volume of air.

Fig. 469   Resected specimen. The lesion measures 14 × 14 mm, and simulates early cancer, type IIc.

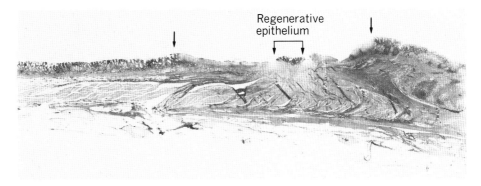

Fig. 470   Cross section of the lesion showing marked involvement of the submucosa and slight involvement of the propria muscle layer. Histologically, it is diagnosed as adenocarcinoma scirrhosum (poorly differentiated adenocarcinoma).

Case 127　Advanced Cancer Simulating Type IIc (ss).

A 56-year-old woman (CIH). (Figs. 471-474)

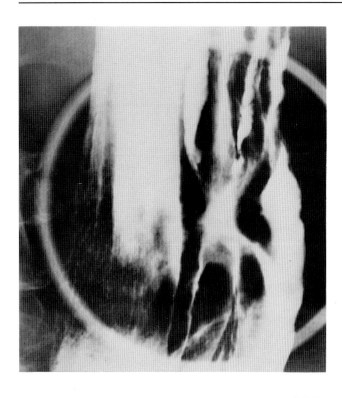

Fig. 471 Advanced cancer, simulating type IIc, with marked involvement of the submucosa and slight involvement of the propria muscle layer and subserosa (ss). Compression film with moderate compression demonstrates irregular depression and surrounding radiolucency.

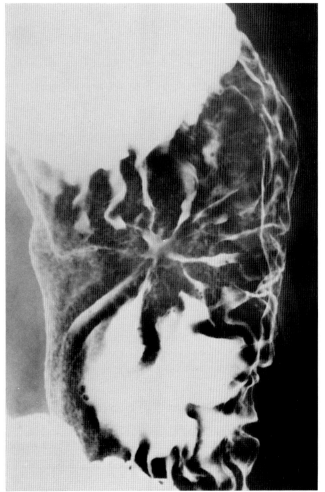

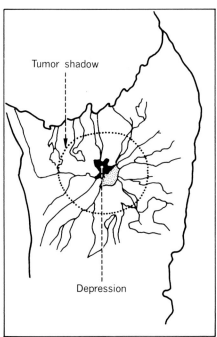

Tumor shadow

Depression

Fig. 472 Double contrast film with a moderate amount of air demonstrates a faint tumor mass. Its outline may correspond to the points where tapering and clubbing of the mucosal convergence begin. Deviation of a converging fold is also visualized.

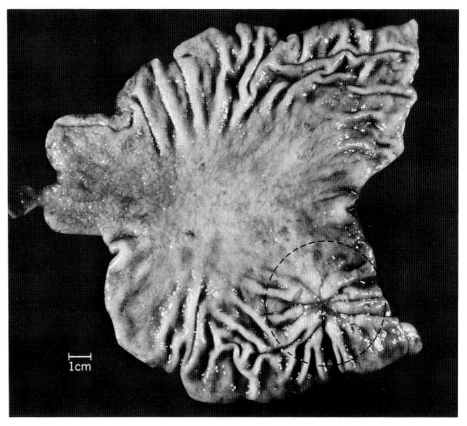

Fig. 473   Resected specimen. The lesion measures 25 × 20 mm, and is completely surround by fundic gland mucosa.

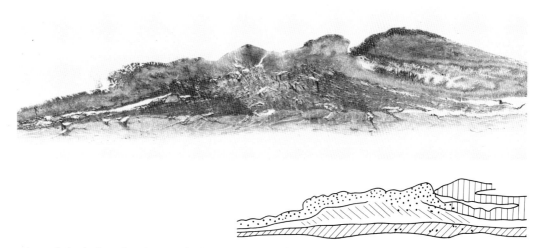

Fig. 474   Cross section of the lesion showing marked involvement of the submocosa and slight involvement of the propria muscle layer and subserosa (ss). Histologically, it is diagnosed as adenocarcinoma scirrhosum (poorly differentiated adenocarcinoma). Schema showing invasion pattern of carcinoma (dots).

Case 128   Advanced Cancer Simulating Type IIc (s).

A 60-year-old woman (CIH). (Figs. 475-481)

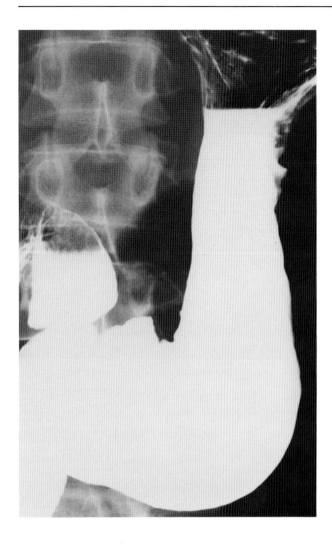

Fig. 475 Advanced cancer simulating type IIc, with marked involvement of the entire thickness of he gastric wall. Upright barium-filled film demonstrates deformed incisura.

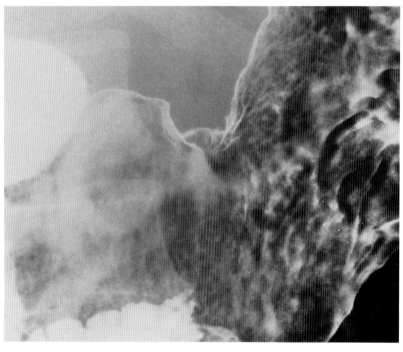

Fig. 476 Supine double contrast film demonstrates retraction of the incisura and a niche.

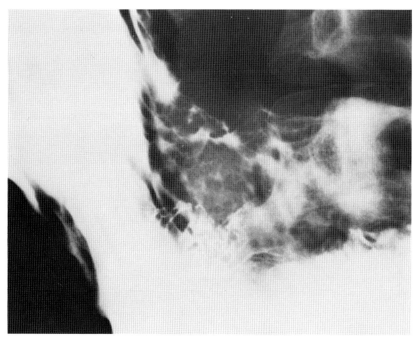

Fig. 477   Prone compression film demonstrates a tumor mass and mucosal irregularity with slight depression.

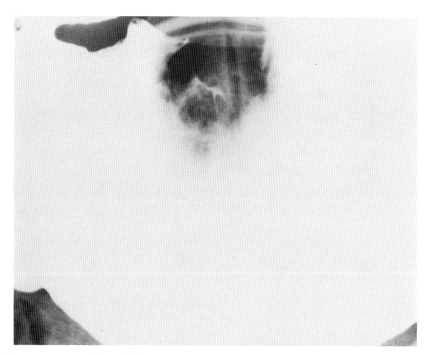

Fig. 478   Upright compression film demonstrates a filling defect and slight mucosal depression of the incisura.

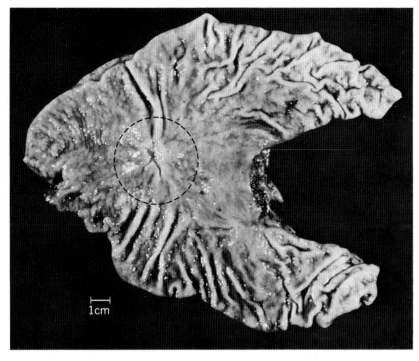

1cm

Fig. 479   Resected specimen.

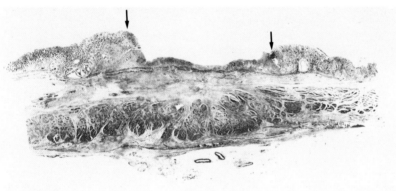

Fig. 480   Cross section of the lesion showing the cancerous involvement of the entire thickness of the gastric wall.

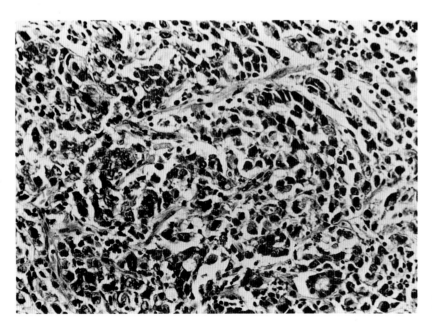

Fig. 481 Histologic findings showing adenocarcinoma scirrhosum (poorly differentiated adenocarcinoma).

Chapter 11

Pattern of Spread of Early Gastric Cancer and Its Radiographic Features

The key in differentiating early gastric cancer from advanced cancer is the degree of invasion through the gastric mucosa, not the size of its horizontal spread. It is the depth of invasion that decides prognosis. Accordingly, horizontal spread of cancer is not directly related to the prognosis. However, the clinical experiences of radiographic and endoscopic diagnosis disclose the difficulty in deciding the extent of spread of a lesion. This results in the difficulty in determining the line of incision, or the necessity of a second operation due to histologic proof of cancer spread to the incision line despite apparent adequate surgical margins. A few cases of stump recurrence have been observed some months or years after operation because of misdiagnosis on the resected specimen. Therefore, the horizontal spread of cancer is an indirect factor of prognosis. In this chapter, the pattern of spread of cancer with its associated problems is discussed in relationship to the size of early cancer.

Type IIb-like Spread of Early Gastric Cancer (Type IIb-simulating Lesion)

Type IIb was initially employed to refer to a cancerous lesion in its incipient phase (refer to Chapter 1). This concept has been justified by the fact that pure type IIb cancers have been discovered only incidentally in operations performed because of some other primary lesions. All of them were smaller than 5 mm (Nakamura et al. 1968). However, there have been many cases which have not been classified as pure type IIb lesion but which simulate type IIb lesion with subtle differences in elevation or depression from the normal surrounding mucosa and consequently without a clear demarcation of the margins. These have been called type IIb-simulating or type IIb-like lesions. This chapter deals with such lesions and excludes pure type IIb. The terms IIb (IIc) and IIb (IIa) are employed to define the types of IIb-simulating lesions as already discussed in Chapter 1, Macroscopic Classification.

In most cases when the largest diameter of depressed early gastric cancer exceeds 20 mm ulceration and converging folds are present, making identification of a lesion easy. In many cases, however, the boundary between a lesion and the normal mucosa is obscure and its borders must be left to the imagination (Fig. 482). Lesion A is expressed as type IIc + IIb (IIc) and lesion B as type IIb(IIc) + IIc, following the principles of macroscopic classification.

Baba et al. (1977) made a detailed study of the radiographic findings of type IIb (IIc). To understand the radiographic findings of type IIb-simulating lesions, remember that histologic types of cancer are initially divided into differentiated and undifferentiated types, as stated in

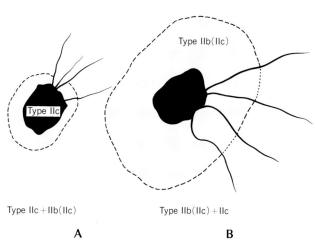

Type IIc + IIb(IIc)   Type IIb(IIc) + IIc

A   B

Fig. 482   Schema showing appearance of type IIb (IIc) lesion.

Chapter 6. According to Baba et al., 60 per cent of type IIb-simulating lesions present radiographic signs characteristic of both. The differentiated type of cancer is characterized by a faint barium shadow which is lacking in granularity (Figs. 483–488). Even though some granularity is observed, it is not distinct and the so-called areae gastricae pattern is mostly unclear (Figs. 489–492). At the estimated border of such a lesion, a translucent shadow gives the impression of areae gastricae and a spiculation is observed.

With undifferentiated types of lesions, in contrast to the differentiated type, the major signs are irregular granularity, tiny barium flecks in regular granularity (Figs. 493–498), reticular shadows and linear cracking shadows. These signs are considered to represent depressions and elevations of the mucosal surface. The above signs are characteristic of each of the histologic types, but such signs as fine granularity or differences in barium coating (Fig. 494) and disarrangement of areae gastricae are common to both.

Case 129   Type IIb (IIc) +IIc Early Cancer.
A 66-year-old man (JU). (Figs. 483-488)

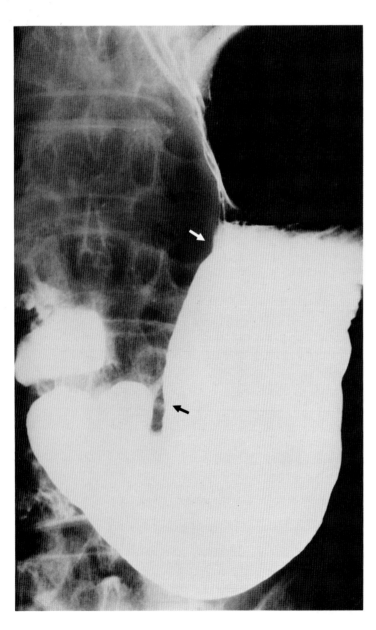

Fig. 483 Upright barium-filled film demonstrates bulging of the lesser curvature (arrows), suggesting the presence of multiple ulcers (cf. Fig. 284).

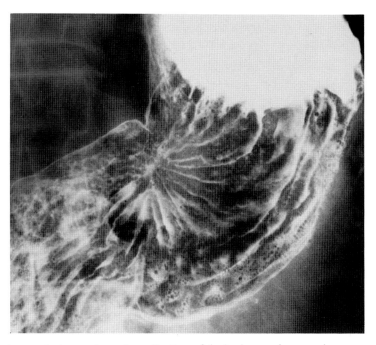

Fig. 484 Supine frontal double contrast film demonstrates an irregular collection of the barium and converging folds in the mid-gastic body near the lesser curvature. The lesion seems to be a typical IIc. However, surrounding the type IIc region, a type IIb simulating lesion is faintly visualized because of a slight abnormality of the folds.

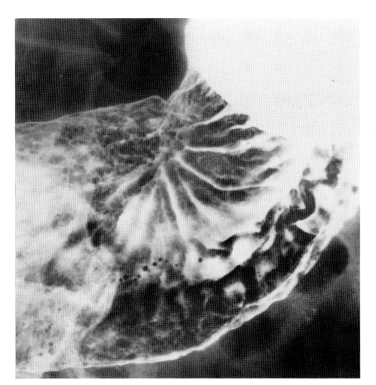

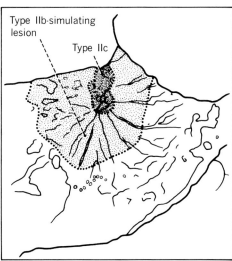

Fig. 485 Another double contrast film demonstrates the type IIc and the large surrounding type IIb-simulating lesion, type IIb (IIc). Schema showing the extent of type IIb (IIc.)

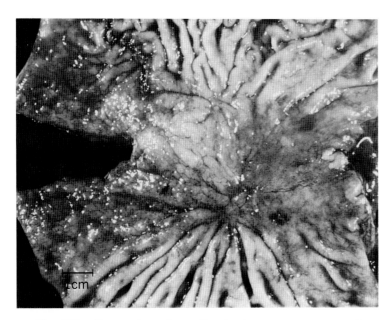
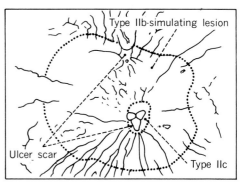

Fig. 486   Resected specimen. Proximal gastrectomy was performed. There are two ulcerations in the lesion. The type IIc part is easily recognized, but the border of the type IIb-simulating lesion is vague. The distal surgical stump was positive for cancer, which eventually led to a total gastrectomy. Schema showing the extent of the type IIb-simulating lesion. The size of he entire lesion was estimated to be 72 x 57 mm histologically. Cancer was limited to the mucosa (m) and was associated with Ul-IIs on the anterior wall and Ul-IIIs on the posterior wall (type IIc part).

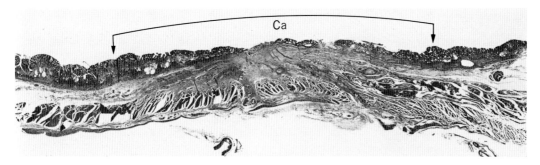

Fig. 487   Cross section of the lesion, showing the type IIb-simulating lesion.

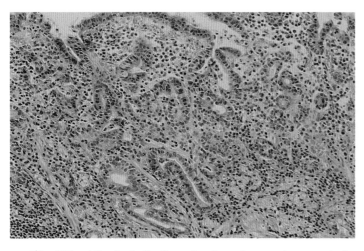

Fig. 488   Histologic findings showing adenocarcinoma tubulare (well differentiated adenocarcinoma).

Case 130 Type IIb (IIa) + IIc Early Cancer.
A 48-year-old man (JU). (Figs. 489-492)

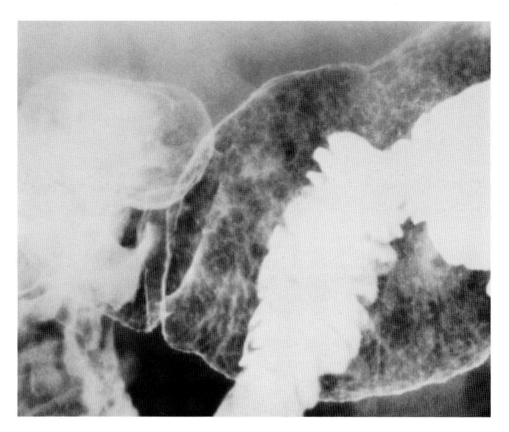

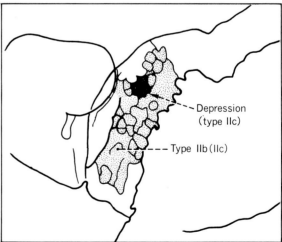

Fig. 489 Double contrast film in the right anterior oblique position demonstrates a faint collection of barium on the posterior wall of the antrum near the lesser curvature representing a slight mucosal depression (erosion). The surrounding mucosa is granular.

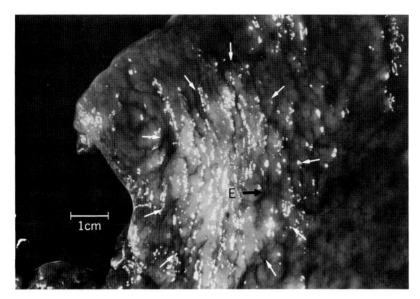

Fig. 490 Resected specimen. An irregular erosion corresponding to the faint collection of barium in Figure 489 is observed at the proximal end of the disolored area of the antrum (➙ E). No marked difference in the thickness of the mucosa or only slight elevation [type IIb (IIa)] compared to the adjacent mucosa is recognized. Cancer was discovered not only in the erosion but also in the surrounding discolored mucosa. The submucosa was slightly involved, and the lesion was not ulcerated. The irregular granularity visualized on the double contrast radiograph may partly corresponds to the discolored area on the resected specimen. This area is diagnosed macroscopically as type IIb (IIa), according to the macroscopic classification of early gastric cancer. Consequently, the entire lesion is diagnosed macroscopically as type IIb (IIa) + IIc.

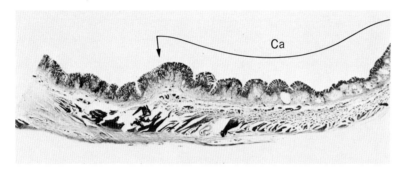

Fig. 491 Cross section of the lesion showing mostly a part of type IIb (IIa).

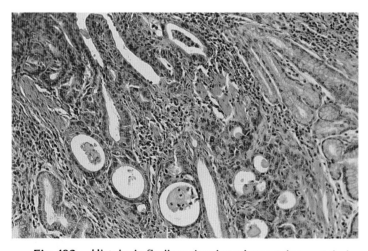

Fig. 492 Histologic findings showing adenocarcinoma tubulare (well differentiated adenocarcinoma).

Case 131   Type IIb (IIc) +IIc Early Cancer.
A 59-year-old man (JU). (Figs. 493-498)   8)

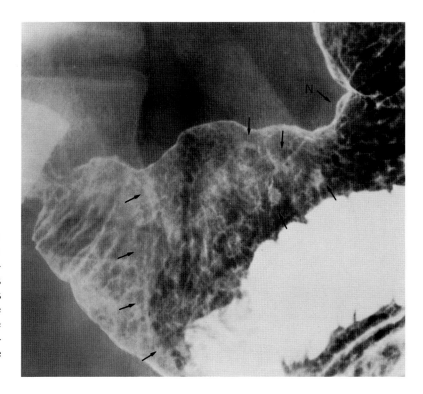

Fig. 493 Supine double contrast film in the right anterior oblique position demonstrates an area of irregular granularity in which some very faint collections of barium are scattered (arrows). Its border on the posterior wall of the antrum is vaguely demarcated, and the lesser curvature of the antrum is deformed. A small niche is noted at the incisura (→ N).

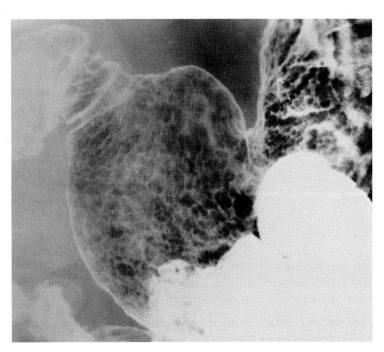

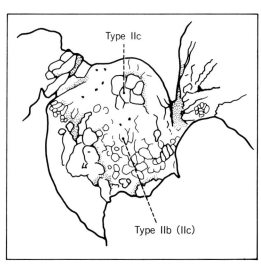

Fig. 494 Another double contrast film in the same position clearly demonstrates the abnormal mucosal pattern of the affected area characterized by irregular granularity and very faint collections of barium. Constant deformity of the lesser curvature is noted.

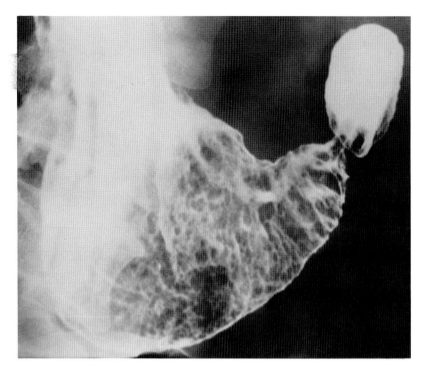

Fig. 495 Prone double contrast film demonstrates the abnormal mucosal pattern of the anterior wall of the antrum consisting of irregular granularity and faint collections of barium.

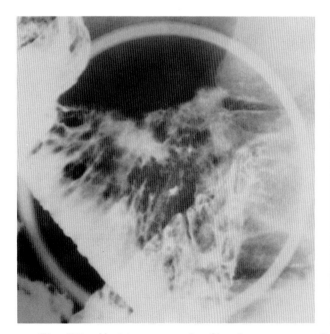

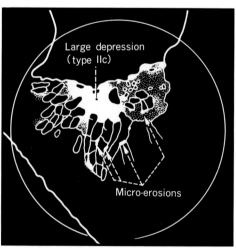

Fig. 496 Upright compression film demonstrates a distinct erosion and surrounding irregular granularity. Based on these radiographs, a distinct erosion (type IIc) is diagnosed, which is probably located on the posterior wall of the antrum near the lesser curvature. A large part of the surrounding antral mucosa is irregularly granulated [type IIb (IIc)] with little difference in thickness compared to the outer normal mucosa. There may be a small ulcer or ulcer scar at the incisura.

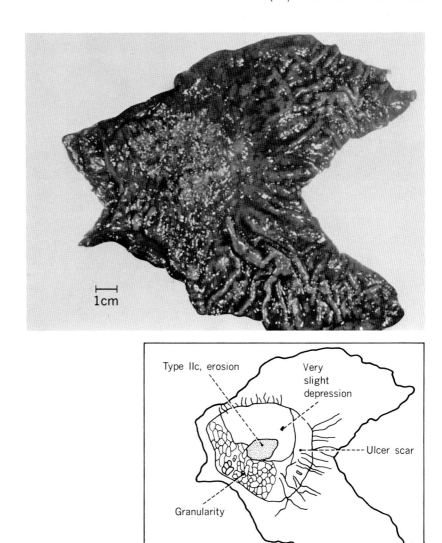

Fig. 497 Resected specimen. The mucosal abnormality is approximately 70 x 45 mm. The distinct erosion (type IIc) is on the posterior wall near the lesser curvature. Most of the lesion reveals very little difference in mucosal thickness compared to the normal adjacent mucosa (type IIb-like lesion), and the entire lesion may be diagnosed as type IIb (IIc) + IIc.

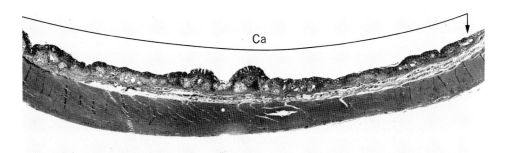

Fig. 498 Cross section of the lesion showing type IIb-simulating lesion. Histologic examination revealed adenocarcinoma mucocellulare (signet ring cell carcinoma) limited to the mucosa (m). The ulcer of the incisura was healed (UI-IIs).

269

Baba et al. (1977) analyzed the differences between the histologic types of type IIb-simulating lesions and the radiographic signs. Among the type IIb-simulating lesions with radiographic signs characteristic of the histologic types of cancer, and with clear borders on radiographs, many lesions are found to have scattered microerosions. On the other hand, among the type IIb-simulating lesions with poor radiographic sings and unclear borders, microerosions were uncommon. Microerosions tend to occur more frequently in undifferentiated than in differentiated types. A lesion affected with fewer microerosions indicates that its surface is mostly covered by normal foveolar epithelium. Such a case makes radiographic diagnosis difficult.

As radiographic diagnosis of type IIb-simulating lesion requires evaluation of extremely fine findings, the diagnosis is apt to be made subjectively. The same findings may not lead other people to the same diagnosis. For more uniformity an endoscopic approach is indispensable, especially when defining the proximal border. This type of lesion is best observed by the dye-spraying method (Ida 1971, Kawai et al. 1972, Suzuki et al. 1973) and best dealt with by carbon ink injection (Ujiie et al. 1971, Takekoshi et al. 1977, Fig. 504) and biopsy.

Superficial Spreading Type of Carcinoma

The first record of this type of lesion is found in Stout's treatise in 1941. Stout observed a type of cancer with depression whose depth of invasion did not involve the propria muscle layer. Since its horizontal spread was wide, he named it superficial spreading type of carcinoma. He reported a case of intramucosal cancer (Case 5) whose horizontal spread measured 90 x 60 mm, but he failed to give a strict definition of superficial spreading type of carcinoma based on the size of its spread. The spread in the second case (Case 14) measured 32 x 30 mm. This is not superficial spreading type of carcinoma, but rather experienced observers classify it as typical type IIc or type IIc + III early cancer. Twenty-two per cent of all cases of superficial spreading type of carcinoma in Stout's series would now be reclassified as early depressed cancer (Figs. 499–502). In Japan the definition of superficial spreading type of carcinoma in the strict sense has not yet been established.

Since Yasui's report (1970), there has been a general concensus that a lesion is superficial spreading type of carcinoma when the product of its longest diameter (a) and the diameter perpendicular to it (b) (S = a x b) exceeds 25 cm^2. The majority of these lesions are indeed superficial early cancer, i.e. type II early cancer. Accordingly, most cases of the type IIb-simulating lesion belong to the superficial spreading type of carcinoma in a wide sense.

Kumakura et al. (1973) reported 65 lesions measuring more than 25 cm^2 comprising 13.4 per cent of the 484 cases of resected early gastric cancer. If divided into differentiated types, elevated lesions comprised 2.5 per cent (12 cases) and depressed lesion 10.9 per cent (53 cases). Fifty-one cases were found to be the largest of the elevated lesions measuring $49 \leqq S < 64$ cm^2, and 3 cases were the largest of the depressed lesions measuring $S \geqq 100$ cm^2 (Figs. 503 and 504).

Stout states that the lesions frequently occurred in the antral portion, but Kumakura (1973) found that the center of the majority of lesions were located near the incisura (44 cases or 67.7%). Fewer occurred in the antral region (14 cases or 21.5%). Kumakura reported a case in the gastric body and 6 cases involving the entire stomach. Most cases of superficial spreading type of carcinoma showed symmetrical spread over the lesser curvature.

Kumakura et al. (1973) made a detailed study of the radiographic diagnosis of superficial spreading type of carcinoma. According to this study, marked deformity of the stomach was the major finding in 23 of 53 depressed lesions. Of the remaining 30 cases, the following occurred: niche in 3 cases, converging folds in 5 cases, marginal irregularity or depression in 4 cases and a slight elevation in 2 cases. Sixteen cases remained. Eight of them were type IIc, enabling diagnosis by double contrast radiography, but the final 8 cases were type IIb-simulating lesions which made them difficult to diagnose.

It is not difficult to radiographically diagnose superficial spreading type of carcinoma. Type IIb-simulating lesions, however, are difficult to diagnose because their borders may be vague. The proximal border is well defined radiographically in lesions of 25 to 36 cm^2, but the difficulty in defining the proximal border increases as the size increases. This may be due to abnormal mucosa affected by type IIc or type IIb-simulating lesions which covers the major area of the mucosal surface revealed in the double contrast image. By inspection it is difficult to differentiate normal from abnormal mucosa.

Case 132   Type IIc Early Cancer.
A 35-year-old man (CIH). (Figs. 499-502)

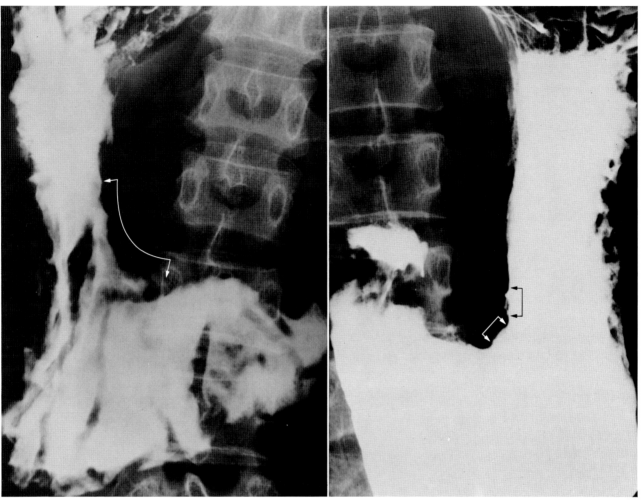

Fig. 499   Fig. 500

Fig. 499   Prone mucosal relief film demonstrates an irregular depression at the incisura and converging folds (arrow line).
Fig. 500   Upright barium-filled film demonstrates two niches, one at and the other above the deformed incisura (arrow lines).

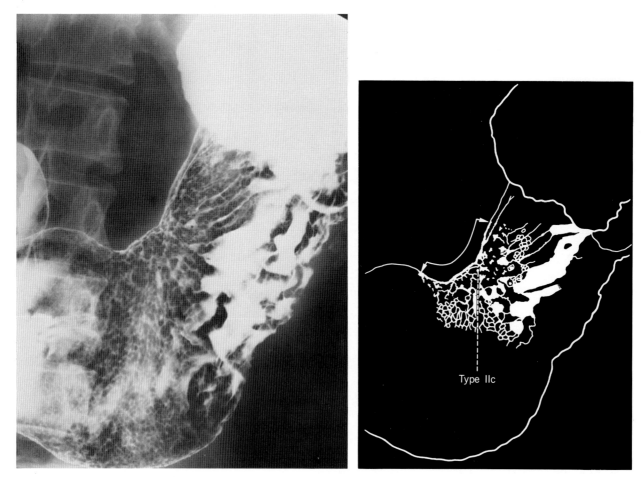

Fig. 501 Supine right anterior oblique double contrast film demonstrates small irregular collections of barium and irregular radiolucencies on the posterior wall of the incisura. These are typical radiographic sign of type IIc lesion, but the border of the lesion is not clearly seen, compared with the macroscopic findings.

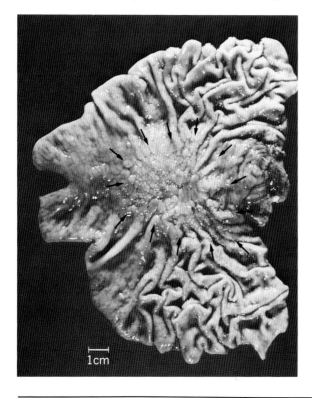

Fig. 502 Resected specimen.

Case 133 Type IIc Early Cancer (Superficial Spreading Type).
A 47-year-old woman (CIH). (Figs. 503 and 504)

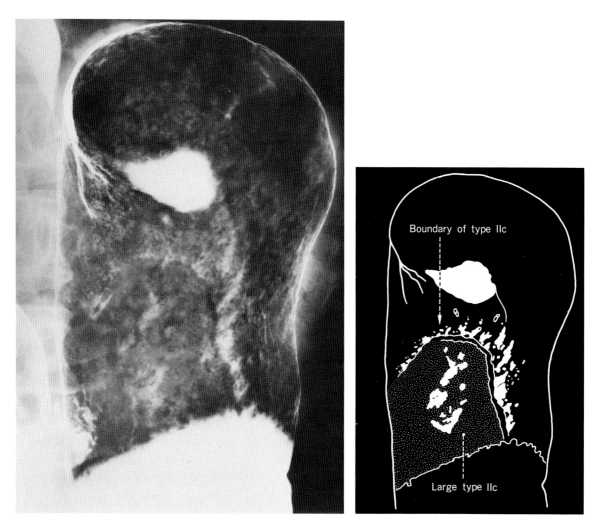

Fig. 503 Upright double contrast film demonstrates a large depression (type IIc) on the posterior wall of the gastric body. The border of the lesion is well defined.

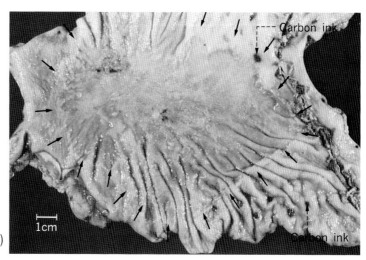

Fig. 504 Resected specimen. The lesion (type IIc) measures 100 x 100 mm.

Chapter 12

Clinical Course of Gastric Cancer

Gastric cancer arises from the glandular epithelium of the gastric mucosa. However, it is unknown how long cancer is confined to the mucosa, what causes it to invade the submucosa, and into what type of advanced cancer it will develop. It is reported that initially most cases of cancer remain confined to the mucosa for from several years to nearly ten years, which is longer than has been generally believed. If this is true, the chance of detecting lesions in their early phases is good. Occasionally, it may be difficult to make the differential diagnosis of whether the lesion is limited to the mucosa or whether it has invaded the submucosa. At the time of discovery, it is almost impossible to determine the time that has elapsed from its evolution as an intramucosal cancer to a cancer invading the submucosa.

Surgery must be performed as soon as a lesion is diagnosed as cancer. However, a knowledge of the development of cancer helps in diagnosing minute cancers, in setting a screening interval to detect cancer before it is untreatable, in judging what type of cancer rapidly invades deeper portions of the gastric wall and in diagnosing the depth of invasion. A prospective study of the course of a lesion is not possible once it is diagnosed as cancer, but a retrospective study of undetected cases offers much information.

Course of Development of Elevated Lesions

Most of the elevated lesions of type I and type IIa consist of differentiated type of cancer. It is reported that the time required to progress into advanced cancer is relatively long. Early cancers of these type are supposed to develop into either Borrmann type 2 via type IIa + IIc or Borrmann type 1 directly.

Figs. 505–511 present a case of supposedly pedunculated intramucosal cancer which may have progressed into a cancer of type IIa + IIc involving the submucosa over a period of five years and four months. During this time the head of the polyp was deformed in relationship to an increase in its size. It will progress into an advanced cancer of typical Borrmann type 2.

Course of Development of Depressed Lesions

Malignant cycle (Murakami et al. 1966)

Depressed lesions indicate types IIc, IIc + III, and III, which are considered similar because ulceration tends to occur on the cancerous tissue. A lesion with an ulcer on type IIc is a type IIc + III or a type III. After healing of the ulcer it returns to a type IIc cancer. This is named the malignant cycle by Murakami owing to the resemblance with the cycle of benign ulcer, i.e. a repetition of ulcer scar formation and recurrence (Figs. 512 and 513).

Figure 511 illustrates the malignant cycle from the histologic point of view, and Figure 513 shows the macroscopic alteration. Many cases repeat the malignant cycle during their long and slow course of development.

Figures 514–520 present a typical case of the malignant cycle. The patient first visited the hospital because of epigastric pain. X-ray examination and endoscopy disclosed a niche suggesting benign ulcer with whitish mucus on the posterior wall of the gastric body (Figs. 513, 515, 518). After two months' treatment the niche almost disappeared and the benign ulcer was thought to be healed (Fig. 518). The patient did not visit the hospital for a while, but a year and eight months later a typical type IIc lesion was visualized by the

274

Case 134 Course of Development of Early Cancer. (Pedunculated Cancer→ Type IIa+IIc). A 70-year-old man (JU). (Figs. 505-511)

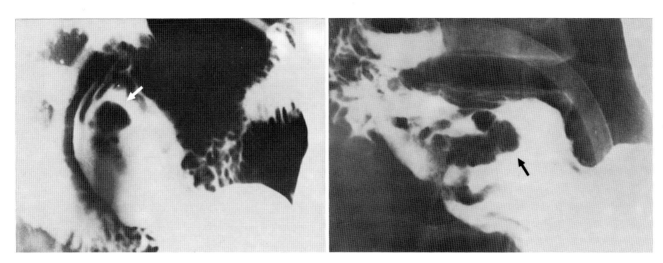

Fig. 505   Fig. 506

Fig. 505   Compression film 5 years and 4 months before surgery demonstrates a pedunculated lesion in the antrum (arrow).
Fig. 506   Compression film 2 years and 11 months before surgery demonstrates that the lesion has enlarged and has a bilobed head (arrow).

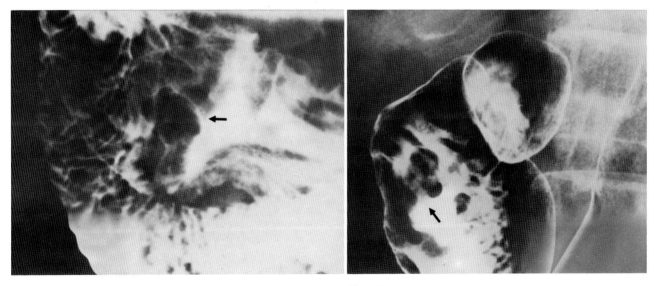

Fig. 507   Fig. 508

Fig. 507   Compression film 1 year and 2 months before surgery demonstrates the enlarged head and stalk of the lesion (arrow).
Fig. 508   Compression film 2 months before surgery demonstrates that the lesion has become sessile and contains a central depression (type IIa + IIc) (arrow).

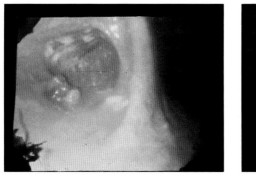
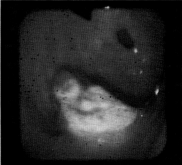

Fig. 509   Fig. 510

Fig. 509 Endoscopic picture 5 years and 4 months before surgery demonstrates a pedunculated lesion.

Fig. 510 Endoscopic picture 2 months before surgery demonstrates a wide-base sessile lesion with central whitish mucus. It looks like a Borrmann type advanced cancer.

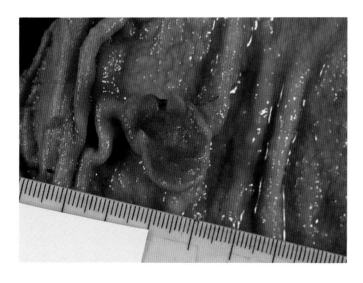

Fig. 511 Resected specimen. The lesion is diagnosed macroscopically as type IIa + IIc early cancer. Histologic examination revealed adenocarcinoma tubulare (moderately differentiated adenocarcinoma) with submucosal invasion (sm).

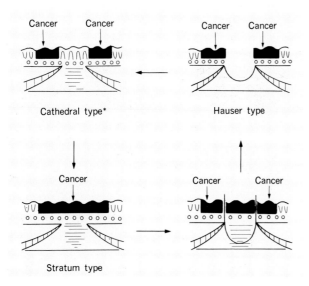

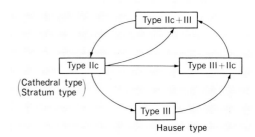

Fig. 513 Changes of macroscopic appearance in the malignant cycle of early gastric cancer.

Fig. 512 Schematic drawing of the malignant cycle (Modified from Murakami 1966).
*This type is literally referred to as sanctuary type in the original article.

276

Case 135   Malignant Cycle of Early Cancer.
A 45-year-old man (CU). (Figs. 514-520)

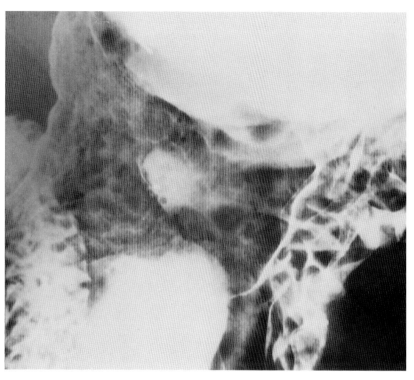

Fig. 514   Type IIc early cancer demonstrating the malignant cycle. Supine double contrast film demonstrates a thick collection of barium. Its outline is sharply demarcated at the lesser curvature aspect but gradually becomes fainter at the greater curvature aspect, which gives the impression of a shallow mucosal depression. The lesion is diagnosed radiographically as type III + IIc early cancer.

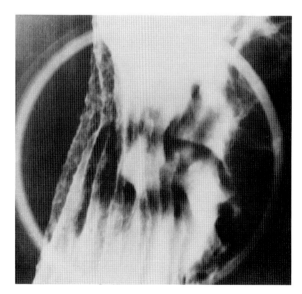

Fig. 515   Upright compression film (on the same date as Figure 514) reveals that the main part of the lesion may be an open ulcer (type III), because a thick collection of barium is still visualized. A faint shadow of barium extending to the greater curvature side may correspond to the part of shallow mucosal depression (erosion) seen in Figure 514.

277

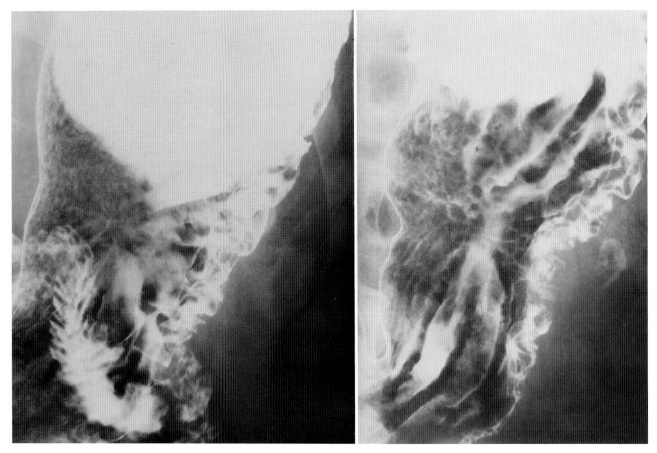

Fig. 516   Fig. 517

Fig. 516   Double contrast film 2 months after the first examination reveals that the lesion has almost completely healed, leaving an ulcer scar. It may be difficult to make the diagnosis of malignancy in this film. Medication has been continued during the interval.

Fig. 517   On the supine double contrast film, it seems that the thick collection of barium is replaced by an irregular shadow containing radiolucencies of various sizes. The surrounding converging folds which are visualized with a moderate amount of air reveal abrupt interruption suggestive of malignancy. The diagnosis of type IIc is now easily made. It may be difficult, however, to define the extent of intramucosal spread. Gastrectomy was performed 4 days after the second examination. Radiographically, the disappearance of an ulcer and its replacement by a cancerous erosion defines the so-called malignant cycle.

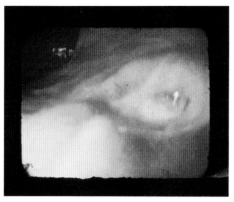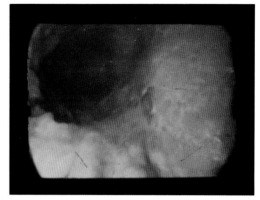

Fig. 518   **Fig. 519**

Fig. 518 Endoscopic picture 1 week after the first radiograph demonstrates large whitish mucus suggesting a benign peptic ulcer.

Fig. 519 Endoscopic picture before surgery demonstrates an irregular redness which is easily diagnosed as a malignant lesion.

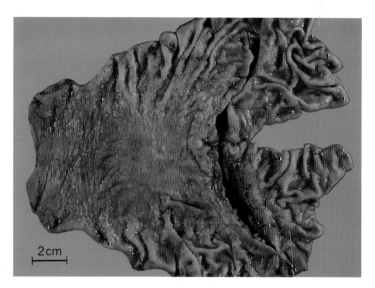

2cm

Fig. 520 Resected specimen. The lesion is diagnosed macroscopically as type IIc with extensive intramucosal spread. Additional resection was performed because cancer was found at the surgical stump.

X-ray examination and endoscopy (Figs. 517 and 519). The lesion increased in size on the mucosal surface. As its border was not discernible, a part of the lesion was left behind at the time of surgery. Following an immediate examination of the stump, additional resection was performed to complete the operation. The lesion was diagnosed as early cancer with a large area of intramucosal spread.

Case 136 Malignant Cycle of Early Cancer.
A 44-year-old woman (CPCC). (Figs. 521 and 522)

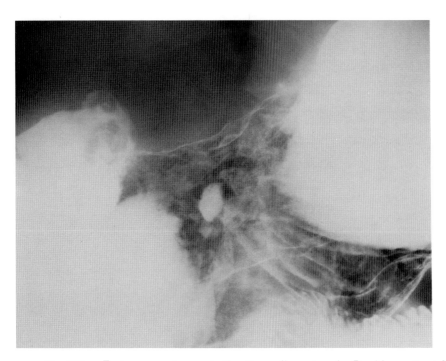

Fig. 521 Early cancer demonstrating the malignant cycle. Double contrast film demonstrates a niche with slight surrounding radiolucency. The diagnosis of benign peptic ulcer was made radiographically, although the niche had an irregularly defined margin on its lesser curvature side.

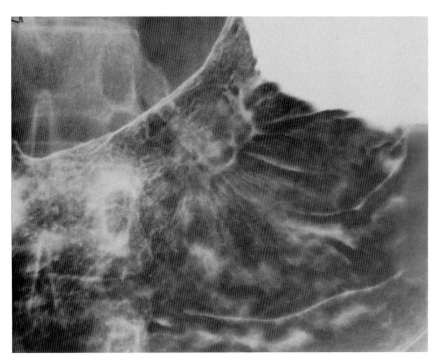

Fig. 522 Double contrast film taken 2 months later demonstrates a large irregular depression. An ulcer scar is visualized in its center. In this case, the surrounding type IIc lesion became prominent as the ulcer (type III) healed.

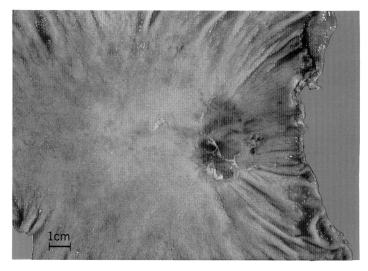

Fig. 523 Macroscopic findings showing the same lesion detected by X-ray films.

Course of development of gastric cancer with vertical invasion

There is a type of cancer that presents a considerable depth of invasion yet the lesion stays small, without forming the malignant cycle. Compared to other types of cancer presenting elevation or the malignant cycle, this type of cancer develops rapidly from an early stage to an advanced stage and is accompanied by deep invasion.

An example is shown in Figures 524–529. This is a small gastric cancer detected in a separate location while an ulcer in the incisura was under observation. Previous X-ray examination and endoscopy failed to detect the subtle change of the cancer a year prior to surgery. At operation the lesion had invaded the submucosa. The mucosa

Case 137   Course of Development of Early Cancer (?→IIc with Submucosal Involvement). A 58-year-old man (CPCC). (Figs. 524-529)

Fig. 524 Early cancer with vertical invasion. Prone mucosal relief film 1 year before operation demonstrates a fleck of barium with marked surrounding radiolucency. This was initially overlooked, probably because the peptic ulcer was in clinical remission.

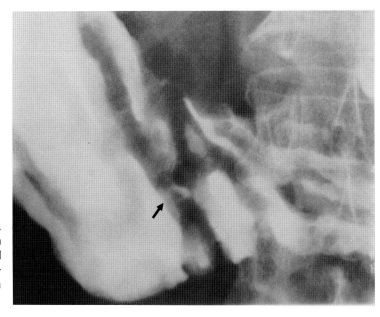

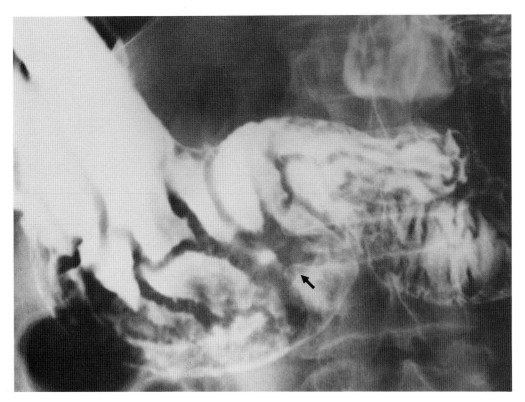

Fig. 525   Prone mucosal relief film 1 year later.

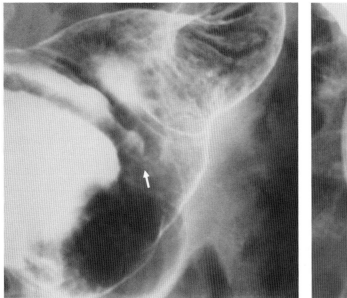

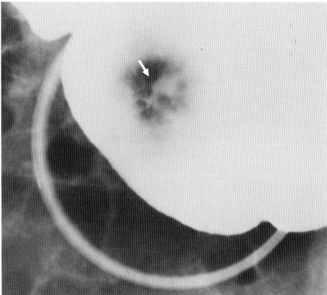

Fig. 526   Fig. 527

Fig. 526   Prone double contrast film with compression 1 year later.
Fig. 527   Upright compression film 1 year later. Figures 525 and 526 reveal that the depression and the surrounding elevation became slightly larger compared to the initial film. Although the details of the depression are not delineated in Figure 526, the diagnosis of malignancy (type IIc) is made with certainty on this film.

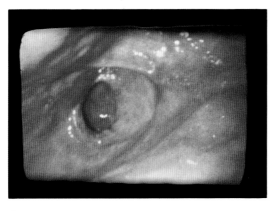 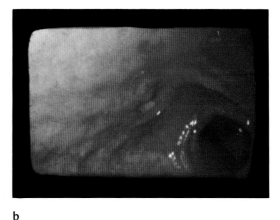

a   b

Fig. 528   Endoscopic findings.
a. Endoscopic picture 1 year before operation demonstrates small whitish mucus on the anterior wall of the gastric antrum, which was initially overlooked.
b. Endoscopic picture 1 year later demonstrates whitish mucus with surrounding elevation.

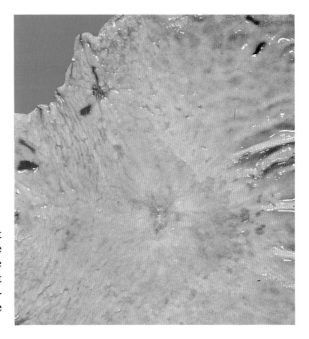

Fig. 529   Resected specimen. There is a benign peptic ulcer at the incisura. The cancer, located on the anterior wall of the antrum is visualized as an irregular mucosal depression. The surrounding elevation is not as marked as demonstrated in the last examination. Histologic diagnosis disclosed adenocarcinoma tubulare (moderately differentiated adenocarcinoma) with extensive submucosal involvement (sm).

surrounding the depression seemed to be elevated more prominently in the X-ray picture than in macroscopic observation.

Figures 530—532 show another example of a lesion in which deep invasion developed fairly rapidly. Findings were almost absent on the radiograph a year and nine months before, except for fine converging folds discerned retrospectively. By the time of operation the lesion developed into type IIc early cancer with the prominent mucosal convergence and had invaded the submucosa.

Case 138 Course of Development of Early Cancer (?→IIc with Submucosal Involvement). A 66-year-old man (CPCC). (Figs. 530-532)

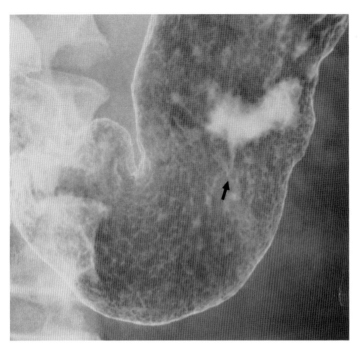 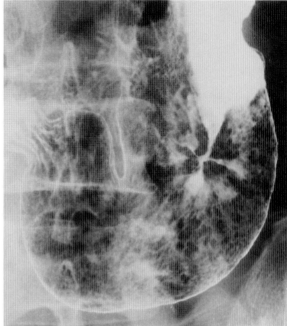

Fig. 530   Fig. 531

Fig. 530 Double contrast film 1 year and 9 months before operation. A very slight mucosal convergence suggesting an ulcer scar is retrospectively seen (arrow).

Fig. 531 Double contrast film immediately before operation demonstrates a small but irregular depression, surrounded by prominent converging folds with tapering, clubbing and fusion.

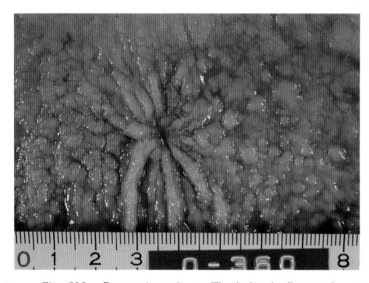

Fig. 532 Resected specimen. The lesion is diagnosed as type IIc with prominent mucosal folds. Histologic examination disclosed adenocarcinoma scirrhosum (poorly differentiated adenocarcinoma) with submucosal invasion (sm).

Development into linitis plastica type cancer

Sometimes a cancer is found that develops with the extreme rapidity of Borrmann type 4 cancers, which supposedly arise from the fundic gland area in the body of the stomach. It is generally called linitis plastica type cancer, yet the mechanism of its evolution and development is uncertain. Type IIc early cancer in the gastric body near the greater curvature is considered to be a precursor of linitis plastica, but its clinical detection is difficult and few cases are found. Most of the cases were detected after rigidity of the wall appeared in both the greater and the lesser curvatures, which formed the "leather-bottle" stomach. These seemed to have developed rapidly.

Such a case is shown in Figs. 533–537. No radiographic signs were discovered at the examinations about a half year and about a year before. The patient complained of epigastric pain at the first X-ray examination and slight rigidity is noticed retrospectively on the margin of the greater curvature. The folds in the greater curvatrue often hinder radiographic and endoscopic diagnosis.

Case 139 **Course of Development into Linitis Plastica Type Cancer.**
A 68-year-old man (CPCC). (Figs. 533-537)

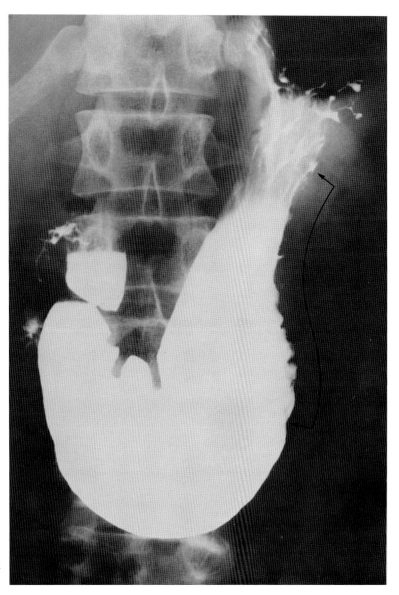

Fig. 533 Linitis plastica type cancer. Upright barium-filled film at the first examination.

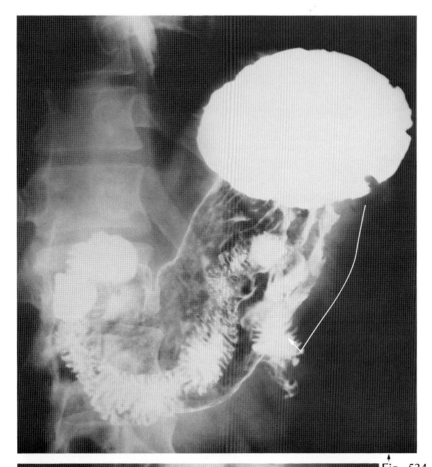

Fig. 534 Supine double contrast film at the first examination. Slight filling defect (Fig. 533, arrow line) and abnormality of the folds in the greater curvature are retrospectively seen.

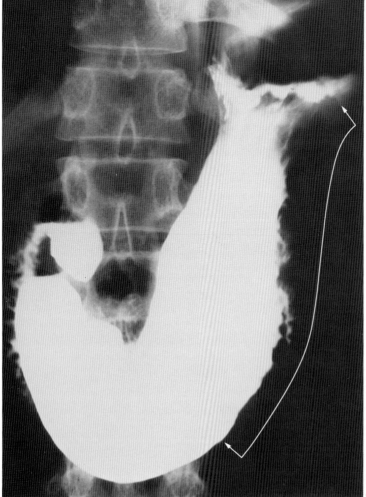

Fig. 535 Upright barium-filled film at the second examination.

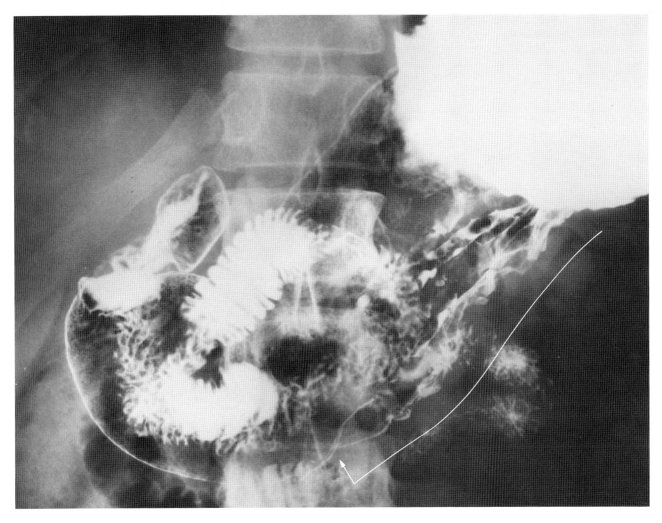

Fig. 536 Supine double contrast film at the second examination. The abnormalities of the greater curvature are more apparent. The diagnosis of linitis plastica should have been made.

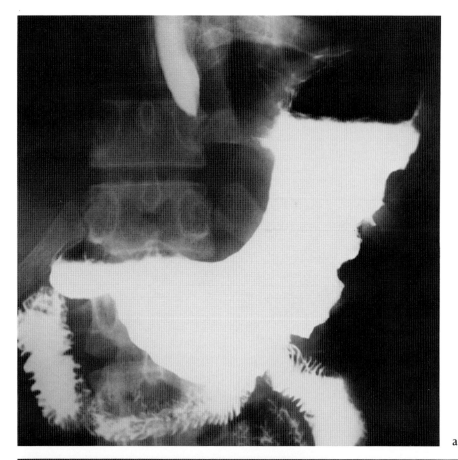

a

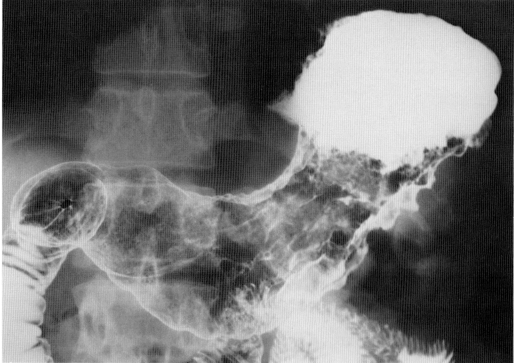

b

Fig. 537 a and b Upright barium-filled film and supine double contrast film at the last examination. Marked contraction of the stomach has taken place. These are typical radiographic features of linitis plastica.

Ulcer-Cancer Sequence and Polyp-Cancer Sequence

Cancer developing from peptic ulcer is called ulcer-cancer. A few depressed early cancers with accompanying ulcer are considered to represent only a certain phase in the malignant cycle. Lately, cancer is interpreted as not developing from peptic ulcer or polyp but rather as arising and developing de novo. Adenoma is rarely found among the cases of polyp of the stomach (see Chapter 4). The fact that most of them are hyperplastic polyps is one of the reasons for their remaining benign, in contrast to polyps in the large bowel. Other evidence is that, clinically, during the

course of observation by X-ray and endoscopy peptic ulcer does not seem to change into cancer. That type IIc early cancer often accompanies ulceration supports the hypothesis that cancer does not generate from ulcer.

In the case presented in Figures 538–543 during the period of three years and four months the configuration of ulcer changed while the size of the lesion remained almost the same. Biopsy was negative at the initial endoscopy, so the lesion was observed. Radiographic and endoscopic evidence on the initial examination did not indicate benign ulcer.

The fact that the ulcer remained and the cancer is developed slowly raises the suspicion that the cancer was preceeded by the ulcer.

Case 140   **Type IIc Early Cancer without Morphologic Alteration during a Long Period of Observation.** 72-year-old man (CPCC). (Figs. 538-543)

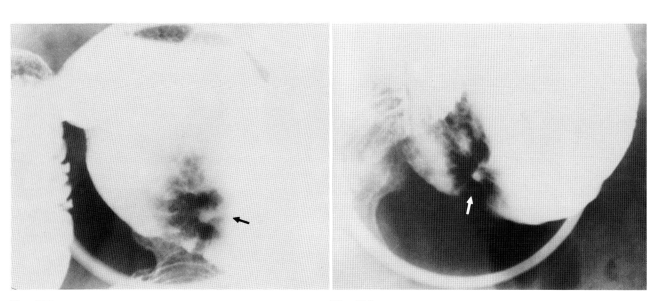

Fig. 538   Fig. 539

Fig. 538   Early cancer which does not show marked morphologic alteration during a long period of observation. Upright compression film at the first examination demonstrates a niche and surrounding radiolucency. The diagnosis of malignancy was made on the basis of the granular appearance of the surrounding radiolucency. Biopsy was negative for cancer and the patient was followed.

Fig. 539   Upright compression film at the second examination demonstrates nearly identical findings.

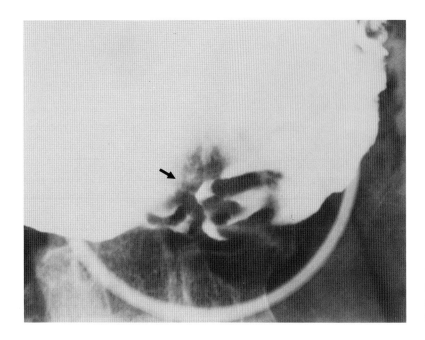

Fig. 540 Upright compression film at the last examination demonstrates irregularity of the niche and converging folds, but the lesion is unchanged in size.

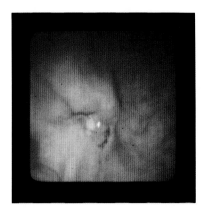
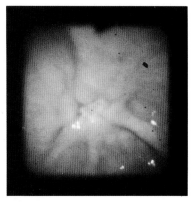

Fig. 541   **Fig. 542**

Fig. 541   Endoscopic picture at the first examination (shortly after the first radiograph).
Fig. 542   Endoscopic picture taken immediately before operation demonstrates marked converging folds. Clubbing and fusion result in the surrounding raised margin. Biopsy was positive for cancer and surgery was performed.

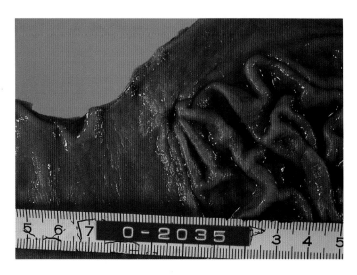

Fig. 543   Resected specimen. There is an ulcerated lesion with converging folds on the posterior wall near the greater curvature of the antrum. Histologic examination revealed adenocarcinoma scirrhosum (poorly differentiated adenocarcinoma) limited to the mucosa (m). In this case, the cancer remained intramucosal for 3 years and 4 months without marked morphologic alteration.

Origin and Development of Cancer

A course of development of cancer is shown in Figure 544. The cancer originates from the glandular epithelium and grows intramucosally, taking either the form of elevation (types II and IIa) or depression (types IIc, IIc + III, and III), or starts from type IIb cancer (partially from the polyp and margin of ulcer), gradually becoming Borrmann type advanced cancer with deep invasion. Cancers of type I and type IIa develop into either Borrmann type 1 or Borrmann type 2 via type IIa + IIc. Some type IIc cancers become Borrmann type 2 via type IIa + IIc, and most of the other depressed type early cancers become either Borrmann type 3 or Borrmann type 4.

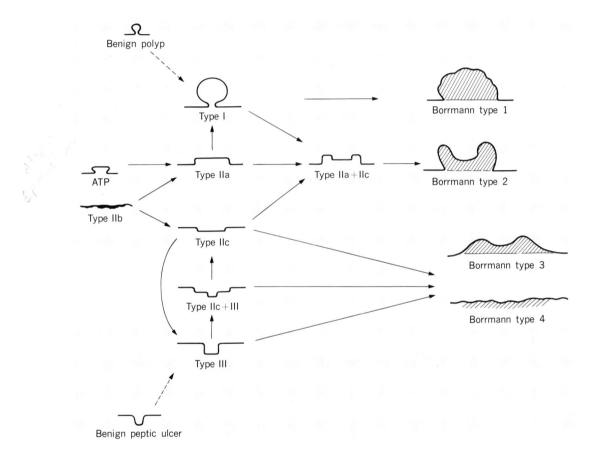

Fig. 544   Development of gastric cancer.

Chapter 13

Multiple Early Cancer and Lesions Coexisting with Early Cancer

Multiple Early Cancer

In the statistics of our research group, multiple early cancer comprises 6.1 per cent of all early cancer cases. Of these, double cancers are most frequent, comprising 4.6 per cent of the multiple cancer cases. Triple cancers occur in 1.2 per cent of cases and there was one case of quadruple cancer. In another case twelve minute cancer foci were discovered histologically. It is characteristic of most multiple cancers that they demonstrate the same morphology (Table 36, Figs. 545–550). A combination of polypoid and depressed lesions is relatively rare.

The radiographic diagnosis of multiple cancer is not difficult if all lesions are larger than 20 mm (Maruyama 1971). If any of the multiple lesions is smaller than 20 mm, it is apt to be overlooked. Frequently, a type IIc lesion which is free of ulcerative change escapes detection. Polypoid early cancers, though small, may be discovered by the compression method, but small depressed lesions which are not associated with converging folds may not be discovered by the double contrast method or the compression method. Baba et al. (1979) reported 21 satellite lesions of early cancer smaller than 10 mm and located within 20 mm of the surgical stump. Most of them could not be detected prior to surgery. He emphasized that particular attention should be paid radiographically to the upper portion of the stomach when determining the surgical stump. Those lesions not associated with converging folds are often discovered by the endoscopic examination. Takekoshi et al. (1978) emphasized the usefulness of the dye-scattering method with Indigocarmine for detecting small type IIc lesions.

Table 36   Multiple early cancer in 740 early gastric cancer cases (Our research group, 1959–1977*).

Two cancers (34 cases)		Three cancers (9 cases)	
Both lesions elevated (Types I, IIa)	9 cases	Two elevated + one depressed	1 case
		Two mixed + one depressed	2 cases
Elevated + mixed (Type IIa + IIc)	1 case	Mixed + depressed + flat	1 case
		All depressed	4 cases
Elevated + depressed (Types IIc, IIc + III, III)	4 cases	Two depressed + one mixed	1 case
Elevated + flat (Type IIb)	1 cases	Four cancers (1 case)	
Both mixed	3 cases	Three type IIa + one type IIc	1 case
Depressed + mixed	5 cases		
Both depressed	11 cases	Twelve cancers (1 case)	
		Four type IIc + eight type IIb	1 case

* Chiba University, 1959–1975.
  Juntendo University, 1968–1977.
  Chiba Prefectural Cancer Center, 1973–1977.
  Tokyo Metropolitan Cancer Detection Center, 1973–1977.

Case 141   Multiple Early Cancer (Type IIc and Type IIc)
A 57-year-old man (CIH). (Figs. 545-550)

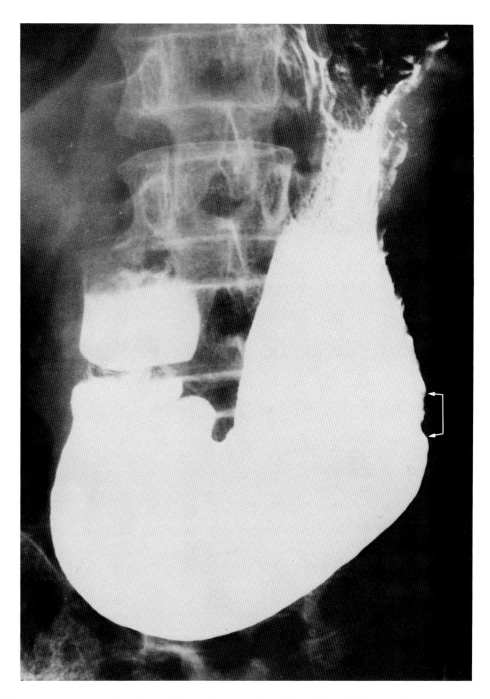

Fig. 545   Barium-filled film demonstrates deformity of the incisura and a slight filling defect of the greater curvature of the lower gastric body (arrow line).

293

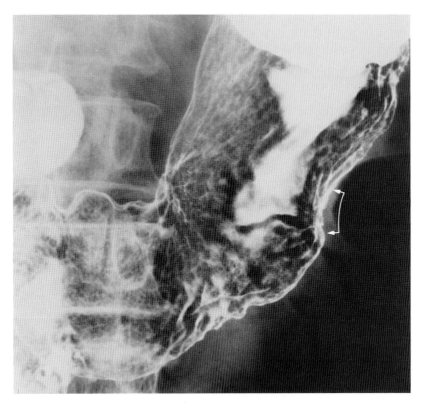

Fig. 546 Supine double contrast film demonstrates localized granularity of the mucosa of the upper part of the incisura with deformity of the lesser curvature. This granularity indicates a type IIc lesion in which barium is not collected. Mucosal convergence is seen at the area of slight indentation of the greater curvature (arrow line).

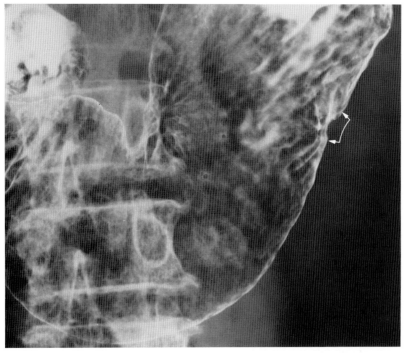

Fig. 547 Supine double contrast film with more air demonstrates a faint collection of barium and fine mucosal convergence at the lower gastric body near the incisura. Note also the greater curvature. In Figure 546 a very slight indentation of the greater curvature with faint convergence of the mucosal folds was visualized and increased distension of the stomach has produced indentation suggestive of malignancy (arrow line).

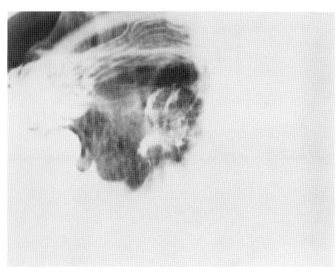 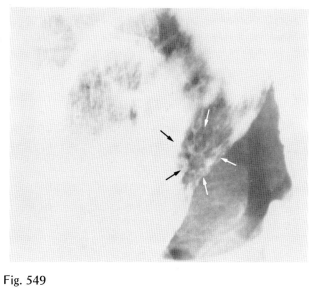

Fig. 548   Fig. 549

Fig. 548   Upright compression film demonstrates the irregular depression (type IIc) of the lesser curvature above the incisura.

Fig. 549   Upright compression film demonstrates faint but irregular depression (type IIc) of the greater curvature (arrows).

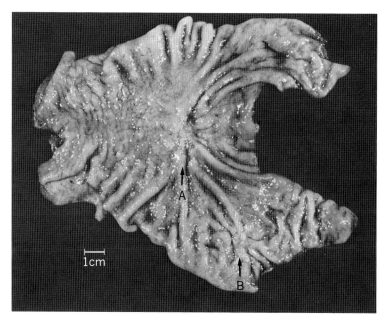

Fig. 550   Resected specimen. Arrow A points to the lesion at the incisura and arrow B points to the lesion on the greater curvature.

Early Cancer Associated with Linear Ulcer

A peculiar association of early cancer and linear ulcer is well known, and it could be evidence for the concept of the ulcer-cancer sequence (Murakami 1973). Murakami, in considering the fact that linear ulcer may have a much longer history than round ulcer, suggested the possibility that cancer is preceded by a linear ulcer and develops at its margin where regenerative change and recurrence usually occur. Based on the analysis of 17 cases of early cancer associated with linear ulcer, Murakami concluded that the ulcer-cancer sequence could not be proved definitively. Concerning the ulcer-cancer sequence, there is a controversial opinion that association of early cancer and linear ulcer merely represents spatial overlapping of ulcer and cancer, regardless of the histological examination (Nakamura et al. 1971).

In most cases, linear ulcer is located perpendicular to the lesser curvature and nearly equidistant between the anterior and posterior wall (see page 142) (Figs. 551–553). In some cases, however, it is located parallel to the lesser curvature (Figs. 554–557) or in the gastric body. Usually, a type IIc lesion surrounds a linear ulcer completely or is located partially at its margin, generally at either end of it. In a series at Juntendo University, cancer was located at either end of a linear ulcer in all cases (Fig. 558).

The radiographic diagnosis of type IIc lesions may be relatively easy when they are large and well defined, but may be difficult when small and located at either end of the linear ulcer. Endoscopic examination and biopsy are necessary in cases of linear ulcer. The margin of both ends of a linear ulcer should be examined.

Case 142 Multiple Type IIc Early Cancer Associated with Linear Ulcer.
A 50-year-old man (JU). (Figs. 551-553)

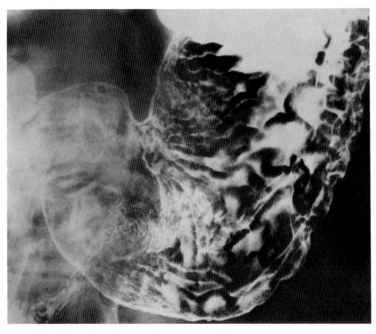 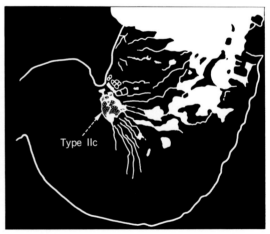

Type IIc

Fig. 551 Supine double contrast film demonstrates an irregular barium-filled erosion with several converging folds.

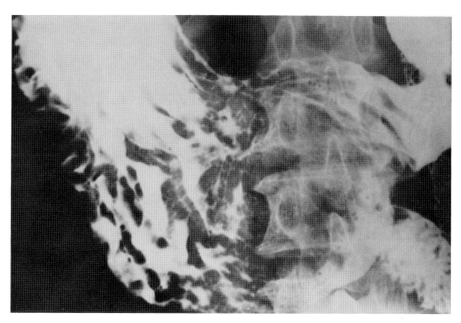

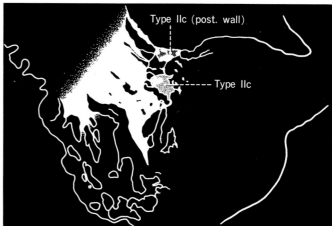

Fig. 552 Prone double contrast film demonstrates irregular collections of barium surrounded by granularity. Thicker collecitons of barium represent deep depressions, and the granularity, which is due to scattered flecks of barium, represents areas of erosion (type IIc). Accordingly, the radiographic diagnosis is type IIc + III.

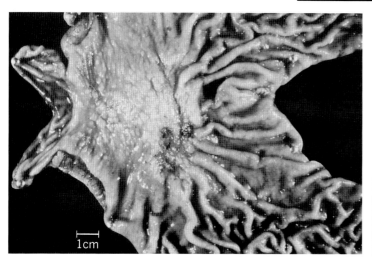

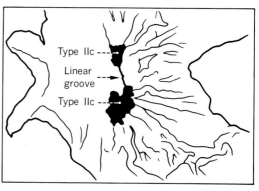

Fig. 553 Resected specimen. There are two erosions, on the anterior and posterior walls of the incisura, and a linear groove is observed between them. The area surrounding the linear groove is discolored and less depressed. The deepest depression in the lesion is on its posterior aspect near the greater curvature. Schematic representation of the macroscopic findings and extent of cancer spread. This case is not included in Figure 558.

Case 143   Type IIc Early Cancer Associated with Linear Ulcer.
A 62-year-old man (JU). (Figs. 554-557)

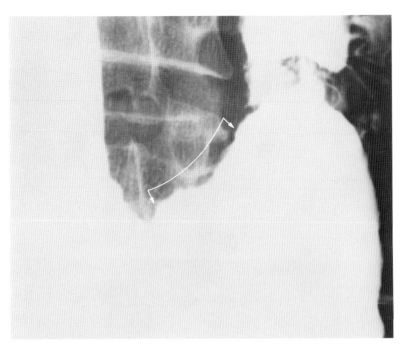

Fig. 554   Prone barium-filled film demonstrates a slight filling defect (arrow line) of the lesser curvature of the antrum.

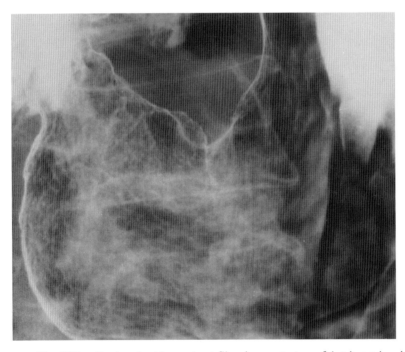 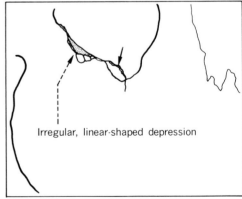

Irregular, linear-shaped depression

Fig. 555   Supine double contrast film demonstrates a faint irregular shadow of barium along the lesser curvature of the antrum.

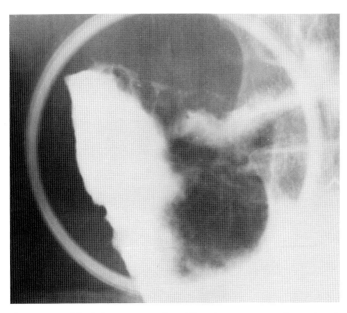
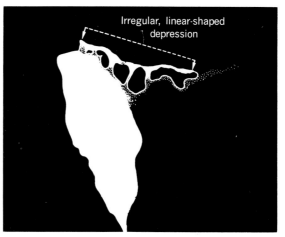

Fig. 556   Upright compression film demonstrates irregular depression surrounded by prominent radiolucencies. These radiographic pictures reveal a several centimeter long, irregular, linear-shaped erosion along the lesser curvature of the antrum. The shape and location of the erosion are very unusual. It is most likely that the erosion is a peculiar form of type IIc. Biopsy disclosed adenocarcinoma tubulare.

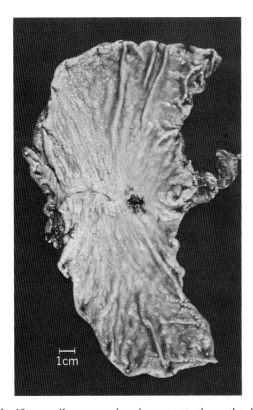
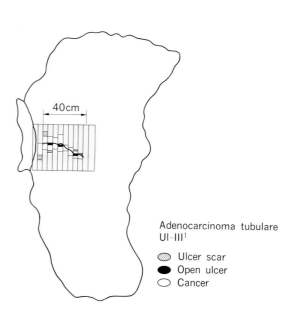

Fig. 557   A 40 mm linear erosion is present along the lesser curvature of the antrum with an ulcer in its proximal part at the incisura Schematic representation of the macroscopic findings and cancer spread.

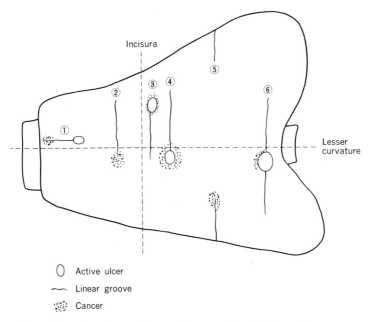

Fig. 558   Location of linear ulcer associated with early cancer.

Lesions Coexisting with Early Gastric Cancer

There is no relationship between early cancer and coexisting lesions of the stomach (Figs. 559 and 560). Atypical epithelium (ATP) or benign hyperplastic polyp often coexists with elevated early cancers (Table 37). Benign peptic ulcer or ulcer scar often coexists with depressed early cancers (Figs. 561—562 and 563—566). A small type IIc lesion is often encountered in the distal part of a peptic ulcer or an ulcer scar, especially in the antrum (Maruyama et al. 1970). Duodenal ulcer rarely coexists with early cancer. It comprises only 6.06 per cent of all early cancer cases (Table 37).

Table 37   Benign lessions coexisting with early cancer (Our research group, 1957—1977).

Coexisting benign lesion Early cancer	Elevated lesion			Depressed lesion			
	Polyp	ATP	Submucosal tumor	Active gastric ulcer	Active duodenal ulcer	RLH	
Types I, IIa, etc.	3	6	—	3	—	—	—
Type IIa + IIc	2	3	—	4	—	—	—
Types IIc, IIc + III, etc.	5	3	2	30	4	1	—

Case 144   Peptic Ulcer Coexisting with Type IIa Early Cancer.

A 68-year-old man (JU). (Figs. 559 and 560)

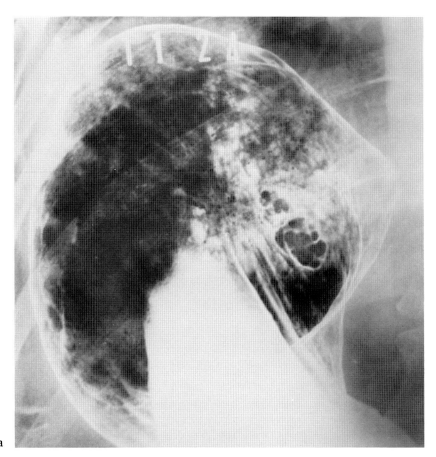

a

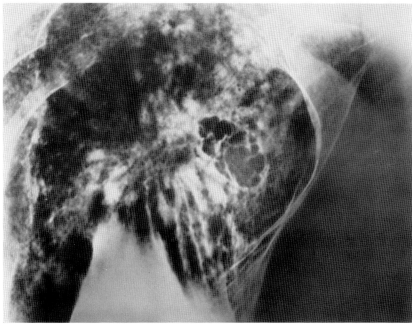

b

Fig. 559 a and b   Prone double contrast film demonstrates a polypoid lesion with surface nodularity at the cardia. This lesion is diagnosed as early cancer (type IIa). In the vicinity of this lesion is a large mucosal convergence. No niche is noted. The converging folds reveal a smooth tapering, compatible with ulcer scar of benign peptic ulcer.

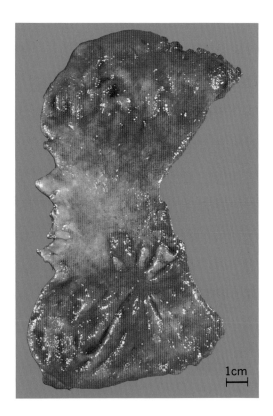

Fig. 560 Resected specimen after cardiectomy. The polypoid lesion (type IIa) measures 25 x 15 mm. The large ulcer is located just above the type IIa lesion on the anterior wall. Histologically, cancer was limited to the mucosa in the type IIa, and the depth of the ulcer scar was UI-IIIs.

Case 145 Peptic Ulcer Coexisting Type IIc Early Cancer.
A 64-year-old man (JU). (Figs. 561-563)

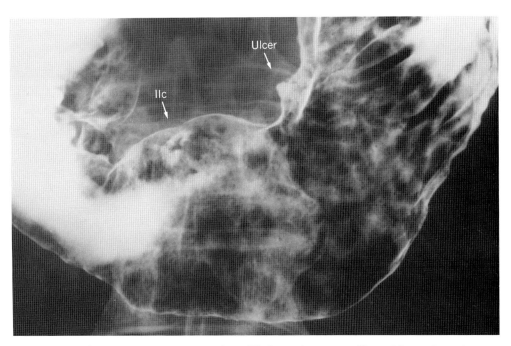

Fig. 561 Supine double contrast film demonstrates a barium-filled erosion, type IIc, with an irregular radiolucency in its center (→ IIc). It is located on the posterior wall of the antrum near the lesser curvature. This is one of the typical radiographic signs of type IIc lesion not associated with an ulceration. A niche at the incisura reveals a benign ulcer (→ Ulcer).

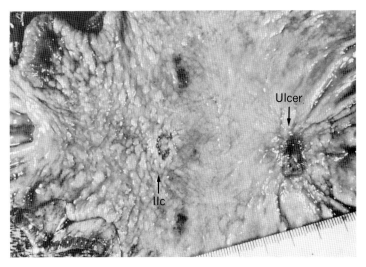

Fig. 562 Resected specimen. The erosion, measuring 10 × 4 mm, is on the posterior wall of the proximal antrum near the lesser curvature. The central part is elevated. This is diagnosed macroscopically as type IIc. Histologically, the lesion was diagnosed as adenocarcinoma tubulare (well differentiated adenocarcinoma), limited to the mucosa (m) and not associated with ulceration. A benign ulcer is seen at the incisura.

Case 146   Multiple Ulcer Scar Coexisting with Type IIc Early Cancer.
A 45-year-old woman (JU). (Figs. 564-567)

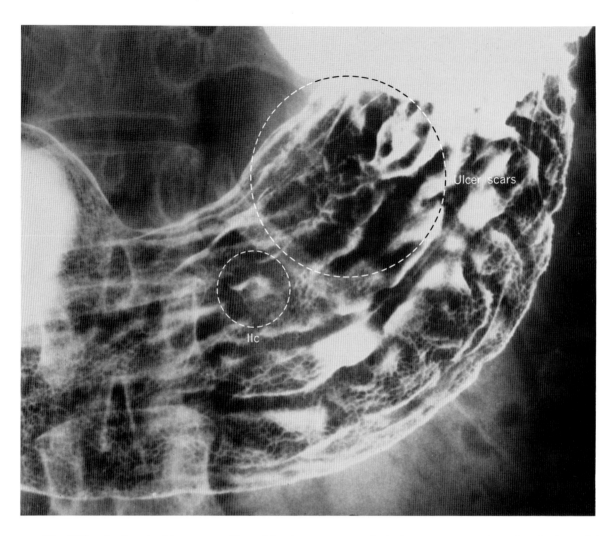

Fig. 563 Supine double contrast film with a large amount of air demonstrates an irregular shadow of barium surrounded by vague radiolucency, toward which two folds are converging from the antral side. They are interrupted at the margin of the radiolucency. At the mid-gastric body an area of mucosal abnormality with some converging folds is observed. In this film overdistension of the stomach has interfered with clear visualization of the lesions.

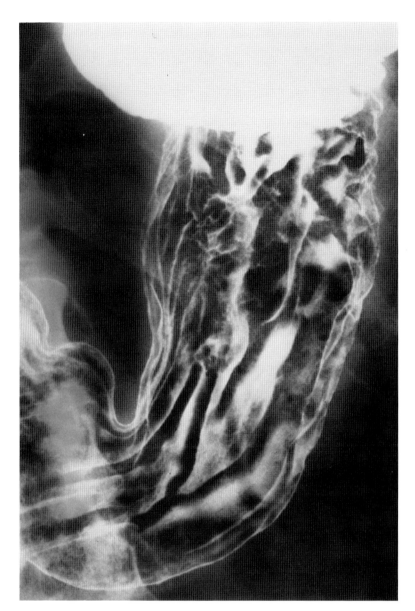

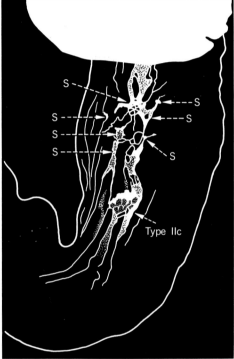

Fig. 564 Supine double contrast film in the right anterior oblique projection with a moderate amount of air demonstrates the details of the mucosal abnormality. The interrupted ends of the two folds and the uneven barium collection in the depression are clearly visualized. The abnormality of the mucosa at the mid-gastic body lacks conclusive signs of malignancy, as multicentric convergence of the fine mucosal folds is sometimes observed in benign multiple ulcers or ulcer scars.

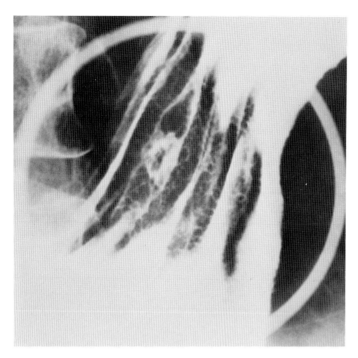

Fig. 565   Upright compression produces the best delineation of barium-filled erosion, type IIc.

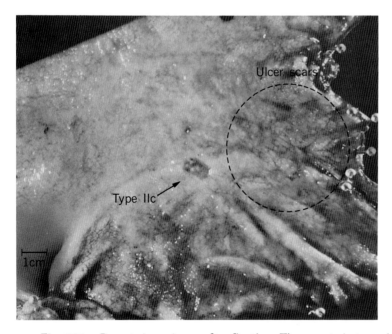

Fig. 566   Resected specimen after fixation. The resected stomach was fixed in such an overdistended stste that the mucosal fold pattern was almost destroyed. There is a small "punched-out" depression of the mucosa on the posterior wall of the lower gastric body, measuring 11 x 5 mm. There is fine nodularity in the bed of the depression, which distinguishes it from a benign erosion. This is a typical macroscopic sign of small early cancer, type IIc. Histologically, the lesion was diagnosed as adenocarcinoma tubulare (well differentiated adenocarcinoma), limited to the mucosa (m) and associated with Ul-IIs.

Chapter 14

Radiographic Diagnosis of Cancer Smaller Than 10 mm

General Considerations

The radiographic diagnosis of cancer smaller than 5 mm (microcarcinoma) was first reported by Kumakura and Maruyama (1969). They searched for radiographic evidence of microcarcinomas which were discovered histologically in stomachs operated on for early and advanced cancer and for peptic ulcer. In several of their cases the microcarcinoma was recognized macroscopically as a very small, irregular depression of the mucosa with a slightly raised margin that was visible on the color photographs of the freshly resected specimen or on the specimen after fixation. In a few cases a very small profile niche was the radiographic sign corresponding to those depressed lesions. In 1969 the limits of endoscopic and radiographic diagnosis of small gastric cancer was discussed in the symposium of Japan Gastroenterological Endoscopy Society, and lesions smaller than 10 mm were defined as microcarcinomas.

Nakamura (1969), using the same cases as Kumakura and Maruyama, discussed the histology of cancer of the stomach smaller than 5 mm. The first clinical report of a cancer smaller than 5 mm was made by Oi in 1970. In this case, biopsy taken from a spotty redness of the mucosa was positive for cancer, but it was not visible on the resected specimen after surgery. Cancer, type IIb, measuring 4 mm in the greatest diameter was eventually diagnosed. Since Oi's report, cancers smaller than 5 mm which were diagnosed prior to surgery have been reported by several authors (Maruyama et al. 1970, Kawamura 1974, Ikeda et al. 1974). However, in most cases detection and diagnosis were possible only by endoscopy and biopsy. In only a few cases did the radiographic examination detect the lesions, which were subsequently confirmed by endoscopy and biopsy (Tsukasa and Nakahara 1974, Ito et al. 1975, Takekoshi et al. 1977, Yarita et al. 1977, 1978). Murohisa et al. (1978) reported two cases of cancer, measuring 1 mm and 2 mm, respectively, whose presence was first suspected by the radiographic examination, but endoscopy did not confirm them. In these cases lavage cytology played a decisive role in establishing malignancy. Tsukasa et al. (1973) also reported a case of cancer smaller than 5 mm which was first detected by the radiographic examination, but which could not be confirmed by endoscopy.

In 1979 the histopathologic and clinical problems of microcarcinoma were discussed in "*I to Cho*" (Stomach and Intestine) (Vol. 14, 1979) and since then radiography and endoscopy has been directed to the detection and diagnosis of cancer smaller than 5 mm.

Histologically, submucosal involvement is sometimes found in cancers which are radiographically undertectable (Nakamura 1972, Takekoshi et al. 1977, Oohara 1979, Hirota et al. 1979). In Nakamura's series submucosal involvement was found in 4 per cent of cancers smaller than 5 mm and these were diagnosed histologically as a microsatellite focus in multiple cancers. Oohara reported submucosal involvement in 50 per cent of single foci smaller than 5 mm and in 3.1 per cent of multiple foci. Extensive distant metastases in a case of multiple minute cancers were reported by Ogata (1969), Yarita et al. (1977), and Sakuma and Kuwahara (1977).

Cancer 6 to 10 mm in Diameter

Gross pathology

All 6 to 10 mm lesions are early cancers. They are the smallest cancers showing radiographic and endoscopic features of malignancy. The macroscopic classification of early gastric cancer applies to the gross pathology of lesions of this size. Depressed lesions (type IIc) predominate over polypoid lesions (type IIa) in single early cancer as well as in multiple early cancers (Hirota 1979). No flat type (type IIb) was encountered in this size lesion. Associated peptic ulcer is found in more than 50 per cent of single lesions but in less than 15 per cent of multiple lesions (Hirota et al. 1979). Maruyama (1971) reported that peptic ulcer was found in 2 of 10 multiple lesions and that 1 of the 2 lesions was detected radiographically. The difference in the frequency of associated peptic ulcer in single and multiple cancers may result from the difficulty in detecting lesions without peptic ulcer in cases of multiple cancer.

Radiographic diagnosis of polypoid early cancer 6 to 10 mm in diameter

Polypoid early cancer, though few in number, is relatively easily detected by the compression or the double contrast method. However, its small size may prevent the analysis of the form and surface pattern which is necessary for the definite diagnosis of malignancy (Chapter 4). Endoscopic polypectomy is performed for diagnosis as well as treatment. In most cases further operation is not required, since submucosal involvement has never been encountered in polypoid early cancers of this size.

Radiographic diagnosis of depressed early cancer 6 to 10 mm in diameter

Depressed early cancer is detected and diagnosed, according to the general principles of the radiographic diagnosis of malignancy. Lesions located in an area where double contrast radiography gives good visualization of the mucosal details and lesions associated with peptic ulcer are easily detected and diagnosed as malignant (Figs. 567–573). Such lesions are always accompanied

---

Case 147   Type IIc Early Cancer.
A 37-year-old woman (JU). (Figs. 568-574)

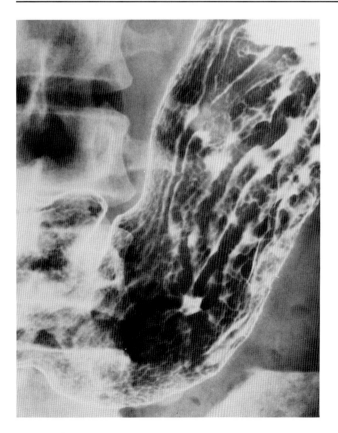

Fig. 567   Early cancer, type IIc, 5 x 6 mm. Double contrast radiograph in the supine position demonstrates a small, irregular depression on the posterior wall of the lower gastric body. It is associated with mucosal convergence, and there is granularity in the depression.

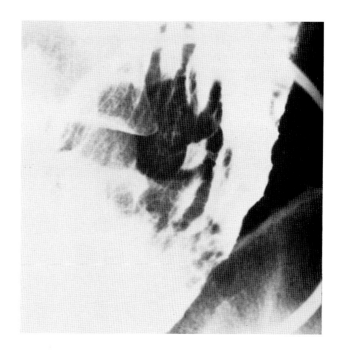

Fig. 568 Compression radiograph demonstrates an irregular depression with granularity.

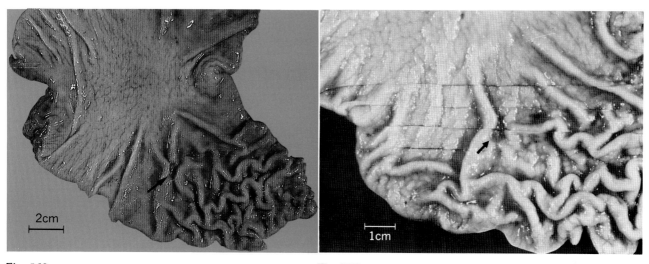

Fig. 569   Fig. 570

Fig. 569   Resected specimen. The lesion was located within the fundic gland mucosa (arrow) and measured 5 x 6 mm.

Fig. 570   Fixed specimen after sectioning. An arrow points to the lesion.

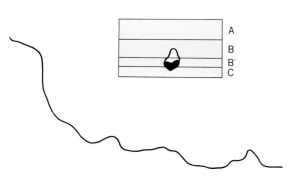

Fig. 571 Schematic representation of the sectioned specimen shows localization of the cancer.

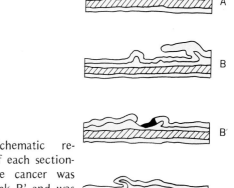

Fig. 572 Schematic representation of each sectioned block. The cancer was present in block B' and was limited to the mucosa (m).

309

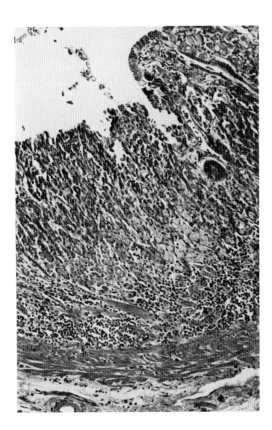

Fig. 573 Histologic findings show adenocarcinoma mucocellulare (signet ring cell carcinoma). No lymph node metastasis was found.

6-10mm (17 cases, 18 lesions) m 14 sm 4

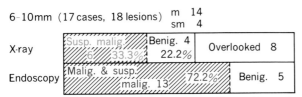

Fig. 574 Sensitivity of the routine radiographic and endoscopic examination for the detection of cancer 6 to 10 mm (From Yarita 1979).

6-10mm (17 cases, 18 lesions) m 14 sm 4

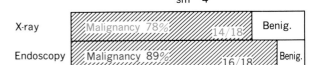

Fig. 575 Comparison of radiography, endoscopy and biopsy in the diagnosis of cancer smaller than 5 mm (From Yarita 1979).

by mucosal convergence, which can suggest malignancy.

Depressed early cancer not accompanied by peptic ulcer is difficult to detect. It may not be seen fluoroscopically, but should be visible on the double contrast radiographs. The diagnosis of malignancy can be established without difficulty, once its location is recognized. In most cases the depression is irregular and its surrounding mucosa is almost always slightly raised (Figs. 576–583 and 584–586). However, sometimes the diagnosis of malignancy cannot be made, even by double contrast radiography with good mucosal coating and an adequate amount of air. In Yarita's series (1979) no lesion was diagnosed as definitely malignant in the first routine radiographic examination. He reported that malignancy was

suspected in 6 of 18 lesions (33.3%). Four lesions (22.2%) were diagnosed as benign, and the remaining 8 lesions (44.4%) were overlooked (Fig. 575). Endoscopy detected the 8 lesions which were missed by the first radiographic examination, and diagnosed 13 of the lesions (72.2%) as malignant or malignancy suspected. In the repeat radiographic examination 14 lesions (78%) were diagnosed as malignant while the remaining 4 lesions were still diagnosed as benign. In the repeat endoscopic examination 19 lesions (89%) were diagnosed as malignant with the remaining 2 lesions still diagnosed as benign. In all cases aimed biopsy was positive for cancer (Fig. 575). It may be possible to diagnose malignancy in 6 to 10 mm lesions if the radiographic examination is carefully repeated.

Case 148   Multiple Type IIc Early Cancer.
A 44-year-old woman (CIH). (Figs. 576-583)

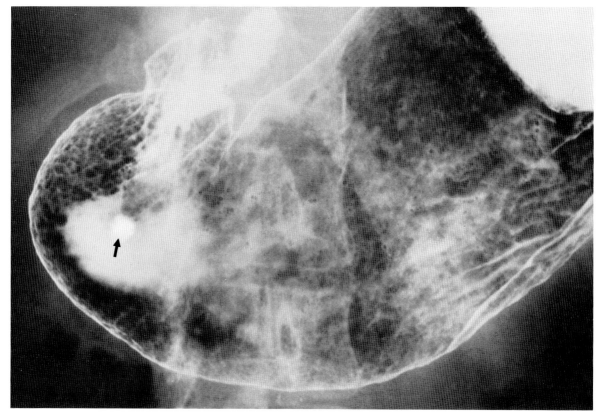

Fig. 576   Multiple early cancers, type IIc, 5 × 7 mm and 4 × 4 mm. Double contrast radiograph at the first routine examination demonstrates a small, irregular depression with surrounding radiolucency (arrow). The lesion is not clearly visualized due to an excess of barium.

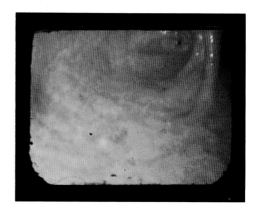

Fig. 577   Endoscopic findings (GTF-A) at the first examination. A shallow, irregular depression with redness is observed in the proximal antrum. The surrounding mucosa is elevated. Biopsy following this examination revealed atypical epithelium (Group III).

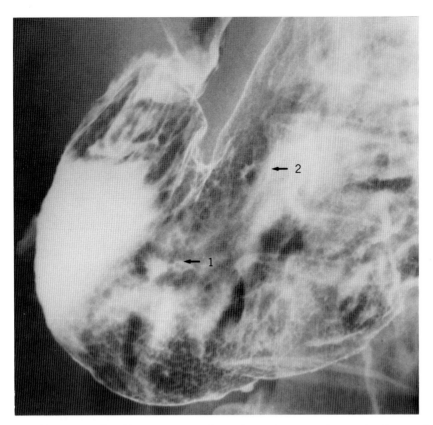

Fig. 578 Double contrast radiograph at the second examination performed 2 months after the first one, demonstrates two small, irregular depressions on the posterior wall of the proximal antrum (arrow 1) and on the posterior wall near the incisura (arrow 2). Radiolucency around the large depression is marked, but is only slightly visualized around the small depression.

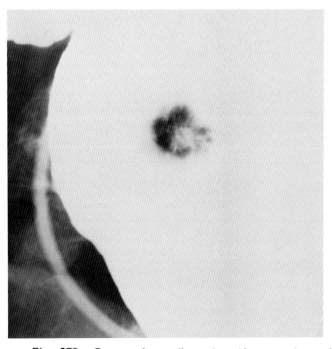

Fig. 579 Compression radiograph at the second examination demonstrates the irregular depression and the marked surrounding radiolucency. The small depression visualized in Figure 578 was not detected at fluoroscopy.

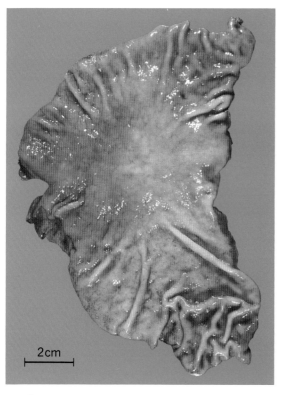

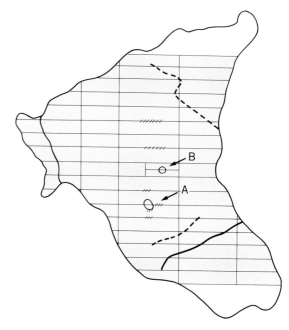

Fig. 580 Resected specimen. The large depression (5 x 7mm) was recognized macroscopically, but the small depression was not.

Fig. 581 Schema showing the location of the two depressions after sectioning of the fixed specimen.

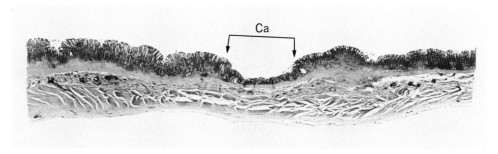

Fig. 582 Cross section of the small depression.

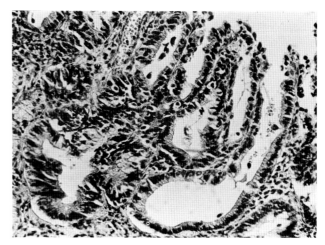

Fig. 583 Histologic findings of the small depression showing adenocarcinoma tubulare (well differentiated adenocarcinoma).

313

Case 149   Multiple Type IIc Early Cancer.
A 68-year-old man (JU). (Figs. 584-586)

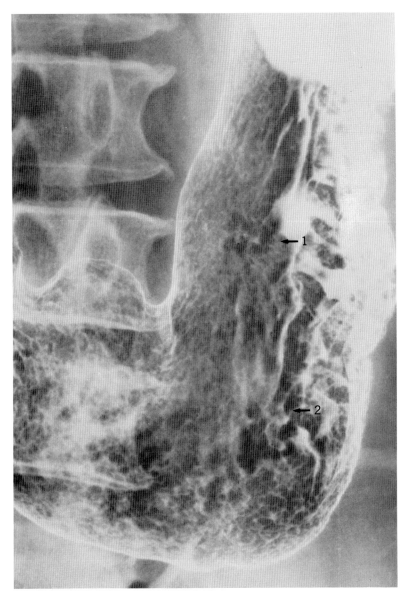

Fig. 584   Multiple early cancers, type IIc, measuring 20 x 25 mm, 4 x 10 mm and 6 x 8 mm. Double contrast radiograph demonstrates a lesion in the lower gastric body (6 x 8 mm, arrow 1) and another on the posterior wall of the incisura (4 x 10 mm, arrow 2). The surrounding radiolucency is clearly visualized in the lower gastric body (arrow 1).

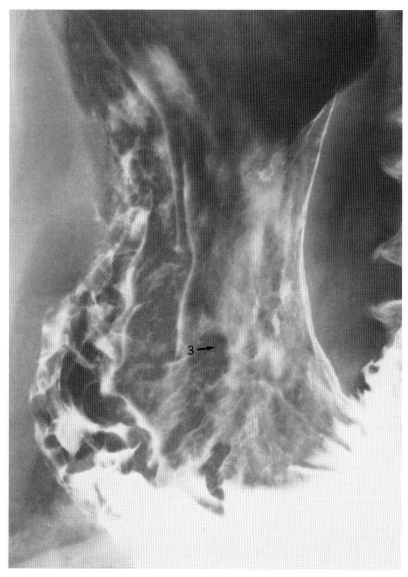

Fig. 585 Prone double contrast radiograph demonstrates the largest (type IIc) in the anterior wall of the lower gastric body (arrow 3).

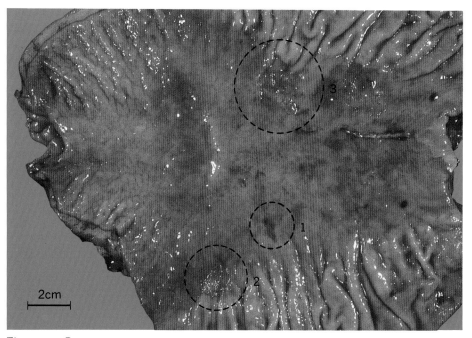

2cm

Fig. 586 Resected specimen.

Cancer Smaller Than 5 mm (Microcarcinoma)

Gross pathology

All lesions of this size are early cancers. In most cases they are one of multiple cancers or are associated with chronic peptic ulcers. The depth of invasion is mostly limited to the mucosa except for Oohara's cases, as mentioned above. Histologically, differentiated cancer predominates over undifferentiated. In Takekoshi's series undifferentiated cancer comprised 13.8 per cent (Table 38). The macroscopic classification was not always applied to the lesions, although Hirota (1979) reported that type IIb was found in 45 per cent of all cancers smaller than 5 mm. In most cases the presence of cancer is only detected histologically, being invisible on color photographs of the fresh or fixed specimen even after careful macroscopic examination. The macroscopic classification is made by the naked eye on the microscopic preparation if it is visible, or on low power magnification under the microscope if it is not.

Table 38 Depth of invasion of cancer smaller than 5mm (From Takekoshi 1978)

Histologic type	Depth of invasion		Total
	Mucosa	Sub-mucosa	
Differentiated* cancer	80 (97.6)	2 (2.4)	82 Lesions
Undifferentiated** cancer	11 (84.6)	2 (15.4)	13
Total	91 (95.8)	4 (4.2)	95 Lesions

* Differentiated carcinoma, tubular and papillotubular.
** Undifferentiated carcinoma, mucocellular and scirrhous.
( ): Per cent
1964—1975. Cancer Institute Hospital, Tokyo.

Table 39 Macroscopic diagnosis of cancer smaller than 5mm visualized on the fixed specimen (From Takekoshi 1978).

Positive diagnosis of cancer	16 lesions	(17.4%)	4*
Presence of lesion recognized	20	(21.7%)	2*
Presence of lesion not recognized	56	(60.9%)	4*

* Discovered endoscopically (excluding 3 lesions of protruded type)
1964—1975. Cancer Institute Hospital, Tokyo.

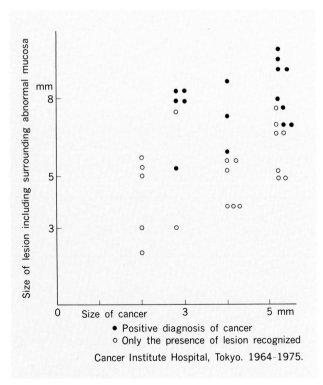

Fig. 587 Comparison of size and macroscopic diagnosis in cancer smaller than 5 mm (Takekoshi 1978).

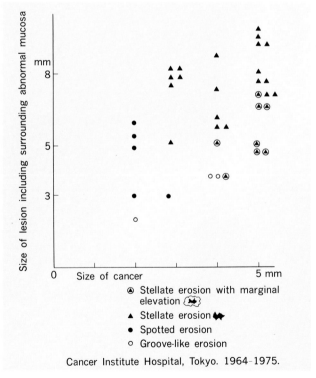

Fig. 588 Comparison of size and macroscopic findings in cancer smaller than 5 mm (From Takekoshi 1978).

Takekoshi et al. (1977, a, b) reported that macroscopic diagnosis of cancer was possible in only 16 of 92 cases (17.4%) of depressed early cancers smaller than 5 mm on retrospective study of the color photographs of the resected stomach after fixation (Table 39). Twenty lesions were recognized, but the remaining 56 lesions (60.9%) were undetected. Takekoshi detected 4 lesions by endoscopy whose location could not be recognized in the resected stomach. Takekoshi compared the size and the macroscopic diagnosis of 36 malignant lesions whose presence was recognized (Fig. 587). According to this analysis, the diagnosis of malignancy was possible when the cancer focus was larger than 3 mm and the size including the surrounding elevation was over 5 mm. On the other hand, the diagnosis of malignancy was impossible when the size including the surrounding elevation, was below 5 mm, even if the cancer focus was larger than 3 mm. Takekoshi et al. (1977a) then compared the macroscopic findings (Fig. 588) with the size of the lesions, including the surrounding elevation. All lessions over 5 mm, incluidng the surrounding elevation, which were diagnosed as malignant revealed a stellate depression with marginal elevation. On the other hand, lesions smaller than 5 mm which could not be diagnosed as cancer revealed a stellate depression without marginal elevation, or spotted or groove-like erosion. The surrounding elevation of the mucosa may be a key for the definitive diagnosis of microcarcinoma.

In Yarita's series (1979) of 19 lesions smaller than 5 mm, no lesion was macroscopically diagnosed as malignant. In his series 32 per cent were diagnosed as benign, and the presence of the remaining 68 per cent of the lesions was not recognized.

Radiographic diagnosis

Yarita et al. (1979) failed to diagnose cancer in the routine radiographic examination (Fig. 589). Only 3 of 19 lesions were diagnosed as benign and the remaining 16 lesions were missed. Endoscopy detected one more lesion and diagnosed it as benign. In that case repeated radiographic examination detected the lesion. The second endoscopy did not increase the detection rate. In 4 lesions cancer was confirmed by biopsy (Fig. 590). Yarita et al.

Smaller than 5mm (8 cases, 19 lesions) m 19

X-ray	Benig. 15.8%	Overlooked
Endoscopy	Benig. 21.1%	Overlooked

Oct. 1968–Feb. 1979.

Fig. 589 Sensitivity of the routine radiographic and endoscopic examination for the detection of cancer smaller than 5 mm (Yarita et al. 1979).

Smaller than 5mm (8 cases, 19 lesions) m 19

X-ray	Benig. 21% 4/19	Overlooked 79%
Endoscopy	Benig.	Overlooked
Biopsy	Malignancy	Not performed

Oct. 1968–Feb. 1979.

Fig. 590 Comparison of radiography, endoscopy and biopsy in the diagnosis of cancer smaller than 5 mm (Yarita et al. 1979).

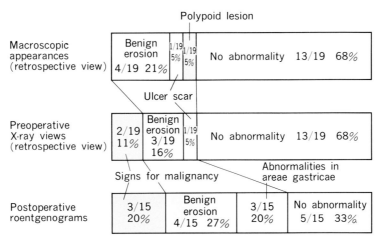

Polypoid lesion

| Macroscopic appearances (retrospective view) | Benign erosion 4/19 21% | 1/19 5% | 1/19 5% | No abnormality 13/19 68% |

Ulcer scar

| Preoperative X-ray views (retrospective view) | 2/19 11% | Benign erosion 3/19 16% | 1/19 5% | No abnormality 13/19 68% |

Signs for malignancy

Abnormalities in areae gastricae

| Postoperative roentgenograms | 3/15 20% | Benign erosion 4/15 27% | 3/15 20% | No abnormality 5/15 33% |

Fig. 591 Comparison of the retroscpective radiographic diagnosis of cancer smaller than 5 mm and its macroscopic findings (From Yarita et al. 1979).

(1979) also reported that some signs of malignancy were present in 2 lesions on retrospective review of the radiographic findings and in 3 lesions by the postoperative roentgenogram of the incised stomach (Fig. 591). In the retrospective review of the radiographic findings, 3 lesions revealed a sign of ulcer scar. In the postoperative roentgenogram the sign of benign erosion was detected in 1 more lesion and abnormalities of the areae gastricae pattern were detected in 3 more lesions. No abnormality was detected in 5 lesions.

Rarely, microcarcinoma may be diagnosed in the routine radiographic examination if the depression is relatively deep and is accompanied by surrounding elevation of the mucosa (Maruyama 1979). Sometimes, careful compression during the detailed radiographic study may demonstrate a depression when the double contrast radiography is unsuccessful (Figs. 592–597). However, in most cases of microcarcinoma the abnormalities are not recognized, even in the detailed examination. Retrospectively, its presence is sometimes recognized as a very small fleck of barium (Figs. 598–600) but this is insufficient for the definite diagnosis of cancer. Moreover, the surrounding elevation of the mucosa is not apparent in the radiographic study as it is on the macroscopic study (Figs. 601–603). The radiographic diagnosis of microcarcinoma is therefore limited.

Case 150   Microcarcinoma.
A 50-year-old woman (CIH). (Figs. 592-597)

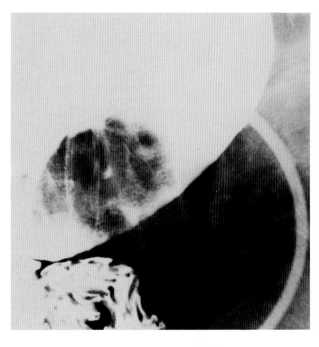

Fig. 592 Compression radiograph of cancer measuring 2 mm.

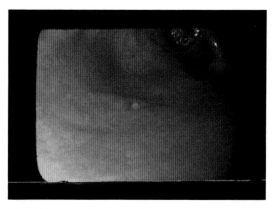

Fig. 593 Endoscopic findings by dye-spraying method with Indigocarmine.

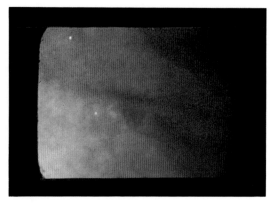

Fig. 594 Close-up view of Figure 594.

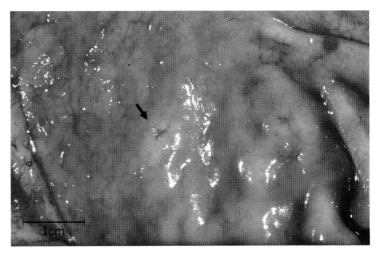

Fig. 595 Resected specimen. An arrow points to the site of cancer measuring 2 mm. There was a type IIc lesion, measuring 50 x 38 mm on the anterior wall of the gastric antrum.

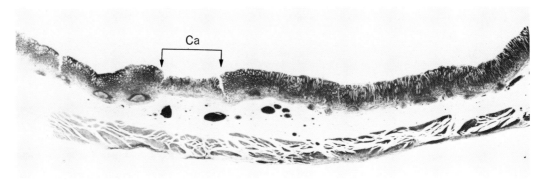

Fig. 596 Cross section of the lesion.

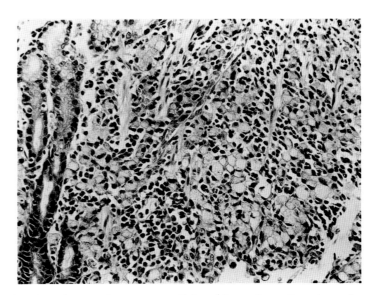

Fig. 597 Histologic findings showing adenocarcinoma mucocellulare (signet ring cell carcinoma).

319

Cace 151   Multiple Microcarcinoma.
A 50-year-old woman (JU). (Figs. 598-601)

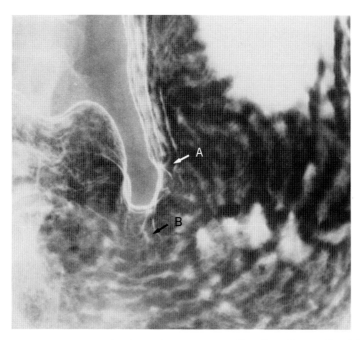

Fig. 598   Multiple early cancers smaller than 5 mm. Double contrast radiograph. Arrows point to the site of cancer which was detected prior to surgery. The lesion indicated by arrow A seems to be an ulcer scar. The lesion indicated by arrow B is a small, irregular depression of the mucosa.

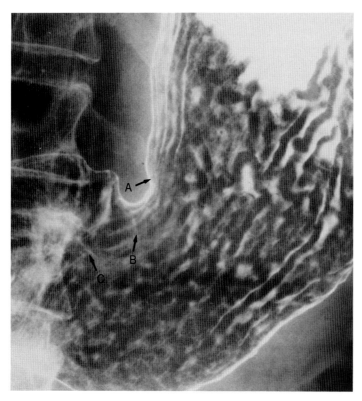

Fig. 599   Additional double contrast radiograph demonstrates the third cancerous lesion smaller than 5 mm (arrow C). This also was detected before surgery.

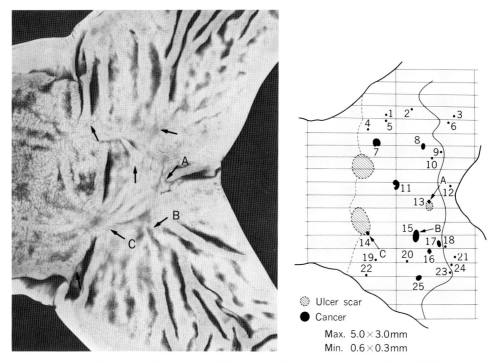

Max. 5.0 × 3.0mm
Min. 0.6 × 0.3mm

Fig. 600 Postoperative roentgenogram of the incised specimen. Three more lesions were detected in addition to those detected before surgery. However, it is difficult to diagnose malignancy in these 6 foci, even in this picture. Schematic representation showing the location of 25 foci of cancers measuring 5 mm. Histologic examination disclosed 25 foci of cancer all of which but one (arrow B) measured smaller than 5 mm. Histologically all foci were signet ring cell carcinoma.

Case 152 Microcarcinoma.
A 75-year-old man (JU). (Figs. 601-603)

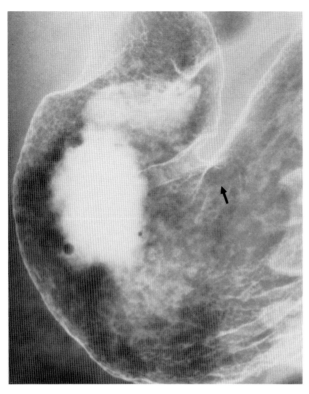

Fig. 601 Cancer measuring 1 mm. Double contrast radiograph demonstrates a faint fleck of barium with slight surrounding radiolucent halo on the posterior wall near the incisura (arrow).

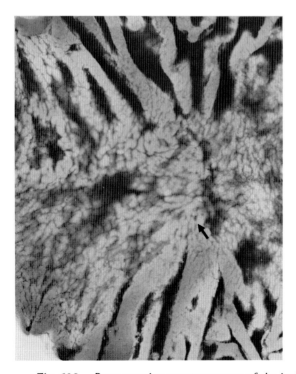

Fig. 602 Postoperative roentgenogram of the incised specimen. An arrow points to the site of the lesion.

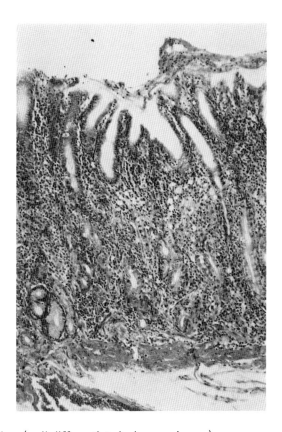

Fig. 603 Histologic findings showing adenocarcinoma tubulare (well differentiated adenocarcinoma).

Chapter 15

Miscellaneous Tumors of the Stomach

General Considerations

Most submucosal tumors can easily be differentiated from the various types of early gastric cancer. They are classified as Yamada-Fukutomi type I or II (refer to Fig. 140 in Chapter 4) and show gradual sloping to the surrounding normal mucosa. The surface of the tumors generally is smooth and not different from that of the surrounding normal mucosa. Radiographically, their outline is not as sharply defined as that of an epithelial tumor. In addition, their size changes to some extent as various degrees of compression are applied. Excessive compression may cause them to disappear. The most definite sign of a submucosal tumor is the presence of a bridging fold. Endoscopically, the above-mentioned findings are more pronounced.

The differential diagnosis is difficult in cases of small submucosal tumors with a central depression simulating a type IIa + IIc early cancer. Some type IIa + IIc lesions reveal mostly submucosal spread, with tumor tissue exposed only in a central depression (refer to Figs. 446—449 in Chapter 10). One must recognize the pattern of invasion of type IIa + IIc lesions as shown in Figure 441 (Chapter 10) and be very careful when obtaining biopsy specimens.

Localized Thickening of the Mucosa

This is seen as a long protuberance of the mucosal folds. Naturally, it occurs most frequently in the area of the mucosal folds, especially in the greater curvature of the gastric body. Compression should be applied and the direction and position of the patient should be changed. The lesion may look like a type IIa + IIc when the contrast medium is retained between the folds (Fig. 604), A frontal view is obtained by changing the position of the patient (Fig. 605). The lesion is usually effaced by strong compression. Localized thickening of a fold may simulate a small submucosal tumor when it is projected tangentially (Fig. 606).

Carcinoid Tumors of the Stomach

Carcinoid tumor is rarely found in the stomach. It arises from the deeper portion of the gastric mucosa and has the appearance of a submucosal tumor in its early phase. As the lesion increases in size, an erosion appears on the central surface, and, finally, an ulceration develops (Fig. 607). It is reported that 20 per cent of gastric carcinoid tumors become malignant (Peskin 1959). Although a few cases have been reported in which flushing attacks were associated with the carcinoid syndrome (Christodoulopoulos and Klotz 1961), this is only rarely seen in cases of small primary carcinoid tumor.

In most cases the surface of the carcinoid tumor has the same mucosal pattern as the normal surrounding mucosa (Fig. 608). In a large carcinoid tumor, the surface may show nodularity similar to that of epithelial tumors. In such cases, however, the characteristics of a submucosal tumor such as bridging folds (Fig. 607, arrows) or gradual sloping of the tumor to the surrounding normal mucosa, usually remain, at least partially.

In most cases radiographic and endoscopic examination is unable to definitively diagnose carcinoid tumor. Endoscopic biopsy plays a decisive role in establishing the diagnosis.

Case 153   Localized Thickening of the Mucosa.
A 39-year-old woman (JU). (Figs. 604 and 605)

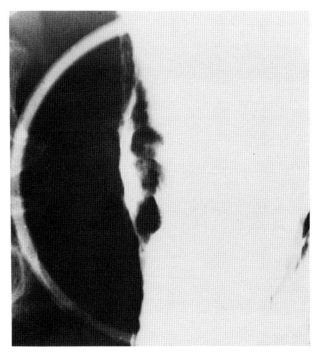

Fig. 604 Upright compression film demonstrates localized thickening of the mucosa at the lesser curvature of the gastric body. The contrast medium retained between the folds looks like an irregular niche.

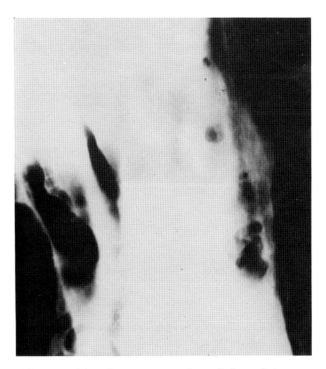

Fig. 605 Upright compression film in the right anterior oblique position demonstrates a frontal view of the lesion.

Case 154 Localized Thickening of the Mucosa.
A 39-year-old man (JU). (Fig. 606)

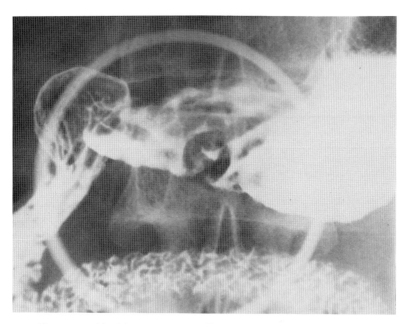

Fig. 606 Upright compression film demonstrates a tangential projection of a thickened fold at the antrum.

Case 155 Carcinoid.
A 61-year-old man (CPCC). (Fig. 607)

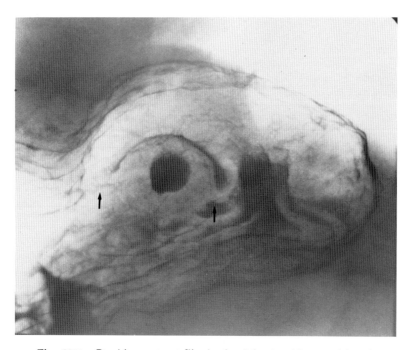

Fig. 607 Double contrast film in the right decubitus position demonstrates a large carcinoid tumor with central depression and bridging folds (arrows) at the upper gastric body.

Case 156　　Carcinoid.

A 52-year-old (JU). (Fig. 608)

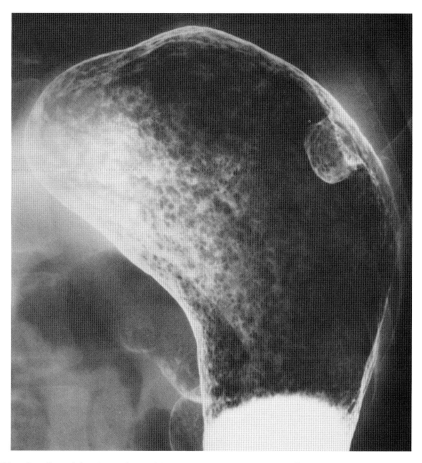

Fig. 608　Upright double contrast film in the right lateral position demonstrating a profile view of small carcinoid tumor on the anterior wall of the gastric fundus.

The lesion looks like a type I early cancer, but the surface pattern, which is the same as that of the normal mucosa, strongly suggests a submucosal origin.

Aberrant Pancreas

Aberrant pancreas usually presents as a submucosal tumor not larger than 2 cm in diameter, but sometimes intramuscular, serosal and intramucosal nodules occur. It consists of some or all of the elements of the normal pancreas and occasionally Brunner's gland (Figs. 609 and 610). The lesion is most frequently found in the gastric antrum.

Radiographically, aberrant pancreas appears as a round or oval tumor with a central depression (Fig. 611), pit or umbilication, and an ectopic excretory duct is rarely visualized. Usually, the central depression or umbilication is delineated as a small collection of barium. The lesion is best demonstrated by the compression method.

Case 157   Aberrant Pancreas.
A 46-year-old man (JU). (Figs. 609 and 610)

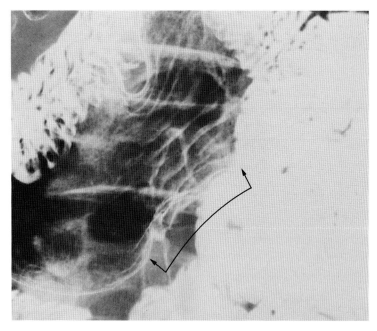

Fig. 609   Double contrast film demonstrates a profile view of Brunneroma at the greater curvature opposite to the gastric angle (arrow line).

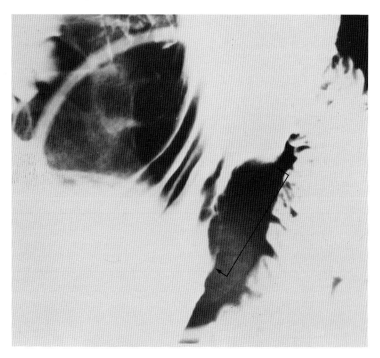

Fig. 610   Upright compression film demonstrating the profile view of the Brunneroma (arow line). Figures 609 and 610 reveal only that the lesion may be submucosal tumor (Yamada-Fukutomi type 2) with irregular surface.

Case 158 Aberrant Pancreas.
A 37-year-old man (CPCC). (Fig. 611)

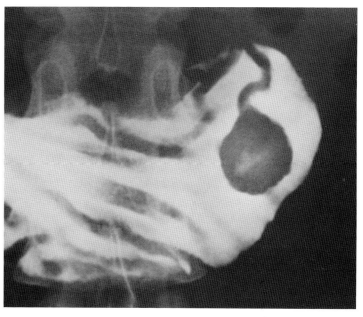

Fig. 611   Prone mucosal relief film demonstrating aberrant pancreas with slight central depression and bridging fold on the antrum.

Leiomyoma and Leiomyosarcoma

Leiomyoma and leiomyosarcoma are the most frequent submucosal tumors of the stomach. They are found most frequently in the upper portion of the stomach, but they can occur in any portion. The gastric fundus is a frequent site. The size of leiomyoma and leiomyosarcoma varies from 20 to 80 mm, and many of them are 30 to 40 mm.

Radiographically leiomyoma and leiomyosarcoma appears as round hemispherial tumor shadows, frequently with a central depression (Fig. 612–617). Their surface is usually smooth. Sometimes the central depression becomes so deep that it simulates a diverticulum. A large ulceration may be seen in leiomyosarcoma, and the lesion seems to be a Borrmann type 2 advanced cancer. The differential diagnosis of leiomyoma and leiomyosarcoma by radiography and endoscopy may be difficult. A bridging fold is a reliable sign of leiomyoma and leiomyosarcoma.

Sometimes, a tumor shadow is observed in a plain film and calcification occasionally may be found (Crummy and Juhl 1962). The tumor is delineated effectively by the double contrast and compression methods. The double contrast method is best able to delineate a lesion in the upper portion of the stomach where the compression method cannot be applied. When a tumor shows extragastric growth, it is better assessed by angiography and computerized tomography.

Neurogenic Tumors

Neurogenic tumors demonstrate the same radiographic features as myogenic tumors (Figs. 618 and 619). They cannot be distinguished from myogenic tumors macroscopically or radiographically. It is also difficult to distinguish benign and malignant forms. The tumor is most frequently found in the gastric body.

329

Case 159   Leiomyosarcoma.
A 55-year-old woman (CIH). (Figs. 612 and 613)

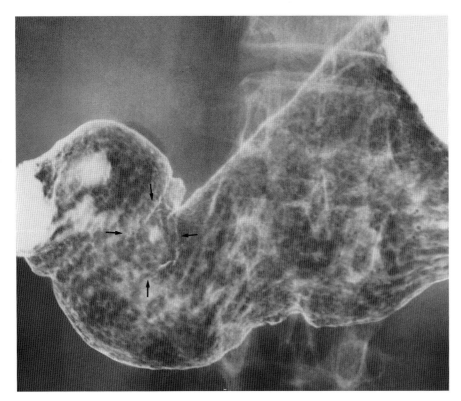

Fig. 612   Double contrast radiograph of a small leiomyosarcoma on the posterior wall of the incisura (arrows). Central depression is present.

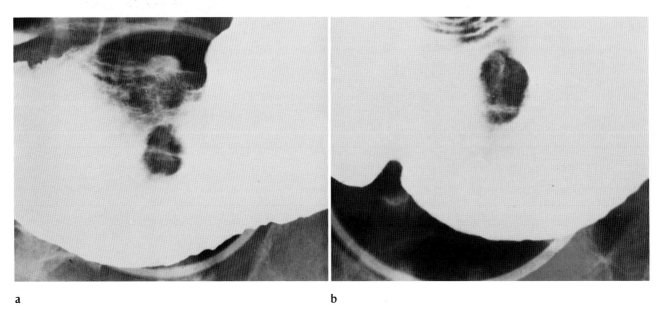

a   b

Fig. 613 a and b   Upright compression film. The central depression is faintly demonstrated in Figure 613 a.

Case 160 Leiomyosarcoma.

A 59-year-old man (RIH). (Fig. 614 and 615)

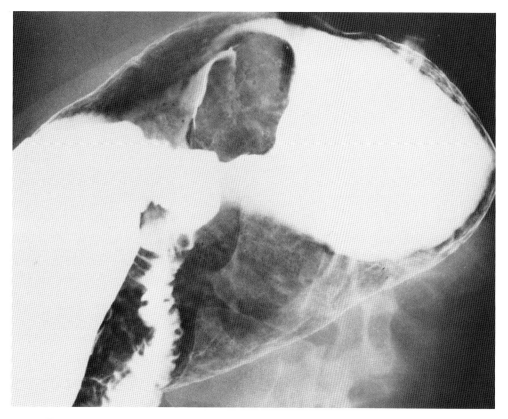

Fig. 614 Double contrast radiograph in the right lateral decubitus positions of a leiomyosarcoma on the cardiac region (en face view).

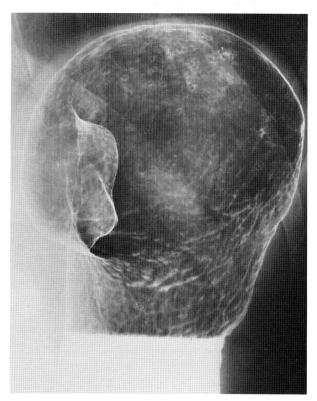

Fig. 615 Upright double contrast radiograph demonstrates a lateral view of the lesion.

Case 161   Leiomyosarcoma.
A 46-year-old woman (CIH). (Figs. 616 and 617)

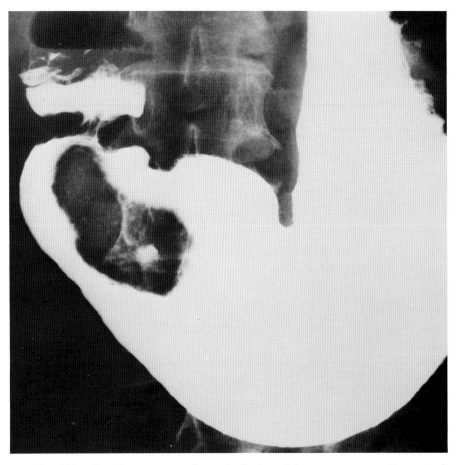

Fig. 616   Double contrast radiograph of a large leiomyosarcoma on the posterior wall of the antrum.

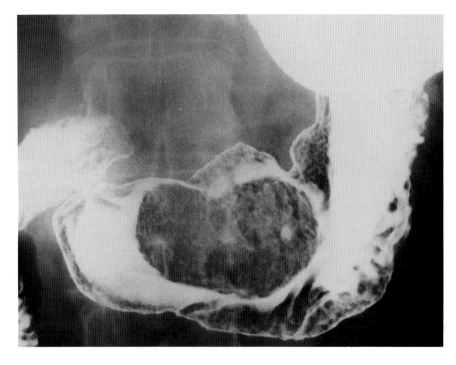

Fig. 617   Compression film.

Case 162 Neurogenic Tumor.
A 72-year-old woman (CPCC). (Figs. 618 and 619)

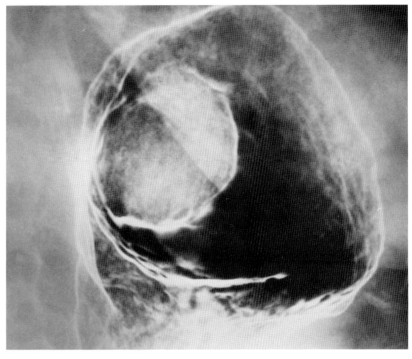

Fig. 618   Upright double contrast film demonstrates a frontal view of neurogenic tumor at the gastric cardia.

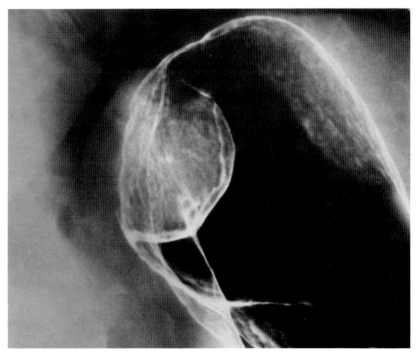

Fig. 619   Upright right anterior oblique double contrast film demonstrates a profile view of the neurogenic tumor.

Eosinophilic Granuloma

A circumscribed type of eosinophilic granuloma should be distinguished from a diffuse type of eosinophilic gastroenteritis.

The circumscribed type of eosinophilic granuloma was described by Vanek in 1949. It is a polypoid lesion arising in the submucosa, characterized by a variable degree of eosinophilic infiltration within fibroelastic tissue, collagen, blood vessels and lymphatic tissue often loosely arranged in whorled patterns. Helwig and Ranier (1953) called this tumor an inflammatory fibroid gastric polyp. Gastric anisakiasis has recently been found to be associated with eosinophilic granuloma of the stomach.

Radiographically, eosinophilic granuloma appears as an oval or round tumor shadow, suggesting a submucosal tumor (Figs. 620 and 621). A central depression is rarely seen.

Case 163   **Eosinophilic Granuloma.**
A 42-year-old man (JU). (Figs. 620 and 621)

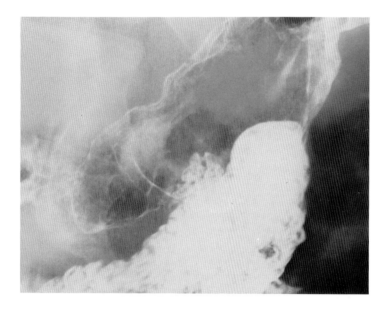

Fig. 620   Double contrast film demonstrating a faint radiolucency of eosinophilic granuloma on the posterior wall of the angular region.

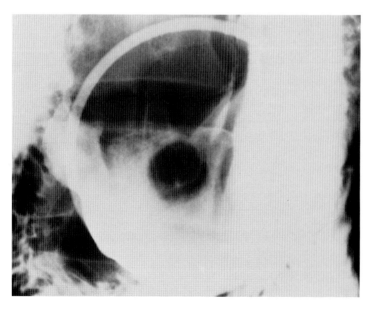

Fig. 621   Upright compression film demonstrating a round defect with smooth surface of eosinophilic granuloma.

References

Chapter 1 Definition and Classification of Early Gastric Cancer

References

Ariga, K.: Statistique sur le cancer de l'estomac a la lumière de la campagne de dépistage faute au Japon. *Ann. Gastroént. Hépatol.*, 6:307, 1970.

Borrmann, R.: Geschwülste des Magens und Duodenums, *in* Henke, F., Lubarsch, O. (eds): *Handbuch der speziellen pathologischen Anatomie und Histologie*, vol 4, part 1. Berlin, Springer-Verlag, 1926, pp 812–1054.

Broders, A.C.: The grading of carcinoma. *Minn. Med.*, 8:726, 1925.

Hayashida, T., Kidokoro, T.: End results of early gastric carcinoma. 4th World Congress of Gastroenterology, Copenhagen, 1970.

Hermanek, P., Rösch, W.: Critical evaluation of the Japanese "early gastric cancer" classification. *Endoscopy*, 5:220, 1973.

Ichikawa, H., *in discussion*: Re-evaluation of the classification of macroscopic findings of early gastric cancer (Panel discussion chaired by T. Murakami).(in Japanese) *I to Cho(Stomach and Intestine)*, 11:30, 1976.

Iwanaga, T., Taniguchi, H.: Klinische Pathologie des Magenfrühkarzinoms. *Leber, Magen, Darm.*, 3:54, 1973.

Japanese Research Society for Gastric Cancer: *The general rules for the gastric cancer study in surgery and pathology*, 10th ed.(in Japanese) Tokyo, Kanehara Shuppan, 1979.

Japanese Research Society for Gastric Cancer: The general rules for the gastric cancer study in surgery and pathology. *Jap. J. Surg.*, 11:127, 1981.

Johansen, A.A.: Early gastric cancer, *in* Morson, B.C. (ed): *Monograph on Pathology of the Gastrointestinal Tract; Current Topics in Pathology 63*. Berlin, Heidelberg, New York, Springer-Verlag, 1976.

Kajitani, T.: Clinical typing of stomach cancer and its significance.(in Japanese) *GANN(Japanese Journal of Cancer Research)*, 41:76, 1950.

Kasugai, T.: Gastric lavage cytology under direct observation with the fibergastroscope, *in* Murakami, T. (ed): *Early Gastric Cancer. GANN Monograph on Cancer Research*, vol 11. Tokyo, University of Tokyo Press, 1971/Baltimore, University Park Press, 1972, pp 207–221.

Kawai, K.: Validity rate of concerted diagnosis using various methods: Concerted diagnosis for type I to III lesions, *in* Murakami, T. (ed): *Early Gastric Cancer. GANN Monograph on Cancer Research*, vol 11. Tokyo, University of Tokyo Press, 1971/Baltimore, University Park Press, 1972, pp 273–282.

Kitaoka, H., Miwa, K.: End-result of the survival rate of early gastric cancer.(in Japanese) *Geka(Surgery)*, 36:1468, 1974.

Kumakura, K., Murayama, M., Sugiyama, N., et al.: Radiological diagnosis of type IIb and IIb-like lesions of the stomach.(in Japanese with English abstract) *I to Cho(Stomach and Intestine)*, 7:21, 1972.

Llorens, P.S.: *Diagnostico Endoscopico del Cancer Gastrico*, 2nd ed. Santiago, Universidad de Chile, 1975.

Maruyama, M., Sugiyama, N., Baba, Y., et al.: Radiodiagnostic possibility of gastric carcinoma involving the proper muscle layer.(in Japanese with English abstract) *I to Cho(Stomach and Intestine)*, 11:855, 1976.

Mochizuki, T., *in discussion*: Reevaluation of the classification of macroscopic findings of early gastric cancer (Panel discussion chaired by T. Murakami).(in Japanese) *I to Cho(Stomach and Intestine)*, 11:30, 1976.

Morson, B.C.: The Japanese classification of early gastric cancer, *in* Yardley, J.H., Morson, B.C., Abell, M.R. (eds): *The Gastrointestinal Tract. International Academy of Pathology Monograph*. Baltimore, The Williams & Wilkins Company, 1977, pp 176–183.

Murakami, T., Yasui, A., Takekawa, H., et al.: Non-cancerous regenerative epithelium in the central portion of scar-carcinoma of the stomach.(in Japanese) *Nippon Byori Gakkai Zasshi(Transactiones Societatis Pathologicae Japonicae)* 55:229, 1966.

Murakami, T.: New concept on ulcer-cancer of the stomach.(in Japanese) *Juntendo Igaku(Juntendo Medical Journal)*, 13:157, 1967.

Murakami, T.: Pathomorphological diagnosis. Definition and gross classification of early gastric cancer, *in* Murakami, T. (ed): *Early Gastric Cancer. GANN Monograph on Cancer Research*, vol 11. Tokyo, University of Tokyo Press, 1971/Baltimore, University Park Press, 1972, pp 53–55.

Murakami, T., *in discussion*: Reevaluation of the classification of macroscopic findings of early cancer. (Panel discussion chaired by T. Murakami).(in Japanese) *I to Cho(Stomach and Intestine)*, 11:30, 1976.

Nakamura, K., Sugano, H., Takagi, K., et al.: Histopathological study on early carcinoma of the stomach: Some

REFERENCES

considerations on the ulcus-cancer by analysis of 144 foci of the superficial spreading carcinomas. *GANN(Japanese Journal of Cancer Research)*, 58:377, 1967.

Nakamura, K.: *Pathology of Gastric Cancer: Microcarcinoma and its Histogenesis.*(in Japanese) Kyoto, Kimpo-do, 1972.

Nakamura, K., Sugano, H., Sugiyama, N., et al.: Clinical and histopathological features of scirrhous carcinoma of the stomach.(in Japanese with English abstract) *I to Cho(Stomach and Intestine)*, 11:1275, 1976.

Nishi, M., Nanasawa, T., Seki, M., et al.: On the five-year survival rate of stomach cancer: with special reference to advanced cancer.(in Japanese with English abstract) *I to Cho(Stomach and Intestine)*, 4:1087, 1969.

Okabe, H.: Growth of early gastric cancer, Clinical study of growth and invasion patterns of early gastric cancer; Its position in the natural history of gastric cancer. *in* Murakami, T. (ed): *Early Gastric Cancer. GANN Monograph on Cancer Research*, vol 11. Tokyo, University of Tokyo Press, 1971/Baltimore, University Park Press, 1972, pp 67—79.

Okabe, H., Mitsui, K., Tamechika, Y., et al.: Endoskopische Differential-diagnose des Magenfrükarzinoms. *Leber, Magen, Darm*, 3:64, 1973.

Okuda, S.: Differential diagnosis of early gastric carcinoma from advanced carcinoma, *in* Murakami, T. (ed): *Early Gastric Cancer. GANN Monograph on Cancer Research*, vol 11. Tokyo, University of Tokyo Press, 1971/Baltimore, University Park Press, 1972, pp 283—301.

Oota, K.: Histogenesis of gastric cancer.(in Japanese) *Nippon Byori Gakkai Zasshi(Transactiones Societatis Pathologicae Japonicae)*, 53:3, 1964.

Palmer, W.L.: Carcinoma of the stomach, *in* Bockus, H.L. (ed): *Gastroenterology*, vol 1. Philadelphia, W.B. Saudnders Company, 1974, pp 949—997.

Sano, R.: Histological studies on evolution site of gastric cancer based on analysis of early gastric cancer; Resent problems on ulcer-cancer sequence of the stomach.(in Japanese) *Nippon Rinsho(Japanese Journal of Clinical Medicine)*, 25:1329, 1967.

Sano, R., Hirota, T., Shimoda, T., et al.: Pathological evaluation of recurrence and mortality in early gastric cancer; Consideration on the pace of depth invasion of gastric cancer.(in Japanese with English abstract) *I to Cho(Stomach and Intestine)*, 5:531, 1970.

Sano, R.: Pathological analysis of 300 cases of early gastric cancer: With special reference to cancer associated ulcers. *in* Murakami, T. (ed): *Early Gastric Cancer. GANN Monograph on Cancer Research*, vol 11. Tokyo, University of Tokyo Press, 1971/Baltimore, University Park Press, 1972, pp 81—89.

Sano, R., *in discussion:* Reevaluation of the classification of macroscopic findings of early gastric cancer (Panel discussion chaired by T. Murakami).(in Japanese) *I to Cho(Stomach and Intestine)*, 11:30, 1976.

Shirakabe, H., Ichikawa, H., Kumakura, K., et al.: *Atlas of X-ray Diagnosis of Early Gastric Cancer.* Tokyo, Igaku-Shoin Ltd., 1966/Philadelphia, J.B. Lippincott Company, 1966.

Takagi, K., Nakada, K.: Lymphnode metastases and surgical results on early gastric cancer.(in Japanese) *Rinsho Geka(Journal of Clinical Surgery)*, 31:19, 1976.

Takagi, K., Nakajima, T., Adachi, H., et al.: A long term follow-up study of gastric cancer cases. (in Japanese) *Shujutsu (Operation)*, 32: 161, 1978.

Takemoto, T., Ichioka, S., Suzuki, S., et al.: The diagnosis of early gastric cancer through fibergastroscopic biopsy, *in* Murakami, T. (ed): *Early Gastric Cancer. GANN Monograph on Cancer Research*, vol 11. Tokyo, University of Tokyo Press, 1971/Baltimore, University Park Press, 1972, pp 233—241.

Ueno, K., Yamagata, S., Masuda, H., et al.: Clinical evaluation of gastric biopsy under direct vision in diagnosis of gastric cancer. 4th World Congress of Gastroenterology, Copenhagen, 1970.

Yamagata, S., Masuda, H.: Magenkarzinom, *in* Demling, L. (ed): *Klinische Gastroenterologie*, vol I. Stuttgart, Georg Thieme Verlag, 1973.

Bibliography

Ayabe, M.: Follow-up examination of carcinoma in situ of the stomach and minor gastric cancer.(in Japanese) *Gan no Rinsho(Japanese Journal of Cancer Clinics)*, 7:99, 1961.

Comfort, M.W., Gray, H.K., Dockerty, M.B., et al.: Small gastric cancer. *Arch. Intern. Med.*, 94:513, 1954.

Comfort, M.W., Priestley, J.T., Dockerty, M.B., et al.: The small benign and malignant lesion. *Surg. Gynec. Obstet.*, 105:435, 1957.

Elster, K., Kolazek, F., Shimamoto, K., et al.: Early gastric cancer: Experience in Germany. *Endoscopy*, 7:5, 1975.

Elster, K., Seifert, E.: *Magenfrühkarzinom*. Baden-Baden, Verlag Gerhard Witzstrock, 1979.

Evans, D.M.D., Craven, J.L., Murphy, F., et al.: Comparison of "early gastric cancer" in Britain and Japan. *Gut*, 19:1, 1978.

Fevre, D.I., Green, P.H.R., Barratt, P.J., et al.: Review of five cases of early gastric cancer. *Gut*, 17:41, 1976.

Finby, N., Eisenbud, M.: Carcinoma of the proximal third of the stomach: A critical study of roentgenographic observations in sixty-two cases. *JAMA*, 154:1155, 1954.

Gloor, F.: Das Oberflächenkarzinom (Frühkarzinom) des Magens. *Schweiz. Med. Wschr.*, 106:21, 1976.

Grogg, E.: Über Frühstudien des Magenkarzionms. *Radiol. Clin.*, 21:10, 1952.

Grundmann, E., Grunze, H., Witte, S.: *Early Gastric Cancer: Current Status of Diagnosis.* Berlin-Heidelberg-New York, Springer-Verlag, 1974.

Hayashida, T., Kidokoro, T.: End results of early gastric cancer collected from twenty-two institutions.(in Japanese with English abstract) *I to Cho(Stomach and Intestine)*, 4:1077, 1969.

Hirschowitz, B.I.: Early gastric cancer. *Gastroint. Endoscopy*, 23:45, 1976.

Inokuchi, K., Furusawa, M., Soejima, K., et al.: Prognosis of gastric cancer as seen from the developmental pattern.(in Japanese) *Gan no Rinsho(Japanese Journal of Cancer Clinics)*, 14:472, 1968.

Inokuchi K., Furusawa, M., Soejima, K.: Features of lymphnode metastases viewed from localization of stomach cancer.(in Japanese) *Gan no Rinsho(Japanese Journal of Cancer Clinics)*, 16:348, 1970.

Inokuchi, K., Ikeda, T., Furusawa, M., et al.: Late results of surgical therapy for stomach cancer.(in Japanese) *Gan no Rinsho(Japanese Journal of Cancer Clinics)*, 18:203, 1972.

Izumoi, S., Takahashi, K., Takagi, K.: The 5-year survival rate in the pm and ss cancer of the stomach with special reference to the analysis of the macroscopic classification.(in Japanese with English abstract) *Gan no Rinsho (Japanese Journal of Cancer Clinics)*, 21:841, 1975.

Jinnai, D., Ono, M., Sakakibara, N.: The necessity of extended radical surgery for gastric carcinoma.(in Japanese) *Geka(Surgery)*, 23:1099, 1961.

Jinnai, D., Tanaka, S., Ono, M., et al.: The necessity of extended radical surgery for gastric carcinoma correlated with lymph node metastasis.(in Japanese) *Geka (Surgery)*, 25:117, 1963.

Kajitani, T., Takagi, K.: Surgical treatment of early gastric carcinoma. *Gastroenterologica Japonica*, 2:294, 1967.

Kajitani, T., Takagi, K.: Cancer of the stomach at Cancer Institute Hospital, Tokyo. *in* Kajitani, T., Koyama, Y., Umegaki, Y. (eds): *Recent Results of Cancer Treatment in Japan, GANN Monograph on Cancer Research*, vol 22. Tokyo, Japan Scientific Societies Press/Baltimore, University Park Press, 1979, pp 77–87.

Kawai, K.: Classification of early gastric cancer.(in Japanese) *I to Cho(Stomach and Intestine)*, 11:25, 1976.

Kidokoro, T.: Frequency of resection, metastasis and five-year survival rate of early gastric carcinoma in a surgical clinic, *in* Murakami, T. (ed): *Early Gastric Cancer. GANN Monograph on Cancer Research*, vol 11. Tokyo, University of Tokyo Press, 1971/Baltimore, University Park Press, 1972. pp 45–49.

Koga, S., Makihara, S., Yamanouchi, Y.: Lymph nodes dessection in operation of gastric cancer and its follow-up result.(in Japanese) *Gan no Rinsho(Japanese Journal of Cancer Clinics)*, 16:316, 1970.

Konjetzny, G.E.: *in* Anschütz, W., Konjetzny, G.E. (eds): *Die Geschwülste des Magens, Deutsche Chirurgie*, vol 46. Stuttgart, Ferdinand Enke Verlag, 1921, p 46.

Konjetzny, G.E.: *Der Magenkrebs.* Stuttgart, Ferdinand Enke Verlag, 1938. pp 139–156.

Konjetzny, G.E.: Der oberflächliche Schleimhautkrebs des Magens: Ein weiter Beitrag zur Kenntnis des Magenkrebses im Beginn. *Chirurg.*, 12:192, 1940.

Konjetzny, G.E.: *Die Geschwürbildung im Magen, Duodenum and Jejunum.* Stuttgart, Ferdinand Enke Verlag, 1947.

Konjetzny, G.E.: Zur Frühdiagnose und Frühoperation des Magenkrebses. *Archiv. Klin. Chir.*, 246:331, 1950.

Muto, M., Maki. T., Majima, S., et al.: Improvement in the end-results of surgical treatment of gastric cancer. *Surgery*, 63:299, 1968.

Nagayo, T.: Microscopical cancer of the stomach: A study on histogenesis of gastric carcinoma. *Inter. J. Cancer*, 16:52, 1971.

Newcomb, W.D.: The relationship between peptic ulceration and gastric carcinoma. *Brit. J. Surg.*, 20:279, 1932.

Nishi, M., Nanasawa, T., Seki, M., et al.: On the five-year survival rate of stomach cancer.(in Japanese with English abstract) *I to Cho(Stomach and Intestine)*, 4:1087, 1969.

Omori, S.: The advanced cancer with good prognosis.(in Japanese with English abstract) *I to Cho(Stomach and Intestine)*, 3:971, 1968.

Prinz, H.: *Frühformen des Magenkrebses.* Hamburg, HH Nölke, 1947.

Rössle, R.: Über einen frühen Oberflächenkrebs der Magenschleimhaut. *Zbl. f. Allg. Pathol. u. Path. Anat.*, 165:82, 1944.

Schindler, R.: Early diagnosis and prognosis of gastric carcinoma. *JAMA*, 115: 1693, 1940.

Takagi, K.: Gastric Cancer.(in Japanese with English abstract) *Gan no Rinsho(Japanese Journal of Cancer Clinics)*, 21:1136, 1975.

Takagi, K., Ohashi, I., Takahashi, T., et al.: Some considerations of operation on early gastric cancer.(in Japanese) *Geka Chiryo(Surgical Therapy)*, 34:61, 1976.

Konjetzny, G.E.: The superficial cancer of the gastric mucosa. *Amer. J. Dig. Dis.*, 20:91, 1953.

Kuhlencordt, F.: Das Carcinoma in situ des Magens und der kleine Magenkrebs. Katamnestische Untersuchungen von 42 Fällen. *Dtsch. Med. Wschr.*, 47:2111, 1959.

Mainetti, J.M.: Cancer Gastrico. Diagnositico y Tratamiento. Buenos Aires, 1967.

Majima, S.: A critical evaluation of super radical gastrectomy (R_3) for cure of carcinoma of the stomach.(in Japanese) *Gan no Rinsho(Japanese Journal of Cancer Clinics)*, 16:340, 1970.

Mallory, T.B.: Carcinoma in situ of the stomach and its bearing on the histogenesis of malignant ulcers. *Arch. Pathol.*, 30:348, 1940.

Miller, G., Kaufmann, M.: Das Magenfrühkarzinom in Europa: 1170 Fälle aus den Jahren 1968–1973. *Dtsch. Med. Wschr.*, 100:1946, 1975.

Murakami, T., Nakamura, S., Suzuki, T.: Macroscopic Diagnosis of Early Ulcer-Cancer and Its Histologic Criteria.(in Japanese) *Rinsho Shokaki Byogaku(Clinical Gastro-enterology)*, 1:7, 1953.

Murakami, T.: Statistics on Ulcer-Cancer of the Stomach. (in Japanese) *Saishin Igaku(Modern Medicine)*, 8:277, 1953.

Murakami, T.: Pathology of Early Cancer of the Stomach. (in Japanese) *Gan no Rinsho(Japanese Journal of Cancer Clinics)*, 3:233, 1957.

Murakami, T., Yasui, A., Nakayama, A., et al.: Problems in early cancer of the stomach from the viewpoint of its histologic diagnosis.(in Japanese) *I to Cho(Stomach and Intestine)*, 1:111, 1966.

Rubio, H.H., Magnanini, F.L., Pardo, R.F. et al.: Cancer Gastrico Tempurano, Premio Cientifico "F. Antonio Rizzuto" Buenos Aires, 1971.

Takagi, K., Adachi, H., Nakajima, T., et al.: Four cases of gastric cancer recurrence with free interval of more than 10 years after gastrectomy.(in Japanese with English abstract) *I to Cho(Stomach and Intestine)*, 12:47, 1977.

Takagi, K., Ohashi, I., Ota, H., et al.: Historical transfiguration in gastric cancer.(in Japanese with English abstract) *I to Cho(Stomach and Intestine)*, 15:11, 1980.

Tasaka, S.: National statistics of early gastric cancer. *Gastroent. Endoscopy*, 4:4, 1962.

Watanabe, H., Enjoji, M., Imai, T.: Gastric carcinoma with lymphoid stroma: Its morphological characteristics and prognostic correlations. *Cancer*, 38:232, 1976.

Chapter 2   Principles and Application of Double Contrast Radiography

References

Frik, W.: Neoplastic diseases of the stomach, *in* Margulis, A.R., Burhenne, H.J. (eds): *Alimentary Tract Roentagenology.* St. Louis, The C.V. Mosby Company, 1973.

Kumakura, K., Fuchigami, A., Takagi, K.: X-ray diagnosis of anterior lesions of the stomach.(in Japanese) *Rinsho Hoshasen(Japanese Journal of Clinical Radiology),* 10:787, 1965.

Kumakura, K.: A guide to double contrast method: X-ray demonstration of type IIc.(in Japanese with English abstract) *I to Cho(Stomach and Intestine),* 4:915, 1969.

Laufer, I., Kressel, H.Y.: *Residents' Manual for Gastrointestinal Radiology,* Gastrointestinal Section, Department of Radiology, Hopsital of the University of Pennsylvania. Philadelphia, 1978.

Laufer, I.: *Double Contrast Gastrointestinal Radiology with Endoscopic Correlation.* Philadelphia, W.B. Saunders Company, 1979.

Maruyama, M.: Early gastric cancer, *in* Laufer, I. (ed): *Double Contrast Radiology.* Philadelphia, W.B. Saunders Company, 1979, pp 241—288.

Nakamura, K., Sugano, H., Takagi, K., et al.: Conception of histogenesis of gastric carcinoma.(in Japanese with English abstract) *I to Cho(Stomach and Intestine),* 6:849, 1971.

Schatzki, R., Gary, J.E.: Face-on demonstration of ulcers in the upper stomach in a dependent position. *Amer. J. Roent.,* 79: 772, 1958.

Shirakabe, H., Ichikawa, H., Kumakura, K., et al.: *Atlas of X-ray Diagnosis of Early Gastric Cancer.* Tokyo, Igaku-Shoin Ltd., 1966/Philadelphia, J.B. Lippincott Company, 1966.

Shirakabe, H. (ed): *Double Contrast Studies of the Stomach.* Tokyo, Bunkodo Co. Ltd., 1971/Stuttgart, Georg Thieme Verlag, 1972.

Bibliography

Bartram, C.I., Kumar, P.: *Clinical Radiology in Gastroenterology.* Oxford, Blackwell Scientific Publications, 1981.

Burhenne, H.J.: Technique of examination of the stomach and duodenum, *in* Margulis, A.R., Burhenne, H.J. (eds): *Alimentary Tract Roentgenology.* St. Louis, The C.V. Mosby Co, 1967, pp 425—449.

Chapman, W.P., Wyman, S.M., Mora, L.O., et al.: Barium studies of comparative action of Banthine, tincture of belladonna and placebos on motility of gastrointestinal tract in man. *Gastroenterology,* 23:234, 1953.

Doi, H.: Clinical and experimental study on the X-ray findings taken by double contrast technique in case of early gastric cancer.(in Japanese) *Nippon Shokaki Byo Gakkai Zasshi(Japanese Journal of Gastroenterology),* 6:502, 1967; 6:595, 1967.

Frik, W., Zeidner, A.: Röntgenuntersuchungen des Magenfeinreliefs. 1 Mitteilung. *Fortschr. Röntgenstr.,* 79:681, 1953.

Frik, W.: The combination of different methods in X-ray diagnosis of stomach cancer and the improvement of cancer detection by the use of intensifying systems. The Proceedings of the 3rd World Congress of Gastroenterology, Tokyo 1:260, 1966.

Frik, W.: Die Röntgenologie des Magens, *in* Boecker, W. (ed): *Speiseröhre-Magen,* Stuttgart, Georg Thieme Verlag, 1967.

Frik, W.: Neoplastic diseases of the stomach, *in* Margulis, A., Burhenne, H.J. (eds): *Alimentary Tract Roentgenology.* St. Louis, The C.V. Mosby Company, 1979.

Gelfand, D.W., Hachiya, J.: The double-contrast examination of the stomach using gas-producing granules and tablets. *Radiology,* 93:1381, 1969.

Golden, R., Cimmino, C.V., Collins, L.C., et al.: *in* Robbins, L.L. (ed): *Golden's Diagnostic Radiology,* Sect 5. Baltimore, Williams & Wilkins Company, 1969.

Goldstein, H.M.: Double-contrast gastrography. *Amer. J. Dig. Dis.,* 21: 797, 1976.

Hedemand, N., Mathiasen, M.S.: Double contrast roentgenography of the stomach. *Danish. Med. J.,* 136:1079, 1974.

Heitzeberg, H., Treichel, J.: Intensivierte Röntgendiagnostik des Magens mittels Doppelkontrast, Erfahrungsbericht über ein neues Zusatzpräparat zur Kontrastmitteluntersuchung. *Fortschr. Röntgenstr.,* 116:529, 1972.

Herlinger, H., Glanville, J.N., Kreel, L.: An evaluation of the double contrast barium meal (DCBM) against endoscopy. *Clin. Radiol.,* 28:307, 1977.

Hilpert, F.: Das Pneumorelief des Magens. *Fortschr. Röntgenstr.,* 38:80, 1928.

Hunt, J.H., Anderson, I.F.: Double contrast upper gastrointestinal studies. *Clin. Radiol.,* 27:87, 1976.

Ichikawa, H., Yamada, T., Doi, H., et al.: X-ray diagnosis of early gastric cancer: Recent progress of diagnositic technique.(in Japanese) *Gan no Rinsho(Japanese Journal of Cancer Clinics),* 9:683, 1963.

Ichikawa, H., Yamada, T., Doi, H.: *Practical Radiology of the Stomach; For the Diagnostis of Early Gastric Cancer.* Tokyo, Bunkodo, 1964.

Kreel, L., Herlinger, H., Glanville, J.: Technique of the double contrast barium meal with examples of correlation with endoscopy. *Clin. Radiol.,* 24:307, 1973.

Kumakura, K., Maruyama, M., Someya, N.: X-ray demonstration of lesions in the anterior wall of the stomach.(in Japanese with English abstract) *I to Cho(Stomach and Intestine),* 3:873, 1968.

Laufer, I.: A simple method for routine double contrast study of the upper gastrointestinal tract. *Radiology,* 117:513, 1975.

Laufer, I., Mullens, J.E., Hamilton, J.: Correlation of endoscopy and double contrast radiography in the early stages of ulcerative and granulomatous colitis. *Radiology,* 118:105, 1976.

Laufer, I.: Assessment of the accuracy of double-contrast gastroduodenal radiology. *Gastroenterology,* 71:874, 1976.

Menkes, B.: Zur Röntgenanatomie der Magenschleimhaut des Menschen; Ein Beitrag zum Problem der Reliefdarstellung. *Fortschr. Röntgenstr.,* 48:17, 1933.

Miller, R.E., Chernish, S.M., Skucas, J., et al.: Hypotonic roentgenography with glucagon. *Amer. J. Roent.,* 121: 264, 1974.

Miller, R.: The air-contrast stomach examination; An overview. *Radiology,* 117:743, 1975.

Obata, W.G.: A double contrast technique for examination

of the stomach using barium sulfate with semithicone. *Amer. J. Roentgen.*, 115:275, 1972.

Op den Orth, J.O.: *Radiological Examination of the Gastrointestinal Tract*, vol. 1. The Standard Biphasic-Contrast Examination of the Stomach and Duodenum. Hauge-Boston-London, Martinus Nijhoff Medical Division, 1979.

Prévôt, R.: *Grundriss der Röntgenologie des Magen-Darm-Kanals.* Hamburg, HH Nölke, 1948.

Prévôt, R.: Roentgenology of the duodenum, *in* Margulis, A.R. and Burhenne, H.J. (eds): Alimentary Tract Roentgenology, vol. 1. St. Louis, The C.V. Mosby Co, 1967, pp 522–545.

Quattromani, F., Finby, N.: Roentgenographic double-contrast examination of stomach and duodenum. N.Y. State J. Med., 72: 1140, 1972.

Sakamoti, T., Igarashi, T., Tsunoda, S., et al.: Radiologic findings of type IIc early gastric cancer.(in Japanese) *Nippon Shokaki Byo Gakkai Zasshi(The Japanese Journal of Gastroenterology)*, 74:696, 1977.

Scott-Harden, W.G.: Evaluation of double contrast gastro-duodenal radiology. *Proc. Brit. Inst. Radiol.*, 46:153, 1973.

Shirakabe, H. (ed): *Double Contrast Studies of the Stomach.*(in Japanese) Tokyo, Bunkodo, 1970.

Solanke, T.F., Kumakura, K., Maruyama, M., et al.: Double-contrast method for evaluation of gastric lesions. *Gut*, 10:436, 1969.

Tanaka, H., Fukumoto, S., Tanaka, M., et al.: Double contrast method for anterior wall lesions with a small amount of air.(in Japanese) *Rinsho Hoshasen(The Japanese Journal of Clinical Radiology)*, 11:952, 1966.

Treichel, J., Oeser, J.: Die Doppelkontrastmethode; Optimale Technik der röntgenologischen Magenuntersuchung. *Dtsch. Med. Wschr.*, 100:2226, 1975.

Teichel, J.: *Doppelkontrastuntersuchung des Magens; Untersuchungs-technik und systematische Morphologie der Magenerkrankungen.* Stuttgart, Georg Thieme Verlag, 1982.

Tsunoda, S., Igarashi, T., Kodama, T., et al.: Radiologic findings of type IIc early cancer of the stomach with special reference to changing aspects of double contrast images by difference in volume of air,.(in Japanese) *Nippon Shokaki Byo Gakkai Zasshi(The Japanese Journal of Gastroenterology)*, 70:997, 1973.

Chapter 3   Diagnosis of Gastric Cancer

Bibliography

Abel, W.: Grenzen der röntgenologischen Magendiagnostik unter besonderer Berücksichtigung der Gastroskopie. *Zschr. Ärtl. Fortbild*, 35:73, 1938.

Albot, G., Toulet, J.: Rapports entre les lésions histologiques et signes radiologiques des cancers de la muqueuse gastrique. *Arch. Mal. Appar. Dig.*, 40:5, 1951.

Albot, G.: Pharmaco-radiography of stomach and duodenum. *Amer. J. Dig. Dis.*, 19:18, 1952.

Albrecht, H.U.: *Die Röntgendiagnostik des Verdauungskanals.* Leipzig, Gerog Thieme Verlag, 1931, (Stuttgart, Georg Thieme Verlag, 1950.)

Amberg, J.R.: Accuracy of roentgen diagnosis in carcinoma of the stomach. *Amer. J. Dig. Dis.*, 5:259, 1960.

Bellin, A.: *Les Gastrites Ulcéreuses; Etude Anatomoclinique et Endoscopique (Thèse).* Paris, 1941.

Benedict, E.B.: The value of gastroscopy in diagnosis. *Radiology*, 29: 480, 1937.

Benedict, E.B.: Correlation of gastroscopic, roentgenologic and pathologic findings in diseases of the stomach; An analysis of 145 proceed cases. *Amer. J. Roentgenol.*, 55: 251, 1946.

Beranbaum, S.L., Stassa, G., Yaghmai, M., et al.: *Fluoroscopy and Radiography of the Gastrointestinal Tract.* Wilmington, Del, duPont Company, 1967.

Berg, H.H.: Beitrag zur röntgenologischen Magendiagnostik. *Chirurg.*, 2:143, 1930.

Berg, H.H.: *Röntgenuntersuchungen am Innenrelief des Verdauungskanals.* Leipzig, Georg Thieme Verlag, 1930.

Berg, H.H.: *Die Frühdiagnose des Magenkrebses.* Vortrag im ärztlichen Verein, Hamburg, 1939.

Brodmerkel, G.L.: Gastroduodenoscopy and X-ray; A comparison, *Gastroenterology*, 62:884, 1972.

Brünner, S., Rahbek, I., Mosbich, J.: Roentgenologic and gastrocamera examinations in the differential diagnosis of gastric ulcer. *Amer. J. Roentgenol.*, 104:598, 1968.

Bücker, J.: Die Frühdiagnose des Magenkrebses im Röntgenbild. *Fortschr. Röntgenstr.*, 63:1, 1941.

Bücker, J.: *Die Diagnose des kleinen Magenkrebses.* Berlin, Springer-Verlag, 1944.

Bücker, J.: *Gastritis, Ulkus und Karzinom.* Stuttgart, Georg Thieme Verlag, 1950.

Buckstein, J.: *The Digestive Tract Roentgenology*, 2nd ed. Philadelphia-London-Montreal, J.B. Lippincott Company, 1953.

Cornet, A.: Confrontation de la radiologie et de la gastrscopie en pathologie gastrique, *in* Albot, G., Poilleux, F. (eds): *L'estomac.* Paris, Masson & Cie, 1954.

del Mazo, J., Korapa, V.S.: Comparison of endoscopy and radiology in the diagnosis of gastric ulcer, *Gastroenterology*, 62:888, 1972.

Doi, H.: Radiologic Diagnosis of small early gastric cancer. (in Japanese) *I to Cho(Stomach and Intestine)*, 2:451, 1967.

Duval, P., Roux, J. -Ch., Béclére, H., et al.: Les plis de la muqueuse gastrique; Etude comparative de leur expression radiologique, des aspects macroscopiques et des lésions histologiques. IIIe Congrès International de Radiologie, Paris, 1931, p 23.

Dyes, O.: Das Röntgenrelief der Magenschleimhaut. *Fortschr. Röntgenstr.*, 43:1, 1931.

Eisler, F.: Zur röntgenologischen Frühdiagnose des Magenkrebses. *Fortschr. Röntgenstr.*, 54:289, 1936.

Fischer, H., Schlotter, H.: Zur Frühdiagnose des Magenkrebses im Beginn. *Zbl. Chir.*, 76: 789, 1951.

Forssell, G.: Über Beziehungen der Röntgenbilder des menschlichen Magens zu seinem anatomischen Bau. *Fortschr. Röntgenstr.*, 30 (suppl), 1913.

Fukuchi, S.: A case of early gastric cancer proved by biopsy but was considered as of benign nature by X-ray and endoscopy.(in Japanese with English abstract) *I to Cho(Stomach and Intestine)*, 4:971, 1969.

Gütemann, R.: *Das Magen- und Kardia-Karzinom.* Stuttgart, Ferdinand Enke Verlag, 1964.

Gutmann, R.A.: Le diagnostic précoce due cancer gastrique. IIe Congrès International de Gastroenterologie, Paris, 1937.

Gutmann, R.A., Bertrand, I.: Le cancer gastrique érosif a marche lente. Press Méd., 46:814, 1938.

Gutmann, R.A., Bertrand, I., Peristiany, T.J.: Le Cancer de l'Estomac au Début. Paris, G. Doin, 1939.

Gutmann, R.A.: Le Diagnostic du Cancer d'estomac à la Période Utile. Paris, G. Doin & Cie, 1959.

Gutmann, R.A., Daoud, J.: Longue évoluation du cancer gastrique. The Proceedings of the 3rd World Congress of Gastroenterology, Tokyo 1: 534, 1966.

Gutmann, R.A.: Le Diagnostic du Cancer d'éstomac Précoce & Avancé, Paris, G. Doin & Cie, 1967.

Gutmann, R.A.: Some problems about gastric cancer. I to Cho(Stomach and Intestine), 5:1337, 1970.

Gutmann, R.A.: Forty years of early diagnosis of gastric cancer, in Grundman, E., Grunze, H. (eds): Early Gastric Cancer, Current Status of Diagnosis. Berlin-Heidelberg-New York, Springer-Verlag, 1974, pp 69–75.

Hafter, E.: Praktische Gastroenterologie, 5th ed. Stuttgart, Georg Thieme Verlag, 1973.

Hanerin, L.G., Margulis, A.R.: Radiologische Diagnostik des Magenkarzinoms. Leber, Magen, Darm, 6:97, 1976.

Henning, N., Heinkel, K., Frik, W.: Röntgenbefund am Feinrelief und bioptischhistologisches Bild der Magenschleimhaut. Dtsch. Med. Wschr., 85:873, 1960.

Henning, N., Kolokussis, H., Heinkel, K., et al.: Die Sicherheit der bioptischen Gastritisdiagnose. Dtsch. Med. Wschr., 87:1029, 1962.

Higurashi, K.: Studies on x-ray diagnosis of early gastric cancer: Especially of the method to find early gastric cancer.(in Japanese) Nippon Shokaki Byo Gakkai Zasshi (Japanese Journal of Gastro-enterology), 64:71, 1967; 64:197, 1967.

Hisamichi, S., Sugawara, N., Fuchigami, A., et al.: False negative rate of stomach cancer in gastric mass survey.(in Japanese) Gan no Rinsho(Japanese Journal of Cancer Clinics), 24:189, 1978.

Holmes, G.W., Schatzki, R.: Examination of the mucosal relief as a diagnostic aid in diseases of the gastrointestinal tract. Amer. J. Roentogenol., 34:145, 1935.

Horikoshi, H.: Studies on mass survey of the stomach; With special reference to the detection of early gastric cancer.(in Japanese) I Gan to Shudan Kenshin(Gastric Cancer and Mass Survey), 7:6, 1965.

Irie, H., Shirakabe, H.: Diagnosis of carcinoma of the upper part of the stomach.(in Japanese) Nippon Igaku Hoshasen Gakkai Zasshi(Nippon Acta Radiologica), 27:799, 1967.

Jutras, A.: L'aasociation des rayons X et de la Gastroscopie dans le diagnostic du cancer de l'estomac. IIe Congrès International de Gastroenterologie, Paris, 1937.

Kalokerinos, J.: Gastro-camera and barium studies of the normal convergence of folds in the gastric fundus and the features distinguishing this from ulceration. Australian Radiol., 13:173, 1969.

Kase, S.: Clinical roentgenological study on carcinoma of the cardiac portion of the stomach.(in Japanese) Nippon Igaku Hoshasen Gakkai Zasshi(Nippon Acta Radiologica), 20:271, 1960.

Kawai, K., Matsuda, I., Seo, I., et al.: Radiologic diagnosis of anterior wall lesions in routine examination.(in Japanese) Rinsho Hoshasen(Japanese Journal of Clinical Radiology), 12:648, 1967.

Kawai, K., Tanaka, H.: Differential Diagnosis of Gastric Diseases. Tokyo, Igaku-Shoin Ltd, 1974/Berlin-Heidelberg-New York, Springer-Verlag, 1974.

Keutner, H.: Die heutige Treffsicherheit der Röntgendiagnose bei Erkrankungen des Magens und Zwölffingerdarmes. Fortschr. Röntgenstr., 60:421, 1939.

Kirklin, B.R.: Relative merits of gastroscopic and roentgenologic examinations. Radiology, 29:492, 1937.

Kirklin, B.R.: Mistakes and misunderstandings in the roentgenologic diagnosis of gastric cancer. Arch. Surg., 46:861, 1943.

Konjetzny, G.E.: Wege zur Frühdiagnose des Magen Krebses. Arch. f. Verdauungskrankh., 62:282, 1938.

Kumakura, K., Maruyama, M., Someya, N., et al.: X-ray diagnosis of the lesion in the greater curvature of the stomach.(in Japanese with English abstract) I to Cho (Stomach and Intestine), 4:5, 1969.

Kumakura, K.: Compression study in demonstrating type IIc on the greater curvature of the stomach.(in Japanese with English abstract) I to Cho(Stomach and Intestine), 6:1063, 1971.

Kurokawa, T., Masuda, H.: Radiographic findings of gastric cancer.(in Japanese) Saishin Igaku(Modern Medicine), 14:35, 1959.

Kurokawa, T., Kajitani, T., Oota, K. (eds): Carcincoma of the Stomach in Early Phase; Clinical Diagnosis, Pathology and Treatment. Tokyo, Nakayama Shoten, 1966.

Kuru, M. (ed): Atlas of Early Carcinoma of the Stomach.(in Japanese) Tokyo, Nakayama Shoten, 1966.

Laufer, I., Mullens, J.E., Hamilton, J.: The diagnostic accuracy of barium studies of the stomach and duodenum; Correlation with endoscopy. Radiology, 115:569, 1975.

Lenk, R.: Die Frühdiagnose des Magenkarzinoms. Wiener Klin. Wschr., 47:818, 1934.

Llorens, P.S.: Diagnostico Endoscopico del Cancer Gastrico, 2nd ed. Santiago, Universidad de Chile, 1975.

Machadao, G., Davies, J.D., Tudway, A.J.C., et al.: Superficial carcinoma of the stomach. Br. Med. J., 2:77, 1976.

Massa, J.: Le Petit Cancer de L'estomac. Paris, Masson & Cie, 1961.

Miller, G., Kaufmann, M.: Magenfrühkarzinoma; Endoskopie oder Radiologie? Dtsch. Med. Wschr., 101:1006, 1976.

Mori, T., Momiyama, T., Kobayashi, S., et al.: A case of early cancer in the greater curvature of the gastric body.(in Japanese) I to Cho(Stomach and Intestine), 2:805, 1967.

Morrissey, J.F.: The diagnosis of early gastric cancer: A survey of experience in the United States. Gastroint. Endoscopy, 23:13, 1976.

Nakano, H., Kumakura, K., Maruyama, M., et al.: Radiologic diagnosis of depressed early cancer in the greater curvature of the stomach.(in Japanese) Rinsho Hoshasen(Japanese Journal of Clinical Radiology), 14:907, 1969.

Prévôt, R.: Der kleine Magenkrebs, in Schinz, H.R., Glauner, R., Uehlingen, E. (eds): Röntgendiagnostik, Ergebnisse 1952–1956. Stuttgart, Georg Thieme Verlag, 1957.

Renshaw, R.J.F.: Correlation of roentgenologic and gastroscopic examination. Amer. J. Roentgen., 51:585, 1944.

Scarrow, G.D., Rad, M.: Radiology of the stomach and the gastric camera. *Brit. J. Radiol.*, 40:23, 1967.

Schindler, R., Templeton, F.: Comparison of gastroscopic and roentgen findings. *Radiology*, 29:472, 1937.

Schlotter, H.: Zur Röntgendiagnose des oberflächlichen Magenschleimhautkrebses. *Bruns Beitr. Klin. Chir.*, 191:269, 1955.

Schwarz, S.: Zur röntgenologischen Frühdiagnose des Carcinoms am Magen-Darmkanal. *Wien Med. Wschr.*, 84:89, 1934.

Schwarz, S.: Grundsätzliches zur röntgenologischen Frühdiagnose der Carcinoms am Magen-Darmtrakt. The Proceedings of the 4th International Congress of Radiology, 2:269, 1934.

Shirakabe, H., Nishizawa, M., Higurashi, K.: X-ray diagnosis of early gastric cancer.(in Japanese) *I to Cho(Stomach and Intestine)*, 1:229, 1966.

Shirakabe, H., Nishizawa, M., Higurashi, K., et al.: Early gastric cancer and some problems on the diagnosis of early gastric cancer.(in Japanese) *Rinsho Hoshasen (Japanese Journal of Clinical Radiology)*, 12:110, 1967.

Shirakabe, H., Nishizawa, M., Higurashi, K., et al.: Differential diagnosis of early gastric cancer by radiology with endoscopic correlation.(in Japanese) *I to Cho(Stomach and Intestine)*, 2:595, 1967.

Shirakabe, H.: X-ray diagnosis or early gastric cancer, *in* Murakami, T. (ed): *Early Gastric Cancer. GANN Monograph on Cancer Research*, vol 11. Tokyo, University of Tokyo Press/Baltimore, University Park Press, 1972, 1971, pp 105—111.

Shirakabe, H., Hayakawa, H., Itai, Y., et al.: Comparison of X-ray, endoscopy and biopsy examinations for the diagnosis of early gastric cancer. *Jap. J. Clin. Oncol.*, 12:93, 1972.

Shirakabe, H.: Röntgendiagnostik des Magenfrühkarzinoms. *Leber, Magen, Darm*, 2:129, 1972.

Shirakabe, H., Nishizawa, M., Hayakawa, H., et al.: Röntgenologisch-endoskopische Diagnostik des Magenfrühkarzinoms. *Leber, Magen, Darm*, 3:60, 1973.

Sokolow, J.N., Antonowitsch, W.B.: Zur Röntgendiagnostik des Karzinoms des oberen Magenabschnitts. *Fortschr. Röntgenstr.*, 95:585, 1960.

Strandjord, N.M., Morseley, R.D., Jr, Schweinefus, R.L.: Gastric carcinoma: Accuracy of radiologic diagnosis. *Radiology*, 74:442, 1960.

Templeton, F.E.: *X-ray Examination of the Stomach.* Chicago, University of Chicago Press, 1944.

Teschendorf, W.: *Lehrbuch der röntgenologischen Differentialdiagnostik*, vol II. Stuttgart, Georg Thieme Verlag, 1964.

Teschendorf, W., Wenz, W.: *Röntgenologische Differentialdiagnostik* Vol II: Erkrankungen der Bauchorgane, 5th ed. Stuttgart, Georg Thieme Verlag, 1978.

von Elischer, J.: Über eine Methode zur Röntgenuntersuchung des Magens. *Fortschr. Röntgenstr.*, 18:332, 1912.

Walder, E.: Zur röntgenologischen Diagnose des früh exulzerierten primären Magenkrebses und der krebsigen Entartung des gewöhnlichen Magengeschwürs im Frühstadium. Schweiz. Med. Wschr., 71:1585, 1941.

Watanabe, N.: Diagnostic accuracy of X-ray TV indirect roentgenography of the stomach with eighteen films.(in Japanese) *Nippon Igaku Hoshasen Gakkai Zasshi(Nippon Acta Radiologica)*, 31:286, 1971.

Chapter 4   Theoretical Basis for the Radiographic Diagnosis of Polypoid Early Cancer

References

Evans, R.W.: *Histological Appearances of Tumour.* London, E & S Livingstone, 1964.

Fukuchi, S., Mochizuki, T.: The significance of FGS biopsy in the diagnosis of polypoid lesions of the stomach.(in Japanese) *Gastroenterological Endoscopy*, 9:105, 1967.

Fujii, A., Funada, A.: On the follow-up after endoscopic polypectomy.(in Japanese) *Progress Digest Endoscopy*, 14:19, 1979.

Furusawa, M.: Endoscopic diagnosis of submucosal tumors of the stomach.(in Japanese) *I to Cho(Stomach and Intestine)*, 1:899, 1966.

Kosaki, G., Iwanaga, T., Kumano, T., et al.: Diagnosis of early gastric cancer.(in Japanese) *Geka Chiryo(Surgical Therapy)*, 16:299, 1967.

Maruyama, M.: Radiologic Diagnosis of Polyps and Carcinoma of the Large Bowel. Tokyo and New York, Igaku-Shoin, 1978.

Ming, S.C., Goldman, H.: Gastric polys. A histogenetic classification and its relation to carcinoma. *Cancer*, 18:1721, 1965.

Nakamura, K., Sugano, H., Takagi, K., et al.: Conception of histogenesis of gastric carcinoma.(in Japanese with English abstract) *I to Cho(Stomach and Intestine)* 6:849, 1971.

Nakamura, K., Takagi, K.: Some considerations on lesion of atypical epithelium of the stomach.(in Japanese with English abstract) *I to Cho(Stomach and Intestine)*, 10:1455, 1975.

Nakamura, K., Takagi, K., Sugano, H.: Pathology of polyp of the stomach and problems on its malignant transformation.(in Japanese) *Nippon Rinsho(Japanese Journal of Clinical Medicine)*, 34:1341, 1976.

Nishizawa, M.: Endoscopic study of early gastric cancer. (in Japanese with English abstract) *Gastroent. Endoscopy*, 8: 203, 1966.

Nishizawa, M., Yoshikawa, Y., Shirakabe, H., et al.: Radiologic diagnosis of polypoid lesions of the stomach. Part 1 Macroscopic classification for the differential diagnosis of polypoid lesions.(in Japanese) *Rinsho Hoshasen(Japanese Journal of Clinical Radiology)*, 13:1, 1968.

Nishizawa, M.: Pre-operative estimation of the depth of invasion in gastric carcinoma with central depression and peripheral elevation (Early carcinoma type IIa+IIc and advanced carcinoma type Borrmann 2).(in Japanese with English abstract) *I to Cho(Stomach and Intestine)*, 12:1217, 1977.

Oota, K.: Genesis of gastric cancer.(in Japanese) *Nippon Byori Gakkai Zasshi(Transactiones Societatis Pathologicae Japonicae)*, 53:3, 1964.

Stout, A.P.: *Tumor of the stomach. Atlas of Tumor Pathology*, Section VI, Fascile 21, Washington DC, Armed Forces Institute of Pathology, 1953.

Sugiyama, N., Ochiai, H., Kumakura, K., et al.: On macroscopic findings and radiologic diagnosis of polypoid lesions of the stomach.(in Japanese) *Nippon Shoka-*

REFERENCES

ki Byo Gakkai Zasshi(Japanese Journal of Gastroenterology), 69:547, 1972.

Takagi, K., Kumakura, K., Sugano, H., et al.: Clinic-pathological study on polypoid lesions of the stomach with special reference to atypical epithelial lesions.(in Japanese) *Gan no Rinsho(Japanese Journal of Cancer Clinics)*, 13:809, 1967.

Takagi, K.: Some problems in diagnosis of early gastric cancer: Type IIa and atypical epithelium.(in Japanese) *I to Cho(Stomach and Intestine)*, 3:15, 1968.

Utsumi, Y.: The limitations of endoscopic diagnosis of early gastric cancer.(in Japanese) *Nippon Rinsho (Japanese Journal of Clinical Medicine)*, 25:1361, 1967.

Watanabe, H., Enjoji, M., Yao, T., et al.: Gastric lesions in familial adenomatosis coli.(in Japanese with English abstract) *Fukuoka Acta Medica*, 67:255, 1976.

Watanabe, H., Enjoji, M., Yao, T., et al.: Gastric lesions in familial adenomatosis coli. Their incidence and histologic analysis. *Human Pathology*, 9:269, 1978.

Yamada, T., Fukutomi, H.: Polypoid lesions of the stomach.(in Japanese) *I to Cho(Stomach and Intestine)*, 1:145, 1966.

Yoshikawa, Y.: X-ray diagnosis of elevated and protruded lesion of the stomach.(in Japanese) *Chiba Igakkai Zasshi(Journal of Chiba Medical Society)*, 43:358, 1967.

Bibliography

Albot, G., Toulet, J.: Substratum histologique des signes radiologiques de suspicion du cancer gastrique au début et des lesions capables de les simuler. The Proceedings of the 3rd World Congress of Gastroenterology, Tokyo 1:267, 1966.

Aoki, N., Fujiwara, M., Iwama, T., et al.: Gastric lesion of familial polyposis coli.(in Japanese with English abstract) *I to Cho(Stomach and Intestine)*, 10:361, 1975.

Berg, J.W.: Histological aspects of the relation between gastric adenomatous polyps and gastric cancer. *Cancer*, 11:1149, 1958.

Heitzeberg, H., Treichel, J.: Intensivierte Röntgendiagnostik des Magens mittels Doppelkontrast: Erfahrungsbericht über ein neues Zusatzpräparat zur Kontrastmitteluntersuchung. *Fortschr. Röntgenstr.*, 116:529, 1972.

Kuramata, H., Unayama, S., Eto, Y., et al.: Case study on IIa type early cancer of the stomach.(in Japanese) *Nippon Shokaki Byo Zasshi(Japanese Journal of Gastroenterology)*, 72:1050, 1975.

Ming, S.C.: *Tumor of the Esophagus and Stomach, The Atlas of Tumor Pathology*, 2nd series, Fasc 7, Washington DC, Armed Forces Institute of Pathology, 1973.

Murakami, T., Hojo, Y., Ohtsuka, K., et al.: Studies on polyps and polypoid cancer of the stomach.(in Japanese) *Gan no Rinsho(Japanese Journal of Cancer Clinics)*, 2:544, 1956.

Murakami, T.: Gastric polyps, *in* Kuru, M. (ed): Surgical Pathology, vol. 2.(in Japanese), Tokyo, Igaku-Shoin, 1963, p 166.

Murakami, T., Shirakabe, H., Ichikawa, H., et al.: Polypoid lesions of the stomach.(in Japanese) *Geka(Surgery)*, 29:1360, 1967.

Muto, T.: Study on polypogenesis and malignant degeneration of adenomatous polyps of the stomach.(in Japanese) *Gan no Rinsho(Japanese Journal of Cancer Clinics)*, 16:95, 1970.

Muto, T., Shimazu, H., Kobori, O., et al.: Malignant transformation of benign gastric polyps: Report of a case.(in Japanese with English abstract) *I to Cho (Stomach and Intestine)*, 10:341, 1975.

Nagayo, T.: Histological criteria of malignant transformation of gastric polyp and its results.(in Japanese with English abstract) *I to Cho(Stomach and Intestine)*, 10:301, 1975.

Nakajima, T.: Radiologic examination of gastric polyp.(in Japanese) *Chiba Igakkai Zasshi(Journal of Chiba Medical Society)*, 35:2620, 1960.

Nakamura, T.: The concept of gastric polyp(in Japanese) *I to Cho(Stomach and Intestine)*, 1:639, 1966.

Nakamura, T.: Malignant transformation of gastric polyps. (in Japanese) *I to Cho(Stomach and Intestine)*, 3:737, 1968.

Nakamura, T.: Gastric polyp resembling adenoma of the colon.(in Japanese) *Nippon Shokaki Byo Gakkai Zasshi (Japanese Journal of Gastroenterology)*, 68:1043, 1971.

Nakamura, T.: Relation between polyps and so-called precancerous lesions of the stomach, *in* Tsuneoka, K. (ed.): *Internal Medicine Series, no. 8. Early Gastric Cancer.*(in Japanese) Tokyo, Nankodo, 1972.

Nakamura, T., Nakano, G.: Malignant change of gastric polyps with special reference to type IV polyp.(in Japanese with English abstract) *I to Cho(Stomach and Intestine)*, 10:369, 1975.

Prévôt, R.: Zur röntgenologischen Diagnostik des sogenannten "Etát mamelonné." *Fortschr. Röntgenstr.*, 71:55, 1949.

Sano, R.: Classification of adenomatous polyp of the stomach and its malignant transformation.(in Japanese) *I to Cho(Stomach and Intestine)*, 1:725, 1968.

Shirakabe, H., Oda, K., Haraikawa, M., et al.: Polypoid lesion of the stomach and its surrounding mucosa.(in Japanese) *Nippon Rinsho(Japanese Journal of Clinical Medicine)*, 34:1350, 1976.

Sugano, H., Nakamura, K., Takagi, K., et al.: Morphogeneses of polyp; polyp-cancer and polypoid cancer and their frequency.(in Japanese) *I to Cho(Stomach and Intestine)*, 3:729, 1968.

Sugiyama, N.: Macroscopic findings and X-ray diagnosis of polypoid lesions of the stomach. XIth Meeting of the Japanese Society of Gastroenterology, 1971.

Tumasulo, J.: Gastric polyps; Histological types and their relationship to gastric carcinoma. *Cancer*, 27:1346, 1971.

Utsunomiya, J., Iwana, T., Watanabe, M.: A case of familial polyposis of the colon associated with multiple polyps of the stomach.(in Japanese with English abstract) *I to Cho(Stomach and Intestine)*, 7:1041, 1972.

Walk, L.: Gastroscopic definition of Etát Mammelonné. *Acta Med. Scand.*, 127:261, 1947.

Yamada, T., Ichikawa, H.: X-ray diagnosis of elevated lesions of the stomach. *Radiology*, 110:79, 1974.

Chapter 5 The concept of Atypical Epithelium (ATP) and Its Radiographic Characteristics

References

Enjoji, M., Watanabe, H.: Adenoma of the stomach; A borderline lesion.(in Japanese with English abstract) *I to Cho(Stomach and Intestine)*, 10:1443, 1975.

Fukuchi, S., Hiyama, M., Mochizuki, T., et al.: Malignant transformation of gastric polyps, based on follow-up study by biopsy.(in Japanese) *Rinsho Kagaku(Journal of Clinical Science)*, 8:1362, 1972.

Ishidate, T.: A borderline lesion of the stomach.(in Japanese) *I to Cho(Stomach and Intestine)*, 10:1465, 1975.

Kino, I., Oota, K., Kobori, O.: Various types of lesions composed of atypical epithelia in the stomach.(in Japanese) *Proceedings of the Japanese Cancer Association*, 28:176, 1969.

Nagayo, T.: Borderline lesion of gastric mucosa; Elevated and excavated type.(in Japanese with English abstract) *I to Cho(Stomach and Intestine)*, 10:1437, 1975.

Nakamura, K., Sugano, H., Takagi, K., et al.: Histogenesis of atypical epithelium of the stomach.(in Japanese) *Gan no Rinsho(Japanese Journal of Cancer Clinics)*, 15:955, 1969.

Nakamura, K., Takagi, K.: Some considerations on lesion of atypical epithelium of the stomach.(in Japanese) *I to Cho(Stomach and Intestine)*, 10:1455, 1975.

Nakamura, T., Iwamaru, M., Takekawa, K.: Pathology (classification) of gastric polyps.(in Japanese) *Nippon Geka Gakkai Zasshi(Journal of Japan Surgical Society)*, 63:949, 1962.

Nakamura, T., Nakano, G.: Problems on adenoma of the stomach.(in Japanese) *Nippon Rinsho(Japanese Journal of Clinical Medicine)*, 34:1368, 1976.

Oota, K.: Genesis of gastric cancer.(in Japanese) *Nippon Byori Gakkai Zasshi(Transactiones Societatis Pathologicae Japonicae)*, 53:3, 1964.

Sano, R.: Borderline lesions of the stomach.(in Japanese) *I to Cho(Stomach and Intestine)*, 10:1433, 1975.

Takagi, K.: Type IIa and ATP; Problems on early gastric cancer.(in Japanese) *I to Cho(Stomach and Intestine)*, 3:15, 1968.

Taniguchi, H., Wada, A., Tateishi, R., et al.: Some considerations on the lesion of the stomach which appeared histologically on the borderline between benignancy and malignancy.(in Japanese with English abstract) *I to Cho(Stomach and Intestine)*, 10:1449, 1975.

Yamada, T., Kimura, T., Keida, Y., et al.: X-ray diagnosis of borderline lesions between malignancy and benignancy.(in Japanese with English abstract) *I to Cho(Stomach and Intestine)*, 10:1479, 1975.

Bibliography

Endo, T.: A clinico-pathological study on comparison between lesions of atypical epithelium and early differentiated carcinomas of the stomach.(in Japanese) *Iwate Igaku Zasshi(Iwate Medical Journal)*, 29:555, 1977.

Fukuchi, S., Hiyama, M., Mochizuki, T.: Endoscopic diagnosis of IIa-subtype of polypoid lesions which belong to borderline lesions between benignancy and malignancy.(in Japanese with English abstract) *I to Cho(Stomach and Intestine)*, 10:1487, 1975.

Morson, B.C.: Gastric polyps composed of intestinal epithelium. *Brit. J. Cancer*, 9:550, 1959.

Nakamura, K., Sugano, H., Takagi, K., et al.: Histological study on early carcinoma of the stomach; Criteria for diagnosis of atypical epithelium. *GANN(Japanese Journal of Cancer Research)*, 57:613, 1966.

Yoshii, T.: Borderline lesion of benign and malignant epithelial cells in stomach.(in Japanese with English abstract) *I to Cho(Stomach and Intestine)*, 10:1471, 1975.

Chapter 6 Theoretical Basis for the Radiographic Diagnosis of Depressed Early Cancer

References

Baba, Y., Narui, T., Ninomiya, T., et al.: A comparative study between radiolobic and macroscopic findings of early gastric carcinoma with IIb-like intramucosal spread; With special reference to radiologic definition of proximal boundary.(in Japanese with English abstract) *I to Cho(Stomach and Intestine)*, 12:1087, 1977.

Kumakura, K., Maruyama, M., Sugiyama, N., et al.: Limitation in radiological diagnosis of malignant ulcer of the stomach.(in Japanese with English abstract) *I to Cho(Stomach and Intestine)*, 8:1183, 1973.

Maruyama, M.: Early gastric cancer, in Laufer, I. (ed): *Double Contrast Radiology*. Philadelphia, W.B. Saunders Company, 1979, pp 241–288.

Murakami, T., Yasui, A., Takekawa, H., et al.: Non-cancerous regenerative epithelium in the central portion of scar-carcinoma of the stomach.(in Japanese) *Nippon Byori Gakkai Zasshi(Transactiones Societatis Pathologicae Japonicae)*, 55:229, 1966.

Murakami, T.: A new concept on ulcer-cancer of the stomach.(in Japanese) *Juntendo Igaku(Juntendo Medical Journal)*, 13:157, 1967.

Nakamura, K., Sugano, H., Takagi, K., et al.: Conception of histogenesis of gastric carcinoma.(in Japanese with English abstract) *I to Cho(Stomach and Intestine)*, 6:849, 1971.

Shirakabe, H., Ichikawa, H.: Early gastric cancer, in Hodes, P.J. (ed): *An Atlas of Tumor Radiology*. Chicago, Year Book Medical Publishers Inc, 1973.

Bibliography

Abel, W.: Grundsätzliches zur Röntgendiagnose des kleinen Magenkrebses. *Bruns Beitr. Klin. Chir.*, 184:1, 1952.

Abel, W.: Oberflächlicher Schleimhautkrebs des Magens. *Fortschr. Röntgenstr.*, 77:743, 1952.

Arai, S., Igarashi, T., Anzai, Y., et al.: Comparison of ulcer scar in IIc type early cancer and ulcer scars of the stomach.(in Japanese) *Nippon Shokaki Byo Gakkai Zasshi(Japanese Journal of Gastroenterology)*, 74:166, 1977.

Baba, Y., Sugiyama, N., Maruyama, M., et al.: A comparative study between histopathological and radiological findings of depressed early carcinoma of the stomach.(in

Japanese with English abstract) *I to Cho(Stomach and Intestine)*, 10:37, 1975.

Dworken, H.J., Roth, H.P., Duber, H.C.: The efficacy of medical criteria in differentiating benign from malignant gastric ulcers. *Ann. Int. Med.*, 47:711, 1957.

Elliot, G.V., Wald, S.M., Benz, R.I.: A roentgenologic study of ulcerating lesions of the stomach. *Amer. J. Roentgenol.*, 77:612, 1957.

Fujiwara, T., Hirokado, H., Yao, T., et al.: Observations on diagnostic problems in depressed type early gastric cancer.(in Japanese with English abstract) *I to Cho (Stomach and Intestine)*, 6:157, 1971.

Fukuchi, S.: Clinical diagnosis and problems of type III early gastric cancer.(in Japanese with English abstract) *I to Cho(Stomach and Intestine)*, 7:171, 1972.

Furusawa, M.: Six cases of type III early gastric cancer.(in Japanese with English abstract) *I to Cho(Stomach and Intestine)*, 7:177, 1972.

Horikoshi, H., Yamada, T., Doi, H., et al.: On the diagnosis of type III early gastric cancer.(in Japanese with English abstract) *I to Cho(Stomach and Intestine)*, 7:145, 1972.

Ichikawa, H.: The differential diagnosis between benign and malignant ulcers of the stomach. *Clin. Gastroent.*, 2:239, 1976.

Igarashi, T.: X-Ray findings of IIc type early cancer: With special reference to comparison of pre- and postoperative images.(in Japanese) *I to Cho(Stomach and Intestine)*, 8:750, 1973; 8:926, 1973; 8:1104, 1973; 8:1334, 1973; 8:1462, 1973.

Kalokerinos, J.: The "distorted spoke" sign of malignant gastric ulceration. *Australian Radiol.*, 11:150, 1967.

Kasugai, T., Aoki, I.: Diagnosis of type III early gastric carcinoma; From endoscopic standpoint.(in Japanese with English abstract) *I to Cho(Stomach and Intestine)*, 7:163, 1972.

Kidokoro, T., Koshikawa, K., Takezoe, K., et al.: A case of type III+IIc early cancer.(in Japanese) *I to Cho(Stomach and Intestine)*, 2:1315, 1967.

Koga, M., Nakata, H., Kiyonari, H., et al.: Roentgen feature of the superficial depressed type of early gastric carcinoma. *Radiology*, 115:289, 1975.

Kumakura, K., Maruyama, M., Sugiyama, N., et al.: Detailed diagnosis of lesions on the anterior wall of the stomach.(in Japanese with English abstract) *I to Cho (Stomach and Intestine)*, 6:1405, 1971.

Kuramata, H., Unayama, S., Eto, S., et al.: Benign lesions of the stomach which appeared malignant: An analysis of gastroscopic findings of the depressed type by gastric biopsy.(in Japanese) *I to Cho(Stomach and Intestine)*, 6:299, 1971.

Lloyd, G.A.S., Morris, J.L.: Malignant gastric ulceration; A review of 26 cases in which there was delay in the diagnosis. *J. Fac. Radiologists*, 7:207, 1956.

Mitsui, K., Okabe, H., Hirokado, K.: Diagnosis of type III early gastric cancer.(in Japanese) *I to Cho(Stomach and Intestine)*, 7:153, 1972.

Nakai, I., Takezono, K., Kenda, T., et al.: A case of III+IIc type early gastric cancer.(in Japanese with English abstract) *I to Cho(Stomach and Intestine)*, 4:995, 1969.

Nakazawa, S., Hayakawa, R., Furuhashi, S., et al.: One case of III+IIb type early gastric cancer.(in Japanese with English abstract) *I to Cho(Stomach and Intestine)*, 3:989, 1968.

Nelson, S.W.: The discovery of gastric ulcers and the differential diagnosis between benignancy and malignancy. *Radiol. Clin. N. Amer.*, 7:5, 1969.

Okabe, H.: Diagnosis of small III+(IIc) early cancer.(in Japanese) *I to Cho(Stomach and Intestine)*, 5:501, 1970.

Ritvo, M., Shauffer, I.A.: Superficial spreading carcinoma of the stomach, *in* Gastrointestinal X-Ray Diagnosis. Philadelphia, Lea & Febiger, 1952.

Ruyeon, W.K., Hoerr, S.O.: The gastric ulcer problem: Prognosis in masked malignancy. *Gastroenterology*, 32:415, 1957.

Schumacher, F.V., Hampton, A.O.: Radiographic differentiation of benign and malignant gastric ulcer. Ciba Clin. Symposia, 8:161, 1956.

Sherman, R.S., Wilner, D.: Superficial spreading gastric carcinoma; Is it detectable roentgenologically? *Amer. J. Roentgenol.*, 79:781, 1958.

Stein, G.N., Paustian, F.F., Finkelstein, A.F., et al.: Accuracy of X-ray diagnosis of ulcerating gastric lesion. *Amer. J. Gastroenterol.*, 36:148, 1961.

Stein, G., Finkelstein, A.: Roentgenologic classification of ulcerating gastric lesions, *in* Bockus, H.L. (ed): *Gastroenterology*, vol 1, 2nd ed. Philadelphia, W.B. Saunders Company, 1963, pp 517–518.

Stein, G.N., Tachdjian, V.O., Magid, N., et al.: Balloon radioautography in differentiation of benign and malignant gastric lesions. *Arch. Intern. Med.*, 115:326, 1965.

Windholtz, F.: Zur Differentialdiagnose gutartiger und bösartiger Schleimhauthyperplasien des Magens. *Radiol. Rundschau.*, 5:93, 1936.

Wolf, B.S.: Observations on roentgen features of benign and malignant gastric ulcers. *Semin. Roentgenol.*, 6:140, 1971.

Chapter 7   Radiographic Diagnosis of Peptic Ulcer

References

Assmann, H.: *Die klinische Röntgendiagnostik der inneren Enkrankungen*, 6th ed. Berlin-Göttingen-Heidelberg, Springer-Verlag, 1949/50.

Baensch, W.E.: Röntgendiagnose des Ulcus. *Fortschr. Röntgestr.*, 35:669, 1926.

Bayer, L.: Über eine neue Möglichkeit therapeutischer Beeinflussung akuter Magengeschwüre. *Dtsch. Med. Wschr.*, 62:636, 1936.

Berg, H.H.: *Röntgenuntersuchungen am Innenrelief des Verdanungskanals*. Stuttgart. Georg Thieme Verlag, 1930.

Bockus, H.L.: *Gastroenterology*, vol 1, 2nd ed. Philadelphia, W.B. Saunders Company, 1963.

Bücker, J.: *Gastritis, Ulkus und Karzinom*. Stuttgart, Georg Thieme Verlag, 1950.

Carman, R.D.: Benign and malignant gastric ulcer from a roentgenologic viewpoint. *Amer. J. Roentgenol.*, 8:695, 1921.

Chaul, H.: Das Schleimhautrelief des Magens im Röntgenbilde. *Dtsch. Zschr. Chir.*, 214:351, 1921.

Chaul, H.: Das Schleimhautrelief des Magens im Röntgen-bilde. *Fortschr. Röntgenstr.*, 39:505, 1929.

Chaul, H., Adam, A.: *Die Schleimhaut des Verdau-ungskanals.* Berlin-Wien, Urban & Schwarzenberg, 1931.

Eisler, R., Lenk, R.: Die Bedeutung der Faltenzeichnung des Magens für die Diagnose des Ulcus ventriculi. *Dtsch. Med. Wschr.*, 47:1459, 1921.

Eschbach, H.: Röntgenstudien zur Geschwürskrankheit. *Fortschr. Röntgenstr.*, 71:436, 1949.

Eschbach, H.: *Röntgenbeurteilung der Ulcuskranheit.* Leipzig, Georg Thieme Verlag, 1949.

Forssell, G.: Normale und pathogische Reliefbilder der Schleimhaut; Ein Überblick über die Autoplastik des Digestionskanals. *Verh. Ges. Verdauungskrkh.*, 7:199, 1927.

Frik, W.: Erosionen der Magenschleimhaut, *in* Schinz, H.R., Baenisch, W.B., Frommhold, W., et al. (eds): *Lehrbuch der Röntgendiagnostik*, vol. V. Stuttgart, Georg Thieme Verlag, 1965, pp 85—104.

Gonoi, T., Igarashi, T., Iino, F., et al.: Radiographic findings of ulcer scar of the stomach.(in Japanese) *Rinsho Hoshasen(Japanese Journal of Clinical Radiology)*, 10:589, 1965.

Gonoi, T., Igarashi, T., Anzai, S.: Scar zone of gastric ulcer and its clinical significance.(in Japanese) *I to Cho (Stomach and Intestine)*, 10:153, 1975.

Gutmann, R.A.: *Le Diagnostic du Cancer D'estomac a la Periode Utile.* Paris, G. Doin & Cie, 1956.

Gutzeit, K.: Die Gastroskopie im Rahmen der klinischen Magendiagnostik. *Erg. Inn. Med.*, 35:1, 1929.

Haenisch, F.: *in* Haenisch, F., Holthusen.(eds): *Einführung in die Röntgenologie.* Leipzig, Georg Thieme Verlag, 1951.

Hampton, A.O.: A safe method for the roentgen demonstration of bleeding duodenal ulcers. Amer. J. Roentgenol., 38:565, 1937.

Haudek, M.: Zur röntgenologischen Diagnose der Ulzerationen in der Pars media des Magens. Münch. Med. Wschr., 57:1587, 1910.

Hauser, F.: Die peptischen Schädigungen des Magens, des Duodenums und der Speiseröhre und des peptische postoperative Jejunalgeschwür, *in* Henke, F., Lubarsch, O. (eds): *Handbuch der Speziellen Pathologischen Anatomie und Histologie*, vol. 4, part 1. Berlin, Julius Springer, 1926, pp 339—811.

Igarashi, I., Gonoi, T.: X-ray findings of gastric ulcerscars. *Jap. J. Clin. Oncol.*, 2: 99, 1972.

Ito, T.: A radiological study of the prognosis of gastric ulcers.(in Japanese) *Chiba Igakkai Zasshi(Journal of Chiba Medical Society)*, 45:920, 1969.

Ivy, A.G., Crossman, M.I., Bachrach, W.H.: *Peptic Ulcer.* Philadelphia and Toronto, The Blakiston Co., 1950.

Katsch, G., Pickert, H.: Das Ulcus des Magens und Zwölffingerdarmes, *in* Bergmann, G., Frey, W., Schwiegk, H. (eds): *Handbuch der Inneren Medizin*, vol. 3, part 1, 4th ed. Berlin, Springer-Verlag, 1953.

Koide, H.: Histopathological studies on the distribution and healing tendency of gastric ulcer.(in Japanese) *Showa Igakkai Zasshi(Showa Medical Journal)*, 20:1700, 1961.

Konjetzny, G.E.: Entzündliche Genese des Magen-Duodenalgeschwürs; Ein Beitrag zur Kenntnis der Ätiologie, Pathogenese und Therapie des Magen-Duodenalgeschwürs. *Arch. Verdauungskrkh.*, 36:189, 1926.

Kuhlmann, F., Rating, B.: Röntgenatlas der Erkrankungen des Magendarmkanals und der Gallenblase. Berlin-Wien, Urban & Schwarzenberg, 1950.

Kumakura, K.: Roentgenological study on gastric ulcer.(in Japanese with English abstract) *Nippon Igaku Hoshasen Gakkai Zasshi(Nippon Acta Radiologica)*, 19:2663, 1960.

Kumakura, K.: Peptic ulcer of the stomach.(in Japanese) *Sogo Rinsho(Clinic All-around)*, 14:1628, 1965.

Kumakura, K., Takagi, K., Nakamura, K., et al.: Radiologic diagnosis of multiple ulcers of the stomach.(in Japanese) *I to Cho(Stomach and Intestine)*, 2:1139, 1967.

Kurokawa, T.: *Radiologic Diagnosis of the Alimentary Tract*, vol. 1.(in Japanese) Tokyo, Nakayama Shoten, 1956.

Meuwissen, T.J.J.H.: *X-Ray Atlas and Manual of Esophagus, Stomach and Duodenum.* Amsterdam, Elsevier, 1955.

Murakami, T., Suzuki, T., Nakamura, S., et al.: Symmetrical ulcer of the stomach.(in Japanese) *Geka(Surgery)*, 16:701, 1954.

Murakami, T., Suzuki, T.: Linear ulcer of the stomach and duodenum.(in Japanese) *Shokaki Byo no Rinsho(Journal of Clinical Digestive Diseases)*, 1:83, 1959.

Murakami, T., Matsui, T., Koide, H., et al.: Surgical indication for gastric ulcer: From the pathological viewpoint.(in Japanese) *Saishin Igaku(Modern Medicine)*, 14:1013, 1959.

Murakami, T.: Healing tendency of peptic ulcer of the stomach and duodenum as seen in resected stomach.(in Japanese) *Nippon Shokaki Byo Gakkai Zasshi(Japanese Journal of Gastroenterology)*, 58:1181, 1961.

Nishizawa, M., Ito, T., Kariya, A.: Stomach, *in* Saitoh, T., Yamashita, H., Tasaka, A., et al. (eds): *Clinical X-Ray Diagnosis*, vol. 4—1, Abdomen.(in Japanese) Tokyo, Igaku-Shoin Ltd, 1970, pp 87—256.

Porcher, P., Stössel, H.U., Mainguet, P.: *Klinische Radiologie des Magens und des Zwölffingerdarms.* Stuttgart, Georg Thieme Verlag, 1959.

Prévôt, R., Lasrich, M.A.: *Röntgendiagnostik des Magen-Darmkanals.* Stuttgart, Georg Thieme Verlag, 1959.

Reiche, F.: Zur Diagnose des Ulcus ventriculi im Röntgenbild. *Fortschr. Geb. Röntgenstr.*, 14:171, 1909.

Rendich, R.A.: The roentgenographic study of the mucosa in normal and pathological states. Amer. J. Roentgenol., 10:526, 1923.

Riedel: Die Entgernung des mittleren Abschnittes vom Magen wegen Geschwür. *Dtsch. Med. Wschr.*, 35:17, 1909.

Schinz, H.R., Baensch, W.E., Friedel, E., et al.: *Lehrbuch der Röntgendiagnostik*, vol. 4. Stuttgart, Georg Thieme Verlag, 1952.

Schmieden, V., Härtel, F.: Röntgenuntersuchung chirurgischer Magenkrankheiten. *Berlin Klin. Wschr.*, 46:669, 1909; 46:721, 1909.

Shirakabe, H., Kumakura, K., Ito, S., et al.: Radiographic study on peptic ulcer of the stomach.(in Japanese) *Nippon Igaku Hoshasen Gakkai Zasshi(Nippon Acta Radiologica)*, 16:471, 1956.

Shirakabe, H., Kumakura, K., Ito, S., et al.: Radiologic diagnosis of symmetrical ulcers of the stomach.(in Japanese) *Rinsho Hoshasen(Japanese Journal of Clinical Radiology)*, 1:535, 1956.

REFERENCES

Shirakabe, H., Kumakura, K., Koyama, R., et al.: Reevaluation of radiologic diagnosis of peptic ulcer of the stomach; Determination of peptic ulcer.(in Japanese) *Nippon Igaku Hoshasen Gakkai Zasshi(Nippon Acta Radiologica)*, 17:615, 1957.

Shirakabe, H., Kumakura, K., Nakajima, T., et al.: Reevaluation of radiologic diagnosis of peptic ulcer of the stomach; Studies on a reasonable method for diagnosis. (in Japanese) *Nippon Igaku Hoshasen Gakkai Zasshi (Nippon Acta Radiologica)*, 18:765, 1958.

Shirakabe, H., Kumakura, K., Koyama, R., et al.: Radiographic study on the healing process of peptic ulcer of the stomach; With special reference to the comparison of limitation of radiographic and gastrocamera diagnoses. (in Japanese) *Rinsho Hoshasen(Japanese Journal of Clinical Radiology)*, 4:42, 1959.

Shirakabe, H., Kumakura, K., Koyama, R., et al.: Radiographic diagnosis of multiple ulcers of the stomach.(in Japanese) *Nippon Igaku Hoshasen Gakkai Zasshi(Nippon Acta Radiologica)*, 19:1823, 1959b.

Shirakabe, H., Kumakura, K., Koyama, R., et al.: X-Ray diagnosis of gastric and duodenal ulcer.(in Japanese) *Nippon Shokaki Byo Gakkai Zasshi(Japanese Journal of Gastro-enterology)*, 58:1187, 1961.

Shirakabe, H., Nishizawa, M., Higurashi, K., et al.: Radiographic diagnosis of peptic gastric ulcer with difficult healing tendency.(in Japanese) *I to Cho(Stomach and Intestine)*, 2:1005, 1967.

Stein, G.N.: X-Ray diagnosis of gastric ulcer, *in* Bockus, H.L. (ed): *Gastroenterology*, vol. I. Philadelphia, W.B. Saunders Company, 1963, pp 482—491.

Stoerk, O.: Zur Pathogenese der akuten Gastritis. Wien Klin. Wschr., 38:1925.

Suzuki, K., Takekawa, H., Tatara, Y., et al.: Surgical treatment of peptic ulcer of the stomach and duodenum. (in Japanese) *Shinryo(Clinical Practice)*, 20:208, 1967.

Tamiya, C.: *Radiographic Diagnosis in Internal Medicine*, vol. 2.(in Japanese) Tokyo, Nanzando, 1923.

Teschendorf, W.: *Lehrbuch der Röntgenologischen Differentialdiagnostik. Erkrankungen der Bauchorgane.* Leipzig, Georg Thieme Verlag, 1949.

Uemura, U.: Statistical, clinical and experimental studies on peptic ulcer of the stomach.(in Japanese) *Nippon Geka Gakkai Zasshi(Journal of Japan Surgical Society)*, 19:833, 1919.

Wolf, B.S., Marshak, R.H.: Profile features of benign gastric niches on roentgen examination. *J. Mt. Sinai Hosp. N.Y.*, 24:604, 1957.

Yokoyama, H.: Limitation of natural healing and indication of surgical resection of gastric and duodenal ulcers.(in Japanese) *Sogo Igaku(Medicine)*, 18:511, 1961.

Bibliography

Amberg, J.R., Zboralske, F.F.: Gastric ulcers after 70. *Amer. J. Roentgenol.*, 96:393, 1966.

Anzai, M., Utsumi, M., Tsunoda, S., et al.: Radiologic and histologic observations of the healing process of peptic ulcers and ulcer scars of the stomach.(in Japanese) *Nippon Shokaki Byo Gakkai Zasshi(Japanese Journal of Gastroenterology)*, 71:1196, 1974.

Aoyama, T.: Diagnosis of a linear ulcer of the stomach by mucosal relief image and gastrocamera.(in Japanese) *Gastroent. Endoscopy*, 3:366, 1962.

Baensch, W.E.: Benign diseases of the stomach, *in* Margulis, A.R., Burhenne, H.J. (eds): *Alimentary Tract Roentgenology*. St. Louis, The C.V. Mosby Company, 1967, pp 457—465.

Berg, H.H.: Grundlagen der Darstellung von Gastritis und Ulcus im Röntgenbild. Med. Klin., 35:1245, 1953.

Bier, A.: Über das Ulcus duodeni. *Dtsch. Med. Wschr.*, 18:836, 1912.

Brügel, C.: Bewegungsvorgänge am pathologischen Magen auf Grund röntgenkinematographischer Untersuchungen. *Münch. Med. Wschr.*, 4:179, 1913.

Bryk, D.: Penetrated ulcer near the cardia of the stomach. *Amer. J. Dig. Dis.*, 11:728, 1966.

Dodd, G.D., Nelson, R.S.: The combined radiologic and gastroscopic evaluation of gastric ulceration. *Radiology*, 77:177, 1961.

Eisler, F.: Zur Röntgendiagnose bei Doppelgeschwüre in Magen un Duodenum. *Med. Klin. Wschr.*, 25:635, 1929.

Elster, K.: Das peptische Ulkus, *in* Der Kranke Magen. München, Urban & Schwarzenberg, 1970, p 24.

Esaki, Y., Yamashiro, M.: Intermediate zone and gastric ulcer; A study on autopsy cases of the aged.(in Japanese with English abstract) *I to Cho(Stomach and Intestine)*, 15:137, 1980.

Forssell, G.: Beobachtungen über die Autoplastik des Digestionskannales. *Fortschr. Röntgenstr.*, 37:393, 1928.

Frik, W.: Peptic ulcer, *in* Schinz, H.R., Baensch, W.E., Frommhold, W., et al. (eds): *Roentgen Diagnosis*, vol. 5, Abdomen, 2nd American ed. New York, Grune & Stratton, 1967, pp 157—177.

Fukuchi, S.: Course of peptic ulcer of the stomach based on follow-up observation by endoscopy.(in Japanese) *Gastroent. Endoscopy*, 6:364, 1965.

Fukuchi, S.: Fibergastroscopic diagnosis of multiple ulcers of the stomach.(in Japanese) *I to Cho(Stomach and Intestine)*, 2:1169, 1967.

Glickman, M.G., Szemes, G., Loeb, P., et al.: Peptic ulcer of the pyloric region. *Amer. J. Roenterol.*, 113:147, 1971.

Goldberg, H.I.: Roentgen diagnosis of ulcerative diseases, *in* Sleisenger, M.H., Fordtran, J.S. (eds): *Gastrointestinal Disease; Pathophysiology, Diagnosis, Management*, vol. 1, 2nd ed. Philadelphia, W.B. Saunders Company, 1978, pp 660—691.

Golden, R.: Gastric ulcer, *in* Robbins, L.L. (ed): *Golden's Diagnostic Radiology*, Section 5: Digestive Tract. Baltimore, The Williams & Wilkins Co, 1969, pp 5, 247.

Gonoi, T., Igarashi, T., Contribution of endoscopy to radiology in the diagnosis of gastric diseases.(in Japanese) *Rinsho Hoshasen(Japanese Journal of Clinical Radiology)*, 10:337, 1965.

Gonoi, T., Igarashi, T.: Peptic ulcer of the stomach, *in* Shirakabe, H., Ichikawa, H. (eds): *Course on Radiographic Interpretation of the Alimentary Tract.*(in Japanese) Tokyo, Kanehara Shuppan, 1969.

Gonoi, T., Igarashi, T.: *Atlas of Radiologic Diagnosis of Peptic Ulcer of the Stomach.*(in Japanese) Tokyo, Kanehara Shuppan, 1975.

Haudek, M.: Ein Typus von schneckenförmiger Einziehung der Pars pylorica, der Karzinom vortauschen kann; Zugleich ein Beitrag zur Antrumgastritis. *Fortschr. Röntgenstr.*, 42:285, 1930.

Hayakawa, H.: A study of X-ray and endoscopic diagnosis

of linear ulcer of the stomach.(in Japanese with English abstract) *Nippon Igaku Hoshasen Gakkai Zasshi(Nippon Acta Radiologica)*, 28:240, 1968.

Hemmeter, J.E.: Neue Methoden zur Diagnose des Magengeschwürs. *Arch. Verdaruungskr.*, 12:357, 1906.

Hinds, S.J., Harper, R.A.: Schortening of the lesser curvature in gastric ulcer. *Brit. J. Radiol.*, 25:451, 1952.

Ichikawa, H., Yamada, T., Doi, H., et al.: Radiologic diagnosis of multiple ulcers of the stomach.(in Japanese) *Rinsho Hoshasen(Japanese Journal of Clinical Radiology)*, 8:391, 1963.

Iino, H., Yoshida, T., Ohishi, H.: Cases of linear ulcer of the stomach.(in Japanese) *Gastroent. Endoscopy*, 3:356, 1962.

Inoue, T., Yokoyama, I., Takeda, M.: A case of linear ulcer.(in Japanese) *I to Cho(Stomach and Intestine)*, 1:561, 1966.

Kawai, K.: Endoscopic follow-up observations of peptic ulcer of the stomach.(in Japanese) *Gastroent. Endoscopy*, 6:354, 1965.

Kawai, K.: X-ray diagnosis on the gastric ulcer.(in Japanese with English abstract) *I to Cho(Stomach and Intestine)*, 2:485, 1967.

Keller, R.J., Wolf, B.S., Khilnani, M.T.: Roentgen features of healing and healed benign gastric ulcers. *Radiology*, 97:353, 1970.

Kirsh, I.E.: Benign and malignant gastric ulcers; Roentgen differentiation. *Radiology*, 64:357, 1955.

Kirsh, I.E.: Radiological aspect of cancer after apparent healing; Veterans Administration Cooperative Study on Gastric Ulcer. *Gastroenterology*, 61:606, 1971.

Konjetzny, G.E.: Über die Beziehung der chronischen Gastritis mit ihren Folgeerscheinungen und des chronischen Magenulcus zur Entwicklung des Magenkrebses. *Bruns Beitr. klin. Chir.*, 85:455, 1913.

Kumakura, K.: *Radiology of Gastric Diseases, Basic Findings and Interpretation.*(in Japanese) Tokyo, Kanehara Shuppan, 1968.

Kurahara, I., Shida, T., Fukumoto, A., et al.: A case of multiple peptic ulcers of the stomach with abnormal radiographic findings.(in Japanese) *I to Cho(Stomach and Intestine)*, 2:817, 1967.

Kusachi, N., Yoshiba, M., Ishigooka, M., et al.: Radiologic diagnosis of multiple peptic ulcers in the pyloric region of the stomach.(in Japanese) *I to Cho(Stomach and Intestine)*, 2:1149, 1967.

Lubert, M., Krause, G.R.: The "ring" shadow in the diagnosis of ulcer. *Amer. J. Roentgenol.*, 90:767, 1963.

Marshak, R.H., Yarnis, H., Friedman, A.I.: Giant benign gastric ulcers. *Gastroenterology*, 24:339, 1953.

Maruyama, M., Kumakura, K., Takekoshi, T., et al.: Radiographic finding of carcinoma in the fundic gland area of the stomach.(in Japanese) *Nippon Gan Chiryo Gakkai Shi(Journal of Japanese Society for Cancer Therapy)*, 7:249, 1972.

Masuda, H., Ohshiba, S.: Relationship between peptic ulcer and carcinoma of the stomach.(in Japanese) *I to Cho(Stomach and Intestine)*, 3:699, 1968.

Masuda, M., Uehara, I., Takada, H., et al.: Gastrocamera diagnosis of linear and symmetrical ulcers of the stomach.(in Japanese) *Gastroent. Endoscopy*, 2:30, 1960.

Masuda, M., Yokota, J., Uehara, I., et al.: Follow-up observations of peptic ulcer of the stomach by endoscopy.(in Japanese) *Gastroent. Endoscopy*, 4:70, 1962.

Masuda, M.: Clinical, fluoroscopic and endoscopic observation on the symmetric ulcer(linear and kissing ulcer) of the stomach. The 2nd World Congress of Gastroenterology, Munich, 1962.

Matsunaga, F., Yamaguchi, T.: Radiologic diagnosis of peptic ulcer in the region around the fornix of the stomach.(in Japanese) *Rinsho Hoshasen(Japanese Journal of Clinical Radiology)*, 10:633, 1965.

Meireles, J.S., Montenegro, M.R., Zatera, S., et al.: Gastric ulcer cicatrization; A comparison of roentgenologic and histologic data. *Amer. J. Dig. Dis.*, 7:661, 1962.

Murakami, T.: Percentage of ulcerocancer in the small pyloric cancers.(in Japanese) *GANN(Japanese Journal of Cancer Research)*, 43:206, 1952.

Murakami, T., Suzuki, T., Nakamura, S., et al.: Clinic and pathology of symmetric ulcer of the stomach and the duodenum.(in Japanese with English abstract) *Nippon Geka Gakkai Zasshi(Journal of Japan Surgical Society)*, 55:731, 1954.

Murakami, T., Suzuki, T., Iwanami, H., et al.: Radiographic findings of peptic ulcer in the upper portion of the stomach.(in Japanese) *Rinsho Hoshasen(Japanese Journal of Clinical Radiology)*, 6:164, 1961.

Nagayo, T.: Statistical, macroscopic and histologic studies on morphogenesis of peptic ulcer of the stomach based on a series of 1,000 surgically resected stomachs.(in Japanese) *Nippon Rinsho(Japanese Journal of Clinical Medicine)*, 16:1272, 1958.

Nakada, H.: Histopathologic study on linear and symmetrical ulcers of the duodenum.(in Japanese) *Osaka Daigaku Igaku Zasshi(Osaka University Medical Journal)*, 9:793, 1957.

Palmer, W.L.: Pathology; Classification, *in* Brockus, H.L. (ed): *Gastroenterology*, 3rd ed, vol. 1, section III, The Stomach. Philadelphia, W.B. Saunders Company, 1974, pp 952–956.

Paustian, F.F., Stein, G.N., Young, J.F., et al.: The importance of the brief trial of rigid medical management in the diagnosis of benign versus malignant gastric ulcer. *Gastroenterology*, 38:155, 1960.

Rønnov-Jessen, V., Ahlgren, P., Qvist, C.F.: Incidence of gastric cancer in medually treated patient with gastric ulcer. Acta Med. Scand., 178:141, 1965.

Saito, M., Igarashi, T., Murai, T., et al.: Rigidity of the gastric wall (der Fibrose) in IIc type early cancer and peptic ulcer scar of the stomach.(in Japanese) *Nippon Shokaki Byo Gakkai Zasshi(Japanese Journal of Gastroenterology)*, 72:1330, 1975.

Sano, K.: Symmetrical and linear ulcers of the stomach and duodenum.(in Japanese) *Rinsho Geka(Journal of Clinical Surgery)*, 12:27, 1957.

Sano, R.: Pathology of multiple ulcers of the stomach.(in Japanese) *I to Cho(Stomach and Intestine)*, 2:1175, 1967.

Sasagawa, M.: Roentgenological study on gastric ulcer scar.(in Japanese) *Nippon Shokaki Byo Gakkai Zasshi (Japanese Journal of Gastroenterology)*, 63:428, 1967.

Schmieden, V.: Differentialdiagnose zwischen Magengeschwür und Magenkrebs; Die pathologische Anatomie dieser Erkrankungen in Beziehung zu ihrer Darstellung im Röntgenbilde. *Arch. Klin. Chir.*, 96:253, 1911.

Shanks, S.C., Kerley, P.: *A Textbook of X-Ray Diagnosis,* 4th ed., London, H.K. Lewis, 1969.

Stein, G.N., Finkelstein, A.K., Markowitz, R.I.: X-Ray diagnosis; Gastric lesions, in Bockus, H.L. (ed): *Gastroenterology,* 3rd ed, vol. 1, section III. Philadelphia, W.B. Saunders Company, 1974, pp 650–665.

Suzuki, T.: Pathological and clinical studies on symmetrical ulcers of the stomach.(in Japanese) *Nippon Geka Gakkai Zasshi(Journal of Japan Surgical Society),* 60:2014–2036, 1959; 60:2133–2151, 1959.

Sydney, J.H., Harper, R.A.K.: Shortening of lesser curvature in gastric ulcers. Brit. J. Radiol., 25:451, 1952.

Takagi, K., Kumakura, K., Maruyama, M., et al.: Acute symmetric ulceration of the antral portion of the stomach; A new concept of hemorrhagic erosion and acute ulceration due to the spasm of the antrum.(in Japanese) *Gan no Rinsho(Japanese Journal of Cancer Clinics),* 15:887, 1969.

Takeuchi, T.: Morphopathological study of multiple gastroduodenal ulcers.(in Japanese) *Nippon Byori Gakkai Zasshi(Transactiones Societatis Pathologicae Japonicae),* 46:855, 1957.

To'th, F., Kelemen, J., Szatai, I.: Methodische Probleme der Röntgenuntersuchung bei Magengeschwülsten der Fornixgegend. *Fortschr. Röntgenstr.,* 97:126, 1962.

Tsugu, Y.: Linear ulcer and pouch-like stomach.(in Japanese) *Rinsho Hoshasen(Japanese Journal of Clinical Radiology),* 6:583, 1961.

Tsukasa, S.: Radiologic diagnosis of multiple peptic ulcers of the gastric body.(in Japanese) *Gastroent. Endoscopy,* 8:387, 1966.

Tsukasa, S.: Studies on ulcers in the body of stomach. Part II, Studies on X-ray diagnosis of ulcers in the body of stomach.(in Japanese with English abstract) *Kagoshima Daigaku Igaku Zasshi(Kagoshima University Medical Journal),* 20:373, 1968.

Tsunoda, T., Shirakabe, H., Kumakura, K., et al.: Reexamination of radiologic diagnosis of gastric ulcers.(in Japanese) *Nippon Shokaki Byo Gakkai Zasshi(Japanese Journal of Gastroenterology),* 53:301, 1956.

Turner, J.C. Jr., Dockerty, M.B., Priestley, J.T., et al.: A clinicopathologic study of large benign gastric ulcers. *Surg. Gynecol. Obstet.,* 104:746, 1957.

Wohl, G.T., Shore, L.: Lesions of the cardiac end of the stomach simulating carcinoma. *Amer. J. Roentgenol.,* 82:1048, 1959.

Yarita, T., Shirakabe, H., Hayakawa, H., et al.: Deformation of the stomach caused by linear ulcer of the gastric body.(in Japanese) *Nippon Shokaki Byo Gakkai Zasshi (Japanese Journal of Gastroenterology),* 71:1050, 1974.

Zaterka, S., Bettarello, A., Meireles Filho, J., et al.: Giant gastric ulcer; Report of 27 cases. Amer. J. Dig. Dis., 7:236, 1962.

Zboralske, F.F.: Gastric ulcer, *in* Margulis, A.R., Burhenne, H.J. (eds): *Alimentary Tract Roentgenology.* St. Louis, The C.V. Mosby Company, 1967, pp 475–487.

Chapter 8 Radiographic Diagnosis of Gastric Erosions

References

Abel, W.: Die Röntgendiagnose der Gastritis erosiva. *Fortschr. Röntgenstr.,* 8:39, 1954.

Aoyama, T.: Gastritis erosiva.(in Japanese) *Nippon Rinsho (Japanese Journal of Clinical Medicine),* 22:1925, 1964.

Berg, H.H.: Grundlagen der Darstellung von Gastritis und Ulcus im Röntgenbild. *Med. Klin.,* 35:1245, 1953.

Bücker, J.: Zur Röntgendiagnostik der Gastritis erosiva. *Radiologie,* 4:78, 1964.

Frik, W., Hesse, R.: Die röntgenologische Darstellung von Magenerosionen; Verbesserte Ergebnisse mit Doppelkontrast-Aufnahmen und Bildverstärker. *Dtsch. Med. Wschr.,* 81:1119, 1956.

Frik, W.: Erosionen der Magenschleimhaut, *in* Schinz, H.R., Baensch, W.E., Frommhold, W., et al. (eds): *Lehrbuch der Röntgendiagnostik,* vol. 5. Stuttgart, Georg Thieme Verlag, 1965, pp 85–104.

Gelfand, D.W.: The Japanese-style double-contrast examination of the stomach. *Gastrointest. Radiol.,* 1:7, 1976.

Henning, N., Schatzki, R.: Gastrophotographisches und röntgenologisches Bild der Gastritis ulcerosa. *Fortschr. Röntgenstr.,* 48:177, 1933.

Hirokado, K., Okabe, H.: Clinical aspects of gastritis erosiva.(in Japanese) *Shokaki Byo no Rinsho(Journal of Clinical Digestive Diseases),* 6:1340, 1964.

Kawai, K., Shimamoto, K., Misaki, F., et al.: Erosion of gastric mucosa; Pathogenesis, incidence and classification of the erosive gastritis. *Endoscopy,* 2:168, 1970.

Koide, H.: Histopathological studies on the distribution and the healing tendency of gastric ulcer.(in Japanese) *Showa Igakkai Zasshi(Showa Medical Journal),* 20:1700, 1961.

Kumakura, K.: Radiologic diagnosis of gastric erosions.(in Japanese) *I to Cho(Stomach and Intestine),* 2:755, 1967.

Laufer, I., Trueman, T.: Multiple superficial gastric erosions due to Crohn's disease of the stomach; Radiologic and endoscopic diagnosis. Brit. J. Radiol., 49:726, 1976.

Nakamura, T., Iwamaru, M., Takekawa, K.: Pathology (classification) of gastric polyps.(in Japanese) *Nippon Geka Gakkai Zasshi(Journal of Japan Surgical Society),* 63:949, 1962.

Sano, R., Hirota, T., Shimoda, T.: Pathological study on early gastric cancer; With special reference to malignant transformation of gastritis verrucosa.(in Japanese) *Nippon Byori Gakkai Zasshi(Transactiones Societatis Pathologicae Japonicae),* 59:136, 1970.

Sano, R.: *Surgical Pathology of Gastric Diseases.*(in Japanese) Tokyo, Igaku-Shoin Ltd, 1974.

Sano, R.: Chronic gastritis in Japanese in a series of operated material due to various pathologies; With special reference to the histological classification of chronic gastritis and its relation to gastric carcinoma.(in Japanese) *Nippon Shokaki Byo Gakkai Zasshi(Japanese Journal of Gastroenterology),* 72:1231, 1975.

Sata, H.: Gastritis erosiva and gastritis verrucosa; Study on morphology and function of varioliform erosions.(in Japanese with English abstract) *Gastroent. Endoscopy,* 16:365, 1974.

Schatzki, R.: The comparative value of gastroscopy and roentgen examination of the stomach. *Radiology*, 29:488, 1937.

Walk, L.: The roentgen signs of gastritis; Clinical analysis. *Amer. J. Roentgenol.*, 74:567, 1955.

Yoshida, T., Okabe, H., Hirokado, K., et al.: Limitations of endoscopic diagnosis of gastric erosions.(in Japanese) *I to Cho(Stomach and Intestine)*, 2:767, 1967.

Bibliography

Akagami, A.: Endoscopic studies of gastric erosion by close-up observation and dying method.(in Japanese) *Gastroent. Endoscopy*, 19:509, 1977.

Akagami, A., Ichioka, S., Suzuki, S.: A study of the gastritis verrucosa from the point of view of the endoscopical dying method.(in Japanese) *Progr. Digest. Endoscopy*, 12:10, 1978.

Ansprenger, A., Kirklin, B.R.: The roentgenologic aspects of chronic gastritis. *Amer. J. Roentgenol.*, 38:533, 1937.

Aono, G., Takezoe, K., Jojima, Y., et al.: Endoscopic study of hemorrhagic erosions of the stomach and review of literature.(in Japanese with English abstract) *I to Cho (Stomach and Intestine)*, 9:1455, 1974.

Auguste, C., Paris, J.: Gastrites érosives et sténose gastrique consécutive à l'absorption de soude caustique. *Arch. Mal. Appar. Dig.*, 37:553, 1948.

Berger, C.: Über Magenerosion. *Münch. Med. Wschr.*, 23:1116, 1907.

Bianchi, P.G.: Gastriti ponfoidi e varioliformi. *Rivista. Anat. Pat. Oncol.*, 1:553, 1948.

Cain, J.C., Jordan, G.L. Jr, Comfort, M.W.: Medically treated small gastric ulcer. *JAMA*, 150:781, 1952.

Calzavara, D.: Gastrite erosiva emorragica acuta dopo resezione gastrica per ulcera. *Arch. Mal. Appar. Dig.*, 2:590, 1933.

D'Aste, G.: Gastriti ponfoidi e varioliformi nell'etiopatogenesi dell'ulcera rotonda. *Rivista. Chir. Med.*, 2:551, 1950.

D'Aste, G.: Neoformazione granulomatosa dell'antro pilorico; In un caso di gastrite varioliforme. *Rivista. Chir. Med.*, 2:579, 1950.

D'Aste, G.: Rilievi anatomo-radiologici caratteristici della gastrite figurata. *Rassegna Ital. Chir. Med.*, 1:1, 1952.

Debray, M.: Les érosions éphémères de l'estomac; Etude clinique et therapeutique. *Progrès. Med.*, 26:933, 1938.

Desmond, A.M., Reynolds, K.W.: Erosive gastritis; Its diagnosis, management, and surgical treatment. *Brit. J. Surg.*, 59:5, 1972.

Dieulafoy, G.: Gastrite ulcéreuse. *Clin. Med. l'Hotel-Dieu*, 3:219, 1898/1899; 4:194, 1901/1902.

Duval, P.: Gastrite érosive hémorragique. Gastrectomie d'urgence. *Guérison Mém. Acad. Chir.*, 66:827, 1940.

Einhorn, M.: Ein klinischer Beitrag zur Kenntniss und Behandlung der "Erosionen des Magens". *Berl. Klin. Wschr.*, 32:435, 1895; 32:457, 1895.

Einhorn, M.: Ein weiterer Beitrag zur Kenntnis der Magenerosionen. *Arch. Verdauungskr.*, 5:317, 1899.

Elsner, H.: Zur Frage der hämorrhagischen Erosionen des Magens. *Dtsch. Med. Wschr.*, 29:735, 1903.

Frik, W., Hesse, R.: The radiological diagnosis of erosion of the gastric mucosa; Improved results with double-contrast pictures and the image-intensifer. *German Med. Month.*, 1:198, 1956.

Furuya, K.: Clinical analysis and new histopathological findings of erosive gastritis observed in the resected stomach with benign ulcer.(in Japanese with English abstract) *Nippon Shokaki Byo Gakkai Zasshi(Japanese Journal of Gastroenterology)*, 67:1115, 1970.

Golden, F.: Mucosal erosions, *in* Robbins, L.L. (ed): *Golden's Diagnostic Roentgenology*, section 5. Baltimore, The Williams & Wilkins Company, 1969, pp 219—220.

Hamperl, H.: Über "Schleimgranulome" und "glanduläre" Erosionene in der Speicheldrüsen und der Magenschleimhaut. *Beitr. Path. Anat.*, 88:193, 1931.

Hamperl, H.: Zur Histologie der akuten Gastritis und der Erosionen der Magenschleimhaut. *Beitr. Path. Anat.*, 90:86, 1932.

Hirashima, T., Oguro, Y., Sasagawa, D., et al.: A case of gastric carcinoma detected during follow-up observation of gastritis erosiva.(in Japanese) *Gastroent. Endoscopy*, 17:52, 1975.

Hirota, T., Itabashi, M., Yamamoto, M., et al.: Pathological study on gastritis verrucosa.(in Japanese) *Progr. Digest. Endoscopy*, 12:36, 1978.

Jankelson, O.M., Jankelson, I.R., Zamcheck, N.: Hemorrhagic (erosive) gastritis. *Amer. J. Dig. Dis.*, 4:603, 1959.

Kalima, T.: Pathologisch-anatomische Studien über die Gastritis des Ulcusmagens nebst einigen Bemerkungen zur Pathogenese und pathologischen Anatomie des Magengeschwürs. *Arch. Klin. Chir.*, 128:20, 1924.

Karasawa, Y., Yamazaki, M., Ohno, M., et al.: Endoscopic observation of so-called hemorrhagic erosions(hemorrhagische Erosionen).(in Japanese) *I to Cho(Stomach and Intestine)*, 2:777, 1967.

Katz, D., Siegel, H.I.: *Erosive Gastritis and Acute Gastrointestinal Mucosal Lesions. Progress in Gastroenterology*. Vol. 1, New York, Grun & Stratton Inc, 1968, pp 67—68.

Kawai, K.: Endoscopic observations of gastric bleeding.(in Japanese) *Gastroent. Endoscopy*, 6:151, 1964.

Kawai, K., Wakabayashi, T., Ida, K.: The process of the erosion.(in Japanese with English abstract) *I to Cho (Stomach and Intestine)*, 2:743, 1967.

Kawai, K., Misaki, F., Murakami, K., et al.: The evolution of the erosion. *Gastroenterologica Japonica*, 3:377, 1968.

Khodadoost, J., Glass, G.B.J.: Erosive gastritis and acute gastrointestinal bleeding in liver cirrhosis. *Digestion*, 7:129, 1972.

Kirklin, B.R.: Bleeding lesions of the gastrointestinal tract and their roentgenologic diagnosis. *Amer. J. Roentgenol.*, 45:171, 1941.

Konjetzny, G.E.: Die entzündliche Grundlage der typischen Geschwürsbildung im Magen und Duodenum. *Ergebn. Inn. Med.*, 37:184, 1930.

Krentz, K.: *Erosions of the Gastric Mucosa. Integrated Atlas of Gastric Diseases*. Lamm, H. (trans). Stuttgart, Georg Thieme Verlag, 1976, pp 30—47.

Kuramata, H., Unayama, S., Etoh, S., et al.: Cases of early carcinoma associated with gastritis verrucosa.(in Japanese) *Gastroent. Endoscopy*, 17:20, 1975.

Kuramata, H., Etoh, S., Miyamoto, S.: On the endoscopic problems of the relationship between gastritis verrucosa and gastric cancer.(in Japanese) *Progr. Digest. Endoscopy*, 12:19, 1978.

349

REFERENCES

Laine, J.: *Des érosions hémorrhagiques de l'estomac (Thèse)*, Paris, 1897.

Mai, M., Morita, H., Watanabe, K., et al.: A case of metastic carcinoma of the stomach in a young girl simulating gastritis erosiva in X-ray and endoscopic findings.(in Japanese with English abstract) *I to Cho(Stomach and Intestine)*, 7:1209, 1972.

Mai, M., Akimoto, R., Ueda, H., et al.: Histopathological studies on atypical epithelial lesion (ATP) and cancer arisen in preexisting gastritis verrucosa.(in Japanese) *Proceedings of the Japanese Cancer Association*, 35:234, 1976.

Mai, M.: Histological aspects of gastric polyps and their relation to gastritis verrucosa.(in Japanese) *Progr. Digest. Endoscopy*, 12:32, 1978.

Metzger, W.H., McAdam, L., Bluestone, R., et al.: Acute gastric mucosal injury during continuous or interrupted aspirin ingestion in humans. *Digest. Dis.*, 21:963, 1976.

Mintz, S.: Über hämorrhagische Magenerosionen. *Dtsch. Zschr. Klin. Med.*, 46:115, 1902.

Miyamoto, S., Etoh, S., Ueda, A., et al.: A IIa aggregation subtype early cancer of the stomach: A case report.(in Japanese) *Progr. Digest. Endoscopy*, 11:157, 1977.

Moszkowicz, L.: Regeneration und Krebsbildung in der Magenschleimhaut. *Arch. Klin. Chir.*, 132:558, 1924.

Moutier, F., Martin, J.: Deux cas de gastrite varioliforme. *Arch. Mal. Appar. Digest.*, 36:155, 1947.

Murashima, Y., Yaoita, T.: Radiologic diagnosis of gastric carcinoma associated with gastritis verrucosa.(in Japanese) *I to Cho(Stomach and Intestine)*, 10:1608, 1975; 11:64, 1976; 11:202, 1976; 11:370, 1976; 11:454, 1976; 11:614, 1976.

Nauwerck, C.: Gastritis ulcerosa chronica. *Münch. Med. Wschr.*, 35:955, 1897.

Nauwerck, C.: Gastritis ulcerosa chronica; Ein Beitrag zur Kenntnis des Magengeschwürs. *Münch. Med. Wschr.*, 36:987, 1897.

Neumaier, F.: La gastrite erosiva: Studio radiologico, *in* Antonietti, L. (ed): *"E Maragliano" de Patologia e Clinica, Collana di Monografie dell'Archivio* No 14. *Genova, Editore A Pesce, 1955*.

O'Brien, T.K., Saunders, D.R., Templeton, F.E.: Chronic gastric erosions and oral aphthae. *Digest. Dis.*, 17:447, 1972.

Ohki, I.: Pursuit and analysis of endoscopic findings of gastritis erosiva in follow-up study.(in Japanese) *Gastroent. Endoscopy*, 12:161, 1970.

Ohki, I., Shimura, M.: A study on verrucose gastritis.(in Japanese) *Progr. Digest. Endoscopy*, 12:15, 1978.

Palmer, E.D.: Erosive gastritis in cirrhosis. *Amer. J. Dig. Dis.*, 2:31, 1957.

Pariser, C.: Über hämorrhagische Erosionen der Magenschleimhaut. *Berlin Klin. Wschr.*, 43:954, 1900.

Poplack, W., Paul, R.E., Goldsmith, M., et al.: Demonstration of erosive gastritis by the double contrast technique. *Radiology*, 117:519, 1975.

Puhl, H.: Über die Bedeutung entzündlicher Prozesse für die Entstehung des Ulcus ventriculi et duodeni. *Virchows Arch. Path.*, 260:1, 1926.

Puhl, H.: Die Veränderungen der Duodenalschleimhaut beim Ulcusleiden. *Virchows Arch. Path.*, 265:160, 1927.

Puhl, H.: Über die Entstehung und Entwicklung des Magen-Duodenal-Geschwürs. *Arch. Klin. Chir.*, 158:1, 1930.

Quintard, E.: Einige Fälle von Magenerosionene (Einhorn). *Arch. Verdauungskrkh.*, 7:81, 1901.

Roch, M., Demole, M., Andereggen, P.: Gastrite varioliforme. *Bull. Mem. Soc. Med. Hôp. Paris*, 13/14:555, 1950.

Rösch, W., Elster, K., Ottenjann, R.: Morbus Crohn des Magens unter dem Bild der "kompletten" Erosionen. *Endoscopy*, 1:178, 1969.

Rösch, W., Ottenjann, R.: Gastric erosions. *Endoscopy*, 2:93, 1970.

Rösch, W.: Diagnose und klinische Bedeutung der Magenerosionen. *Dtsch. Med. Wschr.*, 95:1491, 1970.

Rösch, W.: Erosionen des Magens, *in* Demling, L. (ed): *Handbuch der Inneren Medizin*, 5th ed, vol. 3, Verdauungsorgane, part 3, Magen. Berlin-Heidelberg-New York, Springer-Verlag, 1974, pp 639—657.

Sano, R., Hirota, T., Shimoda, T., et al.: Pathological study on early gastric cancer; Role of gastritis verrucosa in the histogenesis of cancer.(in Japanese) *Nippon Byori Gakkai Zasshi(Transactiones Societatis Pathologicae Japonicae)*, 63:257, 1974.

Sata, H., Kondo, T., Takada, H., et al.: Endoscopic observations and bioptic findings of varioliform erosions of the stomach.(in Japanese with English abstract) *I to Cho(Stomach and Intestine)*, 6:1141, 1971.

Sata, H.: Radiographic findings of gastritis erosiva and gastritis verrucosa.(in Japanese) *I to Cho(Stomach and Intestine)*, 10:596, 1975; 10:800, 1975; 10:876, 1975; 10:1014, 1975; 10:1212, 1975; 10:1316, 1975.

Sata, H.: Follow up study of gastritis verrucosa.(in Japanese) *Progr. Digest. Endoscopy*, 12:27, 1978.

Shirakabe, H., Kumakura, K., Ito, S., et al.: Radiographic and macroscopic findings after surgery of gastritis erosiva.(in Japanese) *Nippon Igaku Hoshasen Gakkai Zasshi(Nippon Acta Radiologica)*, 15:1183, 1956.

Strauszer, T., Castillo, P., Csences, A., et al.: A lesion of chronic gastric erosion resembling IIa+IIc early carcinoma.(in Japanese with English abstract) *I to Cho(Stomach and Intestine)*, 6:481, 1971.

Takasu, S., Inui, Y., Garcia, J.C.: A report of 100 cases of gastritis verrucosa and their long-term follow-up.(in Japanese) *Gastroent. Endoscopy*, 16:763, 1974.

Tamechika, Y., Okabe, H., Hirokado, K., et al.: A case of IIa+IIc type early gastric cancer detected in the course of follow-up of so-called gastritis erosiva.(in Japanese with English abstract) *I to Cho(Stomach and Intestine)*, 5:75, 1970.

Trägårdh, B., Wehlin, L., Ohashi, K.: Radiologic appearance of complete gastric erosions. *Acta Radiol.* [*Diagn*], 19:633, 1978.

Vallebona, A.: Iquadri radiologici delle gastriti, Atti dei congressi della Societa' Italiana di Medicina Interna, 57° Congresso, Milano 15—17 Ottobre 1956. Roma, Luigi Pozzi-Editore, 1956.

Walk, L.: Erosive gastritis. *Gastroenterologia*, 84:87, 1955.

Walk, L.: Erosive gastritis.(in Japanese) *I to Cho(Stomach and Intestine)*, 2:735, 1967.

Walk, L.: Polypous formations caused by gastric erosions. 2nd European Congress of Gastrointestinal Endoscopy. Paris, 1972.

Chapter 9 Radiographic Aspects of Malignant Lymphoma and Reactive Lymphoreticular Hyperplasia (RLH)

References

An article with an asterisk (*) is a case report of early malignant lymphoma mentioned in the text (p 203).

*Akaike, Y., Ushio, K., Tsuboi, R., et al.: A case of primary malignant lymphoma of the stomach.(in Japanese) *I to Cho(Stomach and Intestine)*, 7:925, 1972.

Akazaki, K.: Reticulo-endothelial system and its tumor.(in Japanese) *Nippon Byori Gakkai Zasshi(Transactiones Societatis Pathologicae Japonicae)*, 41:1, 1952.

Akazaki, K., Wakasa, H.: Frequency of lymphoreticular tumors and leukemias in Japan. *J. Natl. Cancer. Inst.*, 52:339, 1974.

Bennet, M.H., Farrer-Brown, G., Henry, K., et al.: Classification of non-Hodgkin's lymphomas. *Lancet*, 2:405, 1974.

Berman, L.: Malignant lymphomas; Their classification and relation to leukemia. *Blood*, 8:195, 1953.

Bockus, H.L. (ed): *Gastroenterology*, vol 2. Philadelphia, W.B. Saunders Company, 1968.

Castleman, B., Iverson, L., Menendez, V.P.: Localized mediastinal lymph node hyperplasia resembling thymoma. *Cancer*, 9:822, 1956.

Culver, G.J., Bean, B.C., Berens, D.L.: Gastric lymphoma. *Radiology*, 65:518, 1955.

Custer, R.P., Bernhard, W.G.: Interrelationship of Hodgkin's disease and other lymphatic tumors. *Amer. J. Med. Sci.*, 216:625, 1948.

Doi, K., Kudo, T., Sasaki, K., et al.: A case of reactive lymphoreticular hyperplasia of the stomach simulating early gastric cancer of type IIa+IIc.(in Japanese with English abstract) *I to Cho(Stomach and Intestine)*, 6:589, 1971.

Dorfman, R.F.: Classification of non-Hodgkin's lymphomas. *Lancet*, 1:1295, 1974.

Faris, T.D., Saltzstein, S.L.: Gastric lymphoid hyperplasia; A lesion confused with lymphosarcoma. *Cancer*, 17:207, 1964.

Feldmann, M.: *Clinical Roentgenology of the Digestive Tract*. Baltimore, W. Wood and Co, 1938.

Frank, A.: Zur Röntgensymptomatologie des Retothelsarkoms des Magens. *Fortschr. Röntgenstr.*, 83:200, 1955.

Franz, P.L.: Roentgenographic features in lymphosarcoma of the stomach. *Radiologe*, 2:139, 1962.

*Furusawa, M., Hayashi, I., Koga, M., et al.: Gastric lymphosarcoma similar to early carcinoma type IIa+IIc. (in Japanese with English abstract) *I to Cho(Stomach and Intestine)*, 15:931, 1980a.

*Furusawa, M., Hayashi, I., Koga, M., et al.: Follicular lymphosarcoma superficially extended in stomach (like IIc+III early carcinoma).(in Japanese) *I to Cho(Stomach and Intestine)*, 15:965, 1980b.

Gall, EA., Mallory, T.B.: Malignant lymphoma; Clinicopathologic survey of 618 cases. Amer. J. Pathol., 18:381, 1942.

Gerard-Marchant, R., Hamlin, I., Lennert, K., et al.: Classification of non-Hodgkin's lymphomas. *Lancet*, 2:406, 1974.

*Goto, N., Goto, K., Yokochi, M., et al.: Recurrent gastric reticulum cell sarcoma in the remnant stomach at five years after operation.(in Japanese with English abstract) *I to Cho(Stomach and Intestine)*, 16:523, 1981.

Guetgemann, A., Schreiber, H.W.: *Die Chirurgie des Magensarkoms*. Stuttgart, Georg Thieme Verlag, 1960.

Herbut, P.A.: Relation of Hodking's disease, lymphosarcoma and reticulum cell sarcoma. *Amer. J. Pathol.*, 21:233, 1945.

Hodgkin, T.: On some morbid appearances of the absorbent glands and spleen. *Trans. Med. Chir. Lond.*, 17:68, 1832.

*Iida, M., Kido, H., Nakamura, Y.: Malignant lymphoma of the stomach in reactive lymphoreticular hyperplasia (RLH), which looked like multiple IIc-type early cancers macroscopically.(in Japanese with English abstract). *I to Cho(Stomach and Intestine)*, 15:981, 1980.

Iida, M., Nanbu, T., Kido, H., et al.: Differential diagnosis between primary malignant lymphoma and reactive lymphoreticular hyperplasia of the stomach;(in Japanese with English abstract) *I to Cho (Stomach and Intestine)*, 16:389, 1981.

*Imai, H., Takita, K., Ejima, K., et al.: A case of early reticulum cell sarcoma.(in Japanese) *I to Cho(Stomach and Intestine)*, 3:43, 1968.

*Ishihara, K., Tanaka, H., Nishio, T., et al.: A case of reticulum cell sarcoma of the stomach difficult to differentiate from IIc type early cancer.(in Japanese) *I to Cho(Stomach and Intestine)*, 1:477, 1966.

Jackson, H., Parker, F.: *Hodgkin's Disease and Allied Disorders*. New York, Oxford University Press, 1947.

Jacobs, D.S.: Primary gastric malignant lymphoma and pseudolymphoma. *Amer. J. Clin. Pathol.*, 40:379, 1963.

Katsumata, T., Takahashi, T., Hiki, Y., et al.: The so-called borderline reactive lymphoid hyperplasia of the stomach, which is difficult to determine whether benign or malignant histologically; Report of a case.(in Japanese with English abstract) *I to Cho (Stomach and Intestine)*, 16:173, 1981.

*Katsumi, K., Ito, M., Inukai, M.: Multiple early malignant lymphoma of the stomach.(in Japanese) *I to Cho(Stomach and Intestine)*, 16:443, 1981.

Kay, S.: Lymphoid tumors of the stomach. *Surg. Gyn. Obst.*, 118:1059, 1964.

Konjetzny, G.E.: Die Entzündungen des Magens, *in* Henke, F., Lubarsch, O. (eds): *Handbuch der Speziellen Pathologischen Anatomie und Histologie*, vol. 4, Partz, Berlin, Springer-Verlag, 1928.

Konjetzny, G.E.: Eine besondere Form der chronischen hypertrophischen Gastritis unter dem klinischen und röntgenologischen Bild eines Carcinomas. *Chirurg.*, 10:260, 1938.

Kumakura, K., Maruyama, M., Takada, R., et al.: X-ray diagnosis of sarcoma of the stomach.(in Japanese with English abstract) *I to Cho(Stomach and Intestine)*, 5:271, 1970.

Laufer, I.: *Double Contrast Gastrointestinal Radiology with Endoscopic Correlation*. Philadelphia, W.B. Saunders Company, 1979.

Lukes, R.J., Collins, R.D.: Immunologic characterization of human malignant lymphomas. *Cancer*, 34:1488, 1974.

Marshall, S.F., Meissner, W.A.: Sarcoma of the stomach. *Ann. Surg.*, 131:824, 1950.

Maruyama, M.: Early gastric cancer, *in* Laufer, I. (ed):

Double Contrast Gastrointestinal Radiology. Philadelphia-London-Toronto, W.B., Saunders Company, 1979, pp 241—288.

Maruyama, Y., Shimizu, H., Rinsho, K., et al.: A case of reactive lymphoreticular hyperplasia of the stomach clinically suspected as early carcinoma.(in Japanese with English abstract) *I to Cho(Stomach and Intestine),* 4:677, 1969.

Mathe, G., et al.: Histological and cytological typing of neoplastic diseases of hematopoietic and lymphatic tissues. *International Histological Classifications of Tumours,* No 14, WHO, Geneva, 1976.

*Mayama, S., Kariya, A., Hayashi, M., et al.: Malignant lymphoma of the stomach with a gross resemblance to early gastric carcinoma of IIc type.(in Japanese with English abstract) *I to Cho(Stomach and Intestine),* 16:537, 1981.

Mochizuki, T.: Pathological aspects of malignant lymphoma of the stomach.(in Japanese) *I to Cho(Stomach and Intestine),* 15:904, 1980.

Mori, S.: Clinical aspects of non-Hodgkin lymphoma; Present status of the histologic classification in Japan.(in Japanese) *Naika(Internal Medicine),* 48:9, 1981.

Morson, B.C., Dawson, I.M.P.: *Gastrointetinal Pathology.* Oxford, Blackwell Scientific Publications, 1972.

Murata, E., Ueda, Y., Kagaya, T., et al.: A case of primary Hodgkin's disease observed by a long-term follow-up study.(in Japanese) *Gastroent. Endoscopy,* 15:713, 1973.

Nakamura, K.: Pathology of reactive lymphoreticular hyperplasia of the stomach.(in Japanese) *I to Cho(Stomach and Intestine),* 2:1293, 1967.

Nakamura, K.: *Pathology of Gastric Cancer: Microcarcinoma and Its Histogenesis.* (in Japanese) Kyoto, Kimpo-do, 1972.

*Nakano, H., Nakazawa, S., Ito, J., et al.: A case of reticulum cell sarcoma of the stomach.(in Japanese with English abstract) *I to Cho(Stomach and Intestine),* 7:375, 1972.

Nakazawa, S., Kawaguchi, S., Yoshino, J., et al.: Malignant lymphoma of the stomach hard to differentiate from the so-called reactive lymphoreticular hyperplasia; Report of a case.(in Japanese with English abstract) *I to Cho (Stomach and Intestine),* 15:297, 1980.

Nakazawa, S., Kawaguchi, S., Yoshino, J., et al.: Malignant lymphoma difficult to differentiate from lymphoid hyperplasia.(in Japanese with English abstract) *I to Cho(Stomach and Intestine),* 16:451, 1981.

*Ninomiya, T., Baba, Y., Ohashi, K., et al.: Multiple IIc-simulating malignant lymphomas limited to the mucosal membrane.(in Japanese with English abstract) *I to Cho(Stomach and Intestine),* 15:927, 1980.

*Ninomiya, T., Baba, Y., Sugiyama, N., et al.: Malignant lymphoma simulating multiple IIc-like advanced carcinomas.(in Japanese with English abstract) *I to Cho(Stomach and Intestine),* 15:969, 1980.

Ninomiya, T., Baba, Y., Maruyama, M., et al.: Macroscopic and radiologic findings of malignant lymphoma of the stomach.(in Japanese with English abstract) *I to Cho (Stomach and Intestine),* 16:371, 1981.

Ninomiya, T., Baba, M., Maruyama, M.: Radiographic and endoscopic aspects of early malignant lymphoma of the stomach, with special reference to its differential diagnosis from early gastric cancer, *in* van Maercke, Y.M.R.,

Van Moer, E.M.J., Pelckmans, P.A.R. (eds): *Stomach Diseases: Current Status. Proceedings of the 13th International Congress on Stomach Disease.* Amsterdam, Excerpta Medica, 1981, pp 262—267.

*Ohashi, Y., Kumakura, K., Sugiyama, N., et al.: Early reticulum cell sarcoma of the stomach; Report of a case showing remarkable changes within a short time.(in Japanese with English abstract) *I to Cho(Stomach and Intestine),* 8:195, 1973.

*Ookado, H., Miyagawa, M., Suko, H., et al.: Early gastric lymphosarcoma; Report of a case.(in Japanese with English abstract) *I to Cho(Stomach and Intestine),* 15:1037, 1980.

Paulson, M.: *Gastroenterologic Medicine.* Philadelphia, Lea & Febriger, 1969.

Rafsky, H.A., Katz, H., Krieger, C.I.: Varied clinical manifestations of lymphosarcoma of the stomach. *Gastroenterology,* 3:297, 1944.

Rappaport, H.: *Tumor pathology of the hematopoietic system. Atlas of Tumor Pathology,* section 3, part 8, Washington DC, Armed Forces Institute of Pathology, 1966,

Sannohe, Y., Araki, H., Takano, S., et al.: Reticulum cell sarcoma of the stomach, a case report; Association of reactive lymphoreticular hyperplasia and death from general metastases shortly after operation.(in Japanese with English abstract) *I to Cho(Stomach and Intestine),* 11:767, 1976.

Schindler, R.: *Gastroscopy; The Endoscopic Study of Gastric Pathology,* 2nd ed. New York, Hafner Publishing Co, 1966.

Shimaoka. K., Sokal, J.E.: Malignant lymphomas, *in* Conn, H.F., Conn, R.B. (eds): *Current Diagnosis.* Philadelphia, W.B. Saunders Company, 1974, p 486.

Smith, J.L., Helwig, E.B.: Malignant lymphoma of stomach; Its diagnosis, distinction to biologic behavior. *Amer. J. Pathol.,* 34:553, 1958.

Suchi, T., Wakasa, H., Mikata, A., et al.: Problems on histologic diagnosis of non-Hodgkin lymphoma; Proposal of new classification.(in Japanese) *Saishin Igaku(Modern Medicine)* 34:2049, 1979.

*Sugiyama, N., Kumakura, K., Maruyama, M., et al.: A case of early reticulum cell sarcoma.(in Japanese with English abstract) *I to Cho(Stomach and Intestine),* 8:187, 1973.

Sugiyama, N.: Radiological diagnosis of malignant lymphoma of the stomach based on its macroscopical classification with special reference to early malignant lymphoma.(in Japanese with English summary) *Nippon Shokaki Byo Gakkai Zasshi(Japanese Journal of Gastroenterology),* 71:1118, 1974.

T- and B-Cell Malignancy Study Group: The Statistical analysis of immunologic, clinical and histopathologic data on lymphoid malignancies in Japan. *Jpn. J. Clin. Oncol.,* 11:15, 1981.

Takasugi, T., Abe, S., Mitsushima, T., et al.: A case of gastric malignant lymphoma having been difficult in differential diagnosis with RLH in its early stage.(in Japanese with English abstract) *I to Cho(Stomach and Intestine),* 13:403, 1978.

Takeuchi, T., Ito, M., Murate, H., et al.: A case of early gastric reticulum-cell sarcoma; Follow-up study with X-ray and gastroendoscope during the early stage.(in Japanese with English abstract) *I to Cho(Stomach and Intestine),* 6:211, 1971.

Takeuchi, T., Ito M., Yazaki, Y., et al.: A case of the gastric RLH (reactive lymphoreticular hyperplasia), to be difficult to differentiate from malignant lymphoma.(in Japanese with English abstract) *I to Cho(Stomach and Intestine)*, 8:1231, 1973.

*Tanehiro, K., Yoshii, Y., Kasugai, K., et al.: Malignant lymphoma of the stomach simulating polypoid carcinoma.(in Japanese with English abstract) *I to Cho(Stomach and Intestine)*, 15:939, 1980.

Tanoue, S., Ida, R., Takesue, T., et al.: A case of gastric reticulum cell sarcoma.(in Japanese) *Igaku Kenkyu(Acta Medica)*, 30:2400, 1960.

Tsugane, Y., Tsune, S., Kitagawa, M., et al.: A case of borderline lymphoma.(in Japanese with English abstract) *I to Cho(Stomach and Intestine)*, 13:249, 1978.

Umezaki, T., Kakimoto, K., Mitsuyasu, Y., et al.: A case of gastric reticulum-cell sarcoma showing rapid growth and spread.(in Japanese) *I to Cho(Stomach and Intestine)*, 6:1569, 1971.

Valdes-Dapena, A.M., Stein, G.N.: *Morphologic Pathology of the Alimentary Canal.* Philadelphia, W.B. Saunders Company, 1970, pp 119–125, 177–223.

Yamashita, H., Sakano, T., Kaneta, K., et al.: Non-Hodgkin's lymphoma in Japan; Trial for TNM clinical staging and histological classification. *Jpn. J. Clin. Oncol.*, 10:3, 1980.

*Yamawaki, Y., Moriyama, N., Ushio, K., et al.: Malignant lymphoma of the stomach showing of superficial spreading form.(in Japanese with English abstract) *I to Cho(Stomach and Intestine)*, 16:447, 1981.

*Yamazaki, S., Nakaizumi, O., Sirasaki, S.: A case of reticulum cell sarcoma of the stomach undergoing changes within a short time.(in Japanese with English abstract) *I to Cho(Stomach and Intestine)*, 9:51, 1974.

*Yoshida, K., Naito, H., Isomura, T., et al.: Non-Hodgkin gastric lymphoma with a 28 months' preoperative course.(in Japanese with English abstract) *I to Cho (Stomach and Intestine)*, 16:555, 1981.

*Yoshida, S., Yamaguchi, H., Oguro, Y., et al.: Malignant lymphoma of the stomach; A characteristic finding for early detection.(in Japanese with English abstract) *I to Cho(Stomach and Intestine)*, 16:465, 1981.

Bibliography

Aoyama, T.: Reactive lymphoreticular hyperplasia.(in Japanese) *I to Cho(Stomach and Intestine)*, 2:1283, 1967.

Azzopardi, J.G., Menzies, T.: Primary malignant lymphoma of the alimentary tract. *Brit. J. Surg.*, 47:358, 1960.

Bond, L.M., Pileggi, J.J.: Primary Hodgkin's disease of the stomach. *Amer. J. Roentgenol. Rad Therapy & Nuclear Med.*, 67:592, 1952.

Kahn, L.B.: Primary gastrointestinal lymphoma; A clinicopathologic study of fiftyseven cases. *Digest. Dis.*, 17:219, 1972.

Kisseler, B., Thurn, P.: Zur Röntgenologie des Magensarkoms. *Fortschr. Röngtenstr.*, 94:571, 1943.

Kurokawa, T.: *Gastroenterology.*(in Japanese) Tokyo, Nanzando, 1959.

Marshak, R.H., Lindner, A.E., Maklansky, D.: Lymphosarcoma of the stomach. *Amer. J. Gastroenterol.*, 66:176, 1976.

Maruyama, M(Michiyoshi)., Watanabe, T., Kobayashi, Y., et al.: Three cases of gastric sarcoma.(in Japanese) *I to Cho(Stomach and Intestine)*, 3:451, 1968.

Matsuura, K., Oshimi, Y., Higuchi, T., et al.: Radiologic findings of lymphoreticular hyperplasia of the stomach. (in Japanese) *Rinsho Hoshasen(Japanese Journal of Clinical Radiology)*, 15:768, 1969.

Menuck, L.S.: Gastric lymphoma; A radiologic diagnosis. *Gastrointest. Radiol.*, 1:157, 1976.

Morris, W.R.: Gastric Hodgkin's disease. *JAMA*, 149:1460, 1952.

Nakamura, K.: Histopathological study on malignant lymphoma of the stomach.(in Japanese) *Gan no Rinsho (Japanese Journal of Cancer Clinics)*, 10:163, 1964.

Nakamura, K., Aoki, M., Sugano, H., et al.: Reactive lymphoreticular hyperplasia of the stomach: Report of 6 surgical cases.(in Japanese) *Gan no Rinsho(Japanese Journal of Cancer Clinics)*, 12.691, 1966.

Nakamura, K., Oonishi, C., Takagi, K., et al.: Double, early reticulum cell sarcoma of the stomach coexisting chronic ulcer; Report of a case.(in Japanese) *Gan no Rincho (Japanese Journal of Cancer Clinics)*, 13:183, 1967.

Palmer, E.D.: Sarcomas of stomach; Review with reference to gross pathology and gastroscopic manifestations. *Amer. J. Digest. Dis.*, 17:186, 1950.

Reed, P.I., Raskin, H.F., Graff, P.W.: Malignant melanoma of the stomach. *JAMA*, 182, 298, 1962.

Rigler, L.G.: Leukemia of stomach producing hypertrophy of gastric mucosa. *JAMA*, 107:2025, 1936.

Schindler, R.: *Gastritis.* New York, Grune & Stratton Inc, 1947.

Sherrick, D.W., Hodgson, J.R., Dockerty, M.B.: The roentgenologic diagnosis of primary gastric lymphoma. *Radiology*, 84:734, 1966.

Shimaoka, K.: Clinical aspects of non-Hodgkin's lymphoma; A new international stage classification and its problems.(in Japanese) *Naika(Internal Medicine)*, 48:21, 1981.

Shirakabe, H., Kumakura, K., Nishizawa, M., et al.: Sarcoma of the stomach.(in Japanese) *Rinsho Hoshasen (Japanese Journal of Clinical Radiology)*, 9:429, 1964.

Shirakabe, H., Kumakura, K., Nishizawa, M., et al.: Sarcoma of the stomach.(in Japanese) *Rinsho Hoshasen (Japanese Journal of Clinical Radiology)*, 9:595, 1964.

Uchita, Y., Kondo, H., Harada, H., et al.: A case report of early lymphosarcoma involving primarily the stomach. (in Japanese with English abstract) *I to Cho(Stomach and Intestine)*, 9:925, 1974.

Valdés-Depena, A., Affolter, H., Vilardell, F.: The gradient of malignancy in lympoid lesions of the stomach. *Gastroenterology*, 50:382, 1966.

Walk, L.: Gastroskopisch untersuchter Fall von diffusem Sarkom des Magens. *Zschr. Klin. Med.*, 142:557, 1943.

Yarnis, H., Colp, R.: Lymphosarcoma of stomach. *Gastroenterology*, 1:1022, 1943.

Chapter 10 Radiographic Diagnosis of Depth of Invasion of Gastric Cancer

References

Maruyama, M., Sugiyama, M., Baba, Y., et al.: Radiological diagnosis of stomach carcinoma involving the proper muscle layer.(in Japanese) *Progr. Digest. Endoscopy*, 7: 15, 1975.

Maruyama, M., Sugiyama, N., Baba, Y., et al.: Radiodiagnostic possibility of gastric carcinoma involving the proper muscle layer.(in Japanese with English abstract) *I to Cho(Stomach and Intestine)*, 11:855, 1976.

Maruyama, M.: Early gastric cancer. *in* Laufer, I. (ed): *Double Contrast Gastrointestinal Radiology.* Philadelphia-London-Toronto, W.B. Saunders Company, 1979, pp 241—288.

Nishizawa, M.: Radiographic demonstration of depressed early cancer of the stomach.(in Japanese) *I to Cho (Stomach and Intestine)*, 6:221, 1971.

Nishizawa, M.: Pre-operative estimation of the depth of invasion in gastric carcinoma with central depression and peripheral elevation; Early carcinoma type IIa+IIc and advanced carcinoma type Borrmann 2.(in Japanese with English abstract) *I to Cho(Stomach and Intestine)*, 12:1217, 1977.

Tsukasa, S., Nishimata, H., Irisa, T., et al.: The estimation of invasion depth and extent of the gastric carcinoma by the use of the roentgenogram of resected specimens: Special reference to invasion depth.(in Japanese with English abstract) *I to Cho(Stomach and Intestine)*, 12:1017, 1977.

Yao, T., Oogushi, H.: Clinicopathological study on the diagnosis of gastric cancer invasion into the deep layer of the gastric wall.(in Japanese with English abstract) *I to Cho(Stomach and Intestine)*, 12:1157, 1977.

Bibliography

Hirokado, K., Okabe, H., Yoshida, T., et al.: Diagnosis of the depth of cancerous invasion in the gastric wall; From the standpoint of quantification of endoscopic diagnosis.(in Japanese with English abstract) *I to Cho(Stomach and Intestine)*, 4:327, 1969.

Igarashi, T., Saito, M., Tsunoda, S., et al.: Radiodiagnostic estimation of the depth of invasion in type IIc cancer; From the view of dynamic observations by double contrast study.(in Japanese with English abstract) *I to Cho(Stomach and Intestine)*, 12:1187, 1977.

Matsunaga, K., Futatsugi, K., Fukuda, H., et al.: Endoscopic study on depressed gastric carcinoma according to histologic type; Estimation of depth of invasion based on converging folds pattern.(in Japanese) *Rinsho to Kenkyu(Japanese Journal of Clinical and Experimental Medicine)*, 53:1116, 1976.

Nakajima, M., Ida, K., Akasaka, Y., et al.: Daignosis of the depth of carcinomatous invasion of the excavated early gastric cancer.(in Japanese) *Kyoto Furitsu Ika Daigaku Zasshi(Journal of Kyoto Prefectural University of Medicine)*, 81:455, 1972.

Nishizawa, M., Nomoto, K., Ito, T., et al.: Development of small gastric cancer and the diagnosis of its invasion depth. *Shinryo(Clinical Practice)*, 24:162, 1971.

Okuda, S., Saegusa, T., Kojima, J., et al.: Depth of involvement and mode of development of early gastric cancer studied by endoscopic method.(in Japanese with English abstract) *I to Cho(Stomach and Intestine)*, 4:313, 1969.

Okuda, S., Imanishi, K., Mimura, S., et al.: Diagnosis for the depth of infiltration in early gastric cancer of depressed type, with reference to an application of multivariate analysis.(in Japanese with English abstract). *I to Cho(Stomach and Intestine)*, 12:1175, 1977.

Sano, R., Hirota, T., Shimoda, T., et al.: Pathological evaluation of recurrences and motality in early gastric cancer; Consideration on the pace of depth invasion of gastric cancer.(in Japanese with English abstract) *I to Cho(Stomach and Intestine)*, 5:531, 1970.

Sasagawa, M., Mitsushima, T., Kimura, T., et al.: The presumable depth of invasion in gastric cancer of the depressed type in radiological diagnosis.(in Japanese with English abstract) *I to Cho(Stomach and Intestine)*, 12:1209, 1977.

Takagi, K., Kumakura, K.: Current issues of gastric cancer; Its further course and the depth of its invasion.(in Japanese with English abstract) *I to Cho(Stomach and Intestine)*, 4:301, 1969.

Ueno, T.: Relationship between the depth of cancer infiltration and abnormal protrusions accompanying with IIc.(in Japanese with English abstract) *I to Cho (Stomach and Intestine)*, 12:1201, 1977.

Watanabe, I., Kato, Y., Haraikawa, M., et al.: Histopathological study on depth invasion of gastric cancer.(in Japanese with English abstract) *I to Cho(Stomach and Intestine)*, 12:1201, 1977.

Yao, T., Fujiwara, T.: Problems on the diagnosis of early gastric cancer correlated with its histologic construction; with special reference to the estimation of depth of invasion.(in Japanese) *Gastroent. Endoscopy*, 18:200, 1976.

Yoshida, K., Ikeuchi, H., Oshibe, M., et al.: Clinicopathological studies of gastric cancers with similar gross findings to early gastric cancer.(in Japanese) *Nihon Shokaki Byo Gakkai Zasshi(Japanese Journal of Gastroenterology)*, 72:725, 1975.

Chapter 11 Pattern of Spread of Early Gastric Cancer and Its Radiographic Features

References

Baba, Y., Narui, T., Ninomiya, T., et al.: A comparative study between radiologic and macroscopic findings of early gastric carcinoma with IIb-like intramucosal spread; With special reference to radiologic definition of proximal boundary.(in Japanese) *I to Cho(Stomach and Intestine)*, 12:1087, 1977.

Ida, K., Kohli, Y.: Endoscopic study on surface pattern of IIb-like lesion of the stomach.(in Japanese) *Gastroent. Endoscopy*, 13:148, 1971.

Kawai, K., Ida, K., Kohli, Y.: On the dye scattering method for endoscopy. New fields in gastrointestinal endoscopy; Urgent endoscopy of digestive and abdominal diseases,

International Symposium, Prague/Carlsbad, 1977. Basel, Karger, 1972. pp 257–260.

Kumakura, K., Maruyama, M., Sugiyama, N., et al.: X-Ray diagnosis of superficial spreading carcinoma of the stomach.(in Japanese with English abstract) *I to Cho (Stomach and Intestine)*, 8:1313, 1973.

Nakai, A., Taniguchi, H., Iwanaga, T. et al.: The limitation of the radiologic method in estimating the extent of carcinomatous invasion into the deep layers of the gastric wall.(in Japanese with English abstract) *I to Cho(Stomach and Intestine)*, 7:739, 1972.

Nakamura, K., Sugano, H., Takagi, K.: Carcinoma of the stomach in incipient phase: Its histogenesis and histological appearnaces. *GANN(Japanese Journal of Cancer Research)*, 59:251, 1968.

Stout, A.P.: Superficial spreading type of carcinoma of the stomach. *Arch. Surg.*, 44: 651, 1942.

Suzuki, S., Suzuki, H., Endo, M., et al.: Endoscopic dyeing method for diagnosis of early cancer and intestinal metaplasia of the stomach. *Endoscopy*, 5:124, 1973.

Takekoshi, T., Maruyama, M., Sugiyama, N., et al.: Significance of endoscopic carbon ink injection method in recognition of boundary of gastric carcinoma, with special reference to defining proximal boundary.(in Japanese with English abstract) *I to Cho(Stomach and Intestine)*, 12:1031, 1977.

Ujiie, T., Takazawa, T., Ikeda, S., et al.: Intramural stomach injection under direct gastrofiberscope observation. *Endoscopy*, 3:73, 1971.

Yasui, A.: Histopathological characteristic of types of gastric cancer.(in Japanese) *Proceedings of the Japanese Cancer Association*, 29:9, 1970.

Yasui, A., Hirase, Y., Miyake, M., et al.: Pathology of superficial spreading type of gastric cancer.(in Japanese) *I to Cho(Stomach and Intestine)*, 8:1305, 1973.

Bibliography

Bralow, S.P., Collins, M.: Relationship of peptic ulceration to superficial spreading carcinoma of the stomach. *Gastroenterology*, 32:1152, 1957.

Fuyuno, S., Yao, T.: Determination of the extent of infiltration in gastric cancer by endoscopic clipping method.(in Japanese with English abstract) *I to Cho (Stomach and Intestine)*, 12:1055, 1977.

Golden, R., Stout, A.P.: Superficial spreading carcinoma of the stomach. Amer. J. Roentgenol. Rad. Ther., 59:157, 1948.

Hara, Y., Maho, T., Tsunoda, H.: A case of superficial flat type (IIb) early gastric cancer.(in Japanese) *I to Cho (Stomach and Intestine)*, 1:569, 1966.

Ida, K., Kubota, Y., Okuda, J., et al.: Diagnosis of the extent of infiltration in gastric carcinoma employing the dye endoscopy.(in Japanese with English abstract) *I to Cho(Stomach and Intestine)*, 12:1043, 1977.

Imai, T., Oota, K., Ayabe, M., et al.: Concept of pre-cancerous conditions and incipient phase of gastric cancer.(in Japanese) *Gan no Rinsho(Japanese Journal of Cancer Clinics)*, 7:91, 1961.

Imai, T.: Peptic ulcer as a site of development of gastric carcinoma, from a histological point of view.(in Japanese) *Nihon Rinsho(Japanese Journal of Clinical Medicine)*, 22:1902, 1964.

Imai, T.: Current topic on histogenesis of gastric cancer;

With special reference to a discussion on ulcer-cancer.(in Japanese) *Shinryo(Clinical Practice)*, 19:1318, 1966.

Inokuchi, K.: Superficial spreading and vertical invasion potential in the development and extension of gastric cancer.(in Japanese) *Gan no Rinsho(Japanese Journal of Cancer Clinics)*, 13:551, 1967.

Inokuchi, K., Furusawa, M., Soejima, K., et al.: Surgical treatment of early gastric cancer; A consideration based on analysis of pattern of invasion.(in Japanese) *Nippon Rinsho(Japanese Journal of Clinical Medicine)*, 25:1378, 1967.

Inui, Y., Kawakita, I., Takei, A., et al.: The diagnostic progress and limitation of gastric carcinoma; The diagnosis of minute cancer type IIb and scirrhous cancer, including a new biopsy method for scirrhous cancer.(in Japanese) *Progr. Dig. Endoscopy*, 10:25, 1977.

Ishiguro, M.: A study of flat type of early gastric carcinoma.(in Japanese) *Nippon Shokaki Byo Gakkai Zasshi(Japanese Journal of Gastroenterology)*, 71:880, 1974.

Kawamura, S., Uchida, T., Omata, N., et al.: A case of IIb+IIc+III type early gastric cancer on the greater curvature as of an extensive superficial spreading type. (in Japanese with English abstract) *I to Cho(Stomach and Intestine)*, 5:87, 1970.

Kiyonari, H., Koga, M., Tanaka, M., et al.: Diagnosis of infiltration of gastric cancer by means of magnified roentgenograms.(in Japanese) *I to Cho(Stomach and Intestine)*, 12:1009, 1977.

Kumakura, K.: Radiologic diagnosis of superficial flat type (IIb) early cancer of the stomach.(in Japanese) *Medicina*, 6:193, 1969.

Kumakura, K., Maruyama, M., Sugiyama, N., et al.: Radiological diagnosis of type IIb and IIb-like lesions of the stomach.(in Japanese with English abstract) *I to Cho(Stomach and Intestine)*, 7:21, 1972.

Mai, M., Takamatsu, O., Asai, T., et al.: Two cases of early gastric cancer diagnosed effectively by endoscopic dye scattering method.(in Japanese with English abstract) *I to Cho(Stomach and Intestine)*, 10:1195, 1975.

Nagayo, T., Sawada, Y., Maruyama, K., et al.: Histological studies on superficially-spreading early carcinoma of the stomach.(in Japanese) *Nippon Byori Gakkai Zasshi (Transactiones Societatis Pathologicae Japonicae)*, 48:29, 1959.

Suzuki, S., Ono, K., Kawada, A., et al.: Studies on endoscopic dye scattering methods.(in Japanese) *Gastroent. Endoscopy*, 15:681, 1973.

Takemoto, T., Kawai, K.(eds): *Gastrointestinal Endoscopy with Application of Dye.*(in Japanese) Tokyo, Igaku-Shoin, 1974.

Tsuda, Y.: A study in the diagnosis of gastric lesions using the fibergastroscope combined with a new staining process.(in Japanese) *Gastroent. Endoscopy*, 9:189, 1967.

Tsukasa, S., Ehira, S., Nakahara, N., et al.: X-Ray diagnosis of type IIb early gastric cancer.(in Japanese with English abstract) *I to Cho(Stomach and Intestine)*, 7:9, 1972.

Ujiie, T., Mikuni, C., Ibayashi, A., et al.: A study on intramural injection of the stomach under direct vision by means of fiberscope.(in Japanese with English abstract) *I to Cho(Stomach and Intestine)*, 5:725, 1970.

Yao, T., Fujiwara, A., Watanabe, H.: Endoscopic diagnosis

of the extent of infiltration in gastric cancer.(in Japanese) *I to Cho(Stomach and Intestine)*, 7:725, 1972.

Zinninger, M.M., Collins, W.T.: Extension of carcinoma of the stomach in to the duodenum. *Ann. Surg.*, 130:557, 1949.

Chapter 12   Clinical Course of Gastric Cancer

References

Murakami, T., Yasui, A., Takekawa, H., et al.: Non-cancerous regenerative epithelium in the central portion of scar-carcinoma of the stomach.(in Japanese) *Nippon Byori Gakkai Zasshi(Transactiones Societatis Pathologicae Japonicae)*, 55:229, 1966.

Murakami, T.: A new concept of ulcer-cancer of the stomach(in Japanese) *Juntendo Igaku(Juntendo Medical Journal)*, 13:157, 1967a.

Murakami, T.: Type IIc+III gastric cancer. *in* Murakami, T., Sano, R., Mochizuki, T., et al. (eds): *Pathology of Gastric Cancer; Diagnosis of Early Gastric Cancer*, vol 5, Tokyo, Bunkodo, 1967b.

Nishizawa, M., Hayakawa, H.: Early gastric cancer. *in* Shirakabe, H., Ichikawa, H. (eds): *Cancer of the Stomach, Lectures on X-ray Interpretation of Digestive Tract*, Part 5, vol 2.(in Japanese) Tokyo, Kanehara Shuppan, 1969.

Bibliography

Abe, M.: Macroscopic changes of gastric cancer (centering on morphologic changes); Macroscopic changes of depressed type gastric cancer (case 19).(in Japanese) *I to Cho(Stomach and Intestine)*, 13:46, 1978.

Abe, M.: Macroscopic changes of gastric cancer (centering on chronologic factors); Cases showing striking changes within a short time, excluding gastric cancer of linitis plastica type (case 28).(in Japanese) *I to Cho(Stomach and Intestine)*, 13:64, 1978.

Aoyama, T.: Clinic in the scirrhous carcinoma of the stomach; Its diagnosis and its course.(in Japanese with English abstract) *I to Cho(Stomach and Intestine)*, 3:935, 1968.

Ashizawa, S.: Cases of gastric carcinoma detected during the course of follow-up examination under the diagnosis of peptic ulcer.(in Japanese) *I to Cho(Stomach and Intestine)*, 3:697, 1968.

Ayabe, M.: Studies on ulcer-cancer of the stomach.(in Japanese) *Igaku(Medicine)*, 6:210, 1949.

Broders, A.C.: Carcinoma in situ contrasted with benign penetrating epithelium *JAMA*, 99:1670, 1932.

Fernet, P., Azar, H.A., Stout, A.P.: Intramural(tubal) spread of linitis plastica along the alimentary tract. *Gastroenterology*, 48:419, 1965.

Fuchigami, A., Kudo, Y., Nishi, M., et al.: A case of early gastric cancer initially simulating xanthoma.(in Japanese with English abstract) *I to Cho(Stomach and Intestine)*, 5:29, 1970.

Fukumoto, S., Hoshijima, S., Tanaka, H., et al.: Macroscopic changes of gastric cancer (centering on morphologic changes); Macroscopic changes of protruding type

gastric cancer (case 6).(in Japanese) *I to Cho(Stomach and Intestine)*, 13:20, 1978.

Fukumoto, S., Miyoshi, Y., Tanaka, H., et al.: Macroscopic changes of gastric cancer (centering on morphologic changes); Macroscopic changes of depressed type gastric cancer (case 15).(in Japanese) *I to Cho(Stomach and Intestine)*, 13:38, 1978.

Gonoi, T., Nakamura, K., Ashizawa, S., et al.: Cases of the gastric cancer showing malignant cycle.(in Japanese) *I to Cho(Stomach and Intestine)*, 7:593, 1972.

Hara, Y., Ogoshi, K., Tobita, Y., et al.: A case of III+IIc type early gastric cancer followed up for 3 years and 1month.(in Japanese with English abstract) *I to Cho (Stomach and Intestine)*, 5:61, 1970.

Hauser, G.: *Das chronische Magengeschwür, sein Vernarbungsprozess und dessen Beziehung zur Entwicklung des Magenkarzinoms.* Leipzig, J.B. Hirschfield, 1883.

Hisamichi, S., Shirane, A.: Macroscopic changes of gastric cancer (centering on morphologic changes); Macroscopic changes of depressed type gastric cancer (case 20).(in Japanese) *I to Cho(Stomach and Intestine)*, 13:48, 1978.

Hisamichi, S., Shirane, A.: Macroscopic changes of gastric cancer (centering on chronologic factors); Cases showing no striking changes for a long time (case 23).(in Japanese) *I to Cho(Stomach and Intestine)*, 13:54, 1978.

Hisamichi, S., Shirane, A.: Macroscopic changes of gastric cancer (centering on chronologic factors); Cases showing striking changes within a short time, excluding gastric cancer of linitis plastica type (case 26).(in Japanese) *I to Cho(Stomach and Intestine)*, 13:60, 1978.

Horinouchi, Y., Koga, Y., Okabe, H.: Clinical and histopathological studies on the course of peptic ulcerations coexisted with gastric carcinoma.(in Japanese with English abstract) *I to Cho(Stomach and Intestine)*, 3:1673, 1968.

Hosoi, T., Yarita, T., Shirakabe, H., et al.: Macroscopic changes of gastric cancer (centering on morphologic changes); Macroscopic changes of protruding type gastric cancer (case 2).(in Japanese) *I to Cho(Stomach and Intestine)*, 13:12, 1978.

Hosoi, T., Yarita, T., Shirakabe, H.: Macroscopic changes of gastric cancer (centering on morphologic changes); Macroscopic changes of protruding type gastric cancer (case 5).(in Japanese) *I to Cho(Stomach and Intestine)*, 13:18, 1978.

Hosoi, T., Yarita, T., Shirakabe, H.: Macroscopic changes of gastric cancer (centering on morphologic changes); Macroscopic changes of depressed type gastric cancer (case 11).(in Japanese) *I to Cho(Stomach and Intestine)*, 13:30, 1978.

Kaneko, E., Utsumi, Y.: A case of early gastric cancer retrospectively investigated for 8 years and 6 months.(in Japanese with English abstract) *I to Cho(Stomach and Intestine)*, 5:55—59, 1970.

Kawai, K.: Peptic ulcer of the stomach as a pre-cancerous lesion.(in Japanese) *I to Cho(Stomach and Intestine)*, 3:713, 1968.

Kawai, K., Takekoshi, T., Ida, K., et al.: Retrograde endoscopical follow-up of depressed type early gastric cancer.(in Japanese with English abstract) *I to Cho (Stomach and Intestine)*, 3:1683, 1968.

Kitaoka, H.: Histopathological considerations on the development of gastric cancer from early into advanced one.(in Japanese with English abstract) *I to Cho (Stomach and Intestine)*, 5:15, 1970.

Kohli, Y., Takeda, H., Toriya, S.: Macroscopic changes of gastric cancer (centering on morphologic changes); Macroscopic changes of depressed type gastric cancer (case 9).(in Japanese) *I to Cho(Stomach and Intestine)*, 13:26, 1978.

Kohli, Y., Takeda, S.: Macroscopic changes of gastric cancer (centering on morphologic changes); Macroscopic changes of depressed typed gastric cancer (case 18).(in Japanese) *I to Cho(Stomach and Intestine)*, 13:44, 1978.

Konjetzny, G.E.: Über die Beziehung der chronischen Gastritis mit ihren Folgerscheinungen und des chronischen Magenulcus zur Entwicklung des Magenkrebses. *Bruns Beitr. Klin. Chir.*, 85:455, 1913.

Konjetzny, G.E.: Die sogenannte Linitis plastica des Magens. *Mitt. Grenzgeb. Med. Chir.*, 31:282, 1919.

Kuru, M.: Site of origin of gastric carcinoma.(in Japanese) *Geka(Surgery)*, 15:1, 1953.

Kuru, M.: Malignant transformation of peptic ulcers of the stomach.(in Japanese) *Saishin Igaku(Modern Medicine)*, 8:180, 1953.

Kuru, M.: Type of gastric carcinoma and its site of origin.(in Japanese) *Nippon Rinsho(Japanese Journal of Clinical Medicine)*, 12 (suppl) 182, 1954.

Kuru, M., Sano, R.: Histological study of gastric carcinomas in the Japanese: Analysis of 150 cases treated in relatively early stages, *in* Harris, R.J.C. (ed): *Ninth International Cancer Congress, UICC Monograph Series*, publication 10. Berlin-Heidelberg-New York, Springer-Verlag, 1967, pp 1–30.

Lauren, P.: The two histological main types of gastric carcinoma; Diffuse and so-called intestinal-type carcinoma: An attempt at a histo-clinical classification. *Acta Pathol. Microbiol. Scand.*, 64:31, 1965.

Lyngborg, K., Nielsen, O.E.: Incidence of gastric cancer in patients treated in medical services for gastric ulcer. *Acta Med. Scand.*, 171, 173, 1962.

MacCarty, W.C.: Chronic ulcer and carcinoma of the stomach. Amer. J. Med. Sci., 173:469, 1927.

Mai, M., Akimoto, R., Nakagawara, G., et al.: Scirrhous carcinoma (linitis plastica type) of the stomach.(in Japanese) *Rinsho Geka(Journal of Clinical Surgery)*, 33:1214, 1978.

Majima, S., Kurakake, S., Hoshi, N., et al.: Ulcer-cancer of the stomach.(in Japanese) *Rinsho Geka(Journal of Clinical Surgery)*, 9:593, 1954.

Majima, S.: Pathology and clinical aspects of ulcer-cancer of the stomach, *in* Shimada, N., Nakatani, H., Urabe, M. (eds): Chronic Gastritis and Peptic Ulcer.(in Japanese) Tokyo, Igaku-Shoin Ltd., 1956, pp 105–124.

Majima, S.: Malignant transformation of peptic ulcer of the stomach.(in Japanese) *Geka Chiryo(Surgical Therapy)*, 3:147, 1960.

Mitsui, H., Okabe, H., Yao, T.: Clinical aspect of Borrmann group 4 gastric cancer.(in Japanese) *I to Cho(Stomach and Intestine)*, 9:437, 1974.

Murakami, T., Nakamura, S.: Relationship between peptic ulcer and cancer of the stomach.(in Japanese) *Naika (Internal Medicine)*, 2:1051, 1958.

Murakami, T., Urushibara, H., Nakamura, S., et al.: Gastric ulcers and gastric carcinoma; On ulcer-cancer in a broad sense.(in Japanese) *Chiryo(Therapy)*, 42:261, 1960.

Murakami, T.: On the ulcerocancer of the stomach.(in Japanese) *Nichidai Igaku Zasshi(Nihon University Medical Journal)*, 24:878, 1965.

Murakami, T., Yasui, A., Nakayama, A., et al.: Concept of early gastric cancer and its development into advanced cancer.(in Japanese) *Nippon Rinsho(Japanese Journal of Clinical Medicine)*, 25:1322, 1967.

Muramatsu, S., Shiohara, M., Nakazawa, S., et al.: Macroscopic changes of gastric cancer (centering on morphologic changes); Macroscopic changes of depressed type gastric cancer (case 17).(in Japanese) *I to Cho(Stomach and Intestine)*, 13:42, 1978.

Nakajima, T.: Gastric cancer with temporary reduction or disappearance of ulcers.(in Japanese with English abstract) *I to Cho(Stomach and Intestine)*, 3:1657, 1968.

Nakamura, K., Sugano, H., Takagi, K., et al.: Histopathological study on early carcinoma of the stomach: Some considerations on the ulcer-cancer by analysis of 144 foci of the superficial spreading carcinomas. *GANN (Japanese Journal of Cancer Research)*, 58:377, 1967.

Nakamura, K., Sugano, H., Takagi, K., et al.: Histogenesis of gastric carcinoma.(in Japanese) *Geka Chiryo(Surgical Therapy)*, 23:435, 1970.

Nakamura, K.: Histogenesis of cancer in the upper segment of the stomach.(in Japanese with English abstract) *I to Cho(Stomach and Intestine)*, 5:1111, 1970.

Nakamura, K., Sugano, H., Maruyama, M., et al.: Histopathological study on primary locus of linitis plastica; Relation between carcinoma arisen from the fundic gland mucosa and linitis plastica.(in Japanese with English abstract) *I to Cho(Stomach and Intestine)*, 10:79, 1975.

Nakamura, K., Sugano, H., Sugiyama, N., et al.: Clinical and histopathological features of scirrhous carcinoma of the stomach.(in Japanese with English abstract) *I to Cho(Stomach and Intestine)*, 11:1275, 1976.

Nakamura, K., Kato, H., Misono, T., et al.: Growing process to carcinoma of linitis plastica type of the stomach from cancer development.(in Japanese) *I to Cho(Stomach and Intestine)*, 15:225, 1980.

Nishizawa, M.: Pre-operative estimation of the depth of invasion in gastric carcinoma with central depression and peripheral elevation; Early carcinoma type IIa+IIc and advanced carcinoma type Borrmann 2.(in Japanese with English abstract) *I to Cho(Stomach and Intestine)*, 12:1217, 1977.

Oguro, Y.: Macroscopic changes of gastric cancer (centering on morphologic changes); Macroscopic changes of protruding type gastric cancer (case 4).(in Japanese) *I to Cho(Stomach and Intestine)*, 13:16, 1978.

Oguro, Y.: Macroscopic changes of gastric cancer (centering on morphologic changes); Macroscopic changes of depressed type gastric cancer (case 12).(in Japanese) *I to Cho(Stomach and Intestine)*, 13:32, 1978.

Ohki, I., Tasaka, S., Murai, T., et al.: A case of IIa type early gastric cancer developing into type I in a fairly short time.(in Japanese with English abstract) *I to Cho(Stomach and Intestine)*, 5:39, 1970.

Ohmori, K(Kohji)., Miwa, T., Kumagai, H.: Follow-up studies on healing ulcer in the early carcinoma of the stomach.(in Japanese with English abstract) *I to Cho (Stomach and Intestine)*, 3:1643, 1968.

Ohmori, K(Kyoji)., Takagi, K., Baba, Y., et al.: Local

recurrence of minute cancer of the stomach, histologically showing spread of linitis plastica type; Report of a case.(in Japanese with English abstract) *I to Cho (Stomach and Intestine)*, 11:1345, 1976.

Okabe, H.: Clinical course of early gastric cancer; As a natural history of early gastric cancer.(in Japanese) *Nippon Rinsho(Japanese Journal of Clinical Medicine)*, 25:1336, 1967.

Okabe, H.: Analysis of gastric cancer followed up under the diagnosis of benign peptic ulcer.(in Japanese) *I to Cho(Stomach and Intestine)*, 3:705, 1968.

Okuda, S.: Tatsuta, M.: A case of early gastric cancer type IIc showing the occurrence and interesting development by endoscopical retrospective study.(in Japanese with English abstract) *I to Cho(Stomach and Intestine)*, 5:47, 1970.

Okuda, S.: Differential diagnosis of early gastric carcinoma from advanced carcinoma, *in* Murakami, T. (ed): *Early Gastric Cancer. GANN Monograph on Cancer Research*, vol 11. Tokyo, University of Tokyo Press, 1971/ Baltimore, University Park Press, 1972, pp 283–301.

Okuda, S., Imanishi, K.: Macroscopic changes of gastric cancer (centering on morphologic changes); Macroscopic changes of ptortuding type gastric cancer (case 1).(in Japanese) *I to Cho(Stomach and Intestine)*, 13:10, 1978.

Okuda, S., Imanishi, K.: Macroscopic changes of gastric cancer (centering on morphologic changes); Macroscopic changes of protruding type gastric cancer (case 7).(in Japanese) *I to Cho(Stomach and Intestine)*, 13:22, 1978.

Okuda, S., Imanishi, K.: Macroscopic changes of gastric cancer (centering on morphologic changes); Macroscopic changes of depressed type gastric cancer (case 10).(in Japanese) *I to Cho(Stomach and Intestine)*, 13:28, 1978.

Okuda, S., Imanishi, K.: Macroscopic changes of gastric cancer (centering on morphologic changes); Macroscopic changes of depressed type gastric cancer (case 14).(in Japanese) *I to Cho(Stomach and Intestine)*, 13:36, 1978.

Olsson, O., Endresen, R.: Ulcer cancer of the stomach. *Acta Chir. Scand.*, 111:16, 1956.

Oota, K.: Histogenesis of gastric cancer.(in Japanese) *Nippon Byori Gakkai Zasshi(Transactiones Societatis Pathologicae Japonicae)*, 53:3, 1964.

Saito, T.: Macroscopic changes of gastric cancer (centering on morphologic changes); Macroscopic changes of depressed type gastric cancer (case 16).(in Japanese) *I to Cho(Stomach and Intestine)*, 13:40, 1978.

Saito, T.: Macroscopic changes of gastric cancer (centering on chronologic factors); Cases showing striking changes within a short time, excluding gastric cancer of linitis plastica type (case 27).(in Japanese) *I to Cho(Stomach and Intestine)*, 13:62, 1978.

Sakita, T., Oguro, Y., Takasu, S., et al.: Observations on the healing of ulcerations in early gastric cancer. *Gastroenterology*, 60:835, 1971.

Sano, R.: Histopathological studies on evolution site of gastric cancer based on analysis of early gastric cancer: Recent problems on ulcer-cancer sequence of the stomach.(in Japanese) *Nippon Rinsho(Japanese Journal of Clinical Medicine)*, 25:1329, 1967.

Sano, R., Hirota, T., Shimoda, T.: Pathologic statistics on 300 cases of early gastric cancer.(in Japanese) *Naika (Internal Medicine)*, 26:15, 1970.

Sano, R., Shimoda, T., Takeuchi, T.: A histopathological and biochemical study on the histogenesis of gastric scirrhous (linitis plastica).(in Japanese) *I to Cho(Stomach and Intestine)*, 9:455, 1974.

Saphir, O., Parker, M.L.: Linitis plastica type of carcinoma. *Surg. Gynec. & Obstet.*, 76:213, 1943.

Sawagawa, M., Kawaguchi, K., Ichikawa, H.: Clinical aspects of scirrhous.(in Japanese with English abstract) *I to Cho(Stomach and Intestine)*, 3:919, 1968.

Sasagawa, M., Okazaki, M., Takasugi, T., et al.: On impeded distensibility of the gastric wall in scirrhous carcinoma studied from changes in roentgenograms.(in Japanese) *I to Cho(Stomach and Intestine)*, 9:445, 1974.

Stromeyer, F.: Die Pathogenese des Ulcus bentriculi, zugleich ein Beitrag zur Frage nach den Beziehungen zwischen Ulcus und Carcinom. *Ziegler Beitr. Path. Anat.*, 65:1, 1912.

Sugiyama, N., Kumakura, K., Maruyama, M., et al.: On radiologic diagnosis and macroscopic observations of carcinoma in the mucosa and glands of the fundus.(in Japanese) *Nippon Shokaki Byo Gakkai Zasshi(Japanese Journal of Gastroenterology)*, 69:949, 1972.

Sugiyama, N., Baba, Y., Maruyama, M., et al.: A clinicopathological study on infiltrating pattern of gastric cancer in relation to its site of origin.(in Japanese with English abstract) *I to Cho(Stomach and Intestine)*, 12:1073, 1977.

Sugiyama, N., Takekoshi, T., Maruyama, M., et al.: Radiologic diagnosis of cancer in fundic gland area.(in Japanese) *I to Cho(Stomach and Intestine)*, 15:145, 1980.

Takeuchi, T., Sano, R., Shimoda, T., et al.: Biochemical study on the mechanism of fibrosis in Borrmann 4 type gastric carcinoma (linitis plastica type); First report.(in Japanese) *Proceedings of the Japanese Cancer Association*, 30:84, 1971.

Takeuchi, T., Ishii, K., Sakita, T., et al.: Studies on the development of Borrmann's type 4 gastric carcinoma (scirrhous). *Nippon Shokaki Byo Gakkai Zasshi (Japanese Journal of Gastroenterology)*, 69:951, 1972.

Takezoe, K.: Macroscopic changes of gastric cancer (centering on morphologic changes); Macroscopic changes of depressed type gastric cancer (case 8).(in Japanese) *I to Cho(Stomach and Intestine)*, 13:24, 1978.

Takezoe, K., Shirane, A., Hisamichi, S., et al.: Macroscopic changes of gastric cancer (centering on chronologic factors); Cases showing no striking changes for a long time (cases 22–24).(in Japanese) *I to Cho(Stomach and Intestine)*, 13:52, 1978.

Taneda, T., Ishii, M., Shimamoto, F.: A case of gastric ulcer scar stationary for 2 years suddenly transforming into advanced cancer of Borrmann type 2 in forty days.(in Japanese with English abstract) *I to Cho(Stomach and Intestine)*, 5:69, 1970.

Tani, K., Nakamura, Y., Watanabe, H.: Macroscopic changes of gastric cancer (centering on chronologic factors); Cases showing striking changes within a short time, excluding gastric cancer of linitis plastica type (case 25).(in Japanese) *I to Cho(Stomach and Intestine)*, 13:58, 1978.

Tone, K., Furusawa, T.: Macroscopic changes of gastric cancer (centering on chronologic factors); Cases showing no striking changes for a long time (case 24).(in

Japanese) *I to Cho(Stomach and Intestine)*, 13:56, 1978.

Utsumi, Y.: Malignant transformation of chronic peptic ulcer of the stomach during its clinical course.(in Japanese) *I to Cho(Stomach and Intestine)*, 3:711, 1968.

Watanabe, H., Yao, T.: Histopathological study on linitis plastica carcinoma of the stomach.(in Japanese) *I to Cho(Stomach and Intestine)*, 11:1285, 1976.

Yao, T.: Carcinoma in fundic gland area of the stomach and its retrospectively observed clinical course.(in Japanese) *Gastroent. Endoscopy*, 17:751, 1975.

Yao, T., Watanabe, H.: Clinico-pathological studies on so-called ulcer-cancer of the stomach.(in Japanese) *I to Cho(Stomach and Intestine)*, 11:573, 1976.

Yao, T., Watanabe, H.: Macroscopic changes of gastric cancer (centering on morphologic changes); Macroscopic changes of protruding type gastric cancer (case 3).(in Japanese) *I to Cho(Stomach and Intestine)*, 13:14, 1978.

Yao, T.: Macroscopic changes of gastric cancer(centering on morphologic changes); Macroscopic changes of depressed type cancer (case 13).(in Japanese) *I to Cho(Stomach and Intestine)*, 13:34, 1978.

Yao, T., Watanabe, H.: Macroscopic changes of gastric cancer (centering on morphologic changes); Macroscopic changes of depressed type gastric cancer (case 21).(in Japanese) *I to Cho(Stomach and Intestine)*, 13:50, 1978.

Yao, T.: Macroscopic changes of gastric cancer (centering on chronologic factors); Cases showing striking changes within a short time, excluding gastristic cancer of linitis plastica type (case 29).(in Japanese) *I to Cho(Stomach and Intestine)*, 13:66, 1978.

Chapter 13 Multiple Early Cancer and Lesions Coexisting with Early Cancer

References

Baba, Y., Kunitake, K., Tajiri, H., et al.: What is the ideal cooperation between radiology and endoscopy in diagnosis of early gastric cancer(in Japanese with English abstract) *I to Cho(Stomach and Intestine)*, 14:323, 1979.

Chen, P-H., Chien, W-H., Su, C-P.: A case of multicentric early gastric cancer.(in Japanese with English abstract) *I to Cho(Stomach and Intestine)*, 3:1593, 1968.

Maruyama, M., Kumakura, K., Takagi, K., et al.: A case of small early gastric cancer.(in Japanese) *I to Cho (Stomach and Intestine)*, 5:56, 1970.

Maruyama, M.: Diagnostic limits for early gastric cancer by radiography, *in* Murakami, T. (ed): *Early Gastric Cancer. GANN Monograph on Cancer Research*, vol 11. Tokyo, University of Tokyo Press, 1971/Baltimore, University Park Press, 1972, pp 119–130.

Murakami, T.: Coexistence of linear ulcer and early cancer in the stomach; From the pathological viewpoint.(in Japanese with English abstract) *I to Cho(Stomach and Intestine)*, 8:1013, 1973.

Nakamura, K., Sugano, H., Takagi, K., et al.: Causality of ulcer and cancer of the stomach.(in Japanese with English abstract) *I to Cho(Stomach and Intestine)*, 6:145, 1971.

Takekoshi, T., Takagi, K., Maruyama, M.: Endoscopic diagnosis of minute stomach cancer. IVth World Congress of Digestive Endoscopy, Madrid, 1978.

Bibliography

Baba, Y., Nakamura, K., Sugano, H., et al.: Multiple gastric cancer; Problem of grossly overlooked synchronous second primary foci near the resection line and their positive evaluation as metachronous second cancer.(in Japanese) *Gan no Rinsho(Japanese Journal of Cancer Clinics)*, 19:912, 1973.

Collins, W.T., Gall, E.A.: Gastric carcinoma; A multicentric lesion. Cancer, 5:62, 1952.

Conover, W.J.: *Practical Nonparametric Statistics; The Kruskal-Wallis Test.* New York, John Wiley & Sons Inc, 1971.

Fukutomi, H., Shiina, H., Sakita, T., et al.: Seventeen cases of coexistence of early gastric cancer and linear ulcer. Case 14: Early gastric cancer (type IIc+III) associated with linear ulcer of the incisura.(in Japanese) *I to Cho(Stomach and Intestine)*, 8:1068, 1973.

Hashimoto, M., Kohli, Y., Kawai, K.: Seventeen cases of coexistence of early gastric cancer and linear ulcer. Case 6: Early gastric cancer (type IIc) adjacent to linear ulcer scar in the antrum.(in Japanese) *I to Cho(Stomach and Intestine)*, 8:1044, 1973.

Hayakawa, H., Takeda, Y., Yarita, T., et al.: Seveteen cases of coexistence of early gastric cancer and linear ulcer. Case 8: Early gastric cancer in the antrum coexisting with linear ulcer in the body.(in Japanese) *I to Cho (Stomach and Intestine)*, 8:1050, 1973.

Ikeda, S., Takazawa, T., Mikuni, C., et al.: A case of early gastric cancer associated with lymphangioma.(in Japanese with English abstract) *I to Cho(Stomach and Intestine)*, 6:1543, 1971.

Kitaoka, H., Oguro, Y., Shimada, M., et al.: Seventeen cases of coexistence of early gastric cancer and linear ulcer. Case 12: Multiple early gastric cancer associated with two linear ulcers.(in Japanese) *I to Cho(Stomach and Intestine)*, 8:1062, 1973.

Kodama, T., Tsunoda, S., Arai, S., et al.: Seventeen cases of coexistence of early gastric cancer and linear ulcer. Case 10: Early gastric cancer (type IIc+III) associated with linear ulcer of the incisura.(in Japanese) *I to Cho (Stomach and Intestine)*, 8:1056, 1973.

Kodama, T., Kamio, Y., Suzuki, S., et al.: Seventeen cases of coexistence of early gastric cancer and linear ulcer. Case 11: Early gastric cancer (type IIc) associated with linear ulcer of the incisura.(in Japanese) *I to Cho (Stomach and Intestine)*, 8:1059, 1973.

Kohli, Y., Miyaoka, T., Kawai, K., et al.: Seventeen cases of coexistence of early gastric cancer and linear ulcer. Case 4: Small early gastric cancer (type IIc) associated with long linear ulcer in the incisura.(in Japanese) *I to Cho(Stomach and Intestine)*, 8:1038, 1973.

Kohli, Y., Kawai, K., Ida, K., et al.: Position of linear ulcer of the stomach as a precancerous lesion.(in Japanese with English abstract) *I to Cho(Stomach and Intestine)*, 8:1085, 1973.

Mai, M., Watanabe, K.: A case of double cancers of the stomach demonstrated by biopsy.(in Japanese with

English abstract) *I to Cho(Stomach and Intestine)*, 9:64, 1974.

Matsue, H., Miwa, T., Oyama, Y., et al.: Seventeen cases of coexistence of early gastric cancer and linear ulcer. Case 15: Early gastric cancer associated with linear ulcer of the incisura.(in Japanese) *I to Cho(Stomach and Intestine)*, 8:1071, 1973.

Nemoto, T., Okano, I., Takayama, T., et al.: Coexistence of IIc with polypoid lesions (ATP) existing independently of each other.(in Japanese with English abstract) *I to Cho(Stomach and Intestine)*, 5:81, 1970.

Nimura, Y., Shichino, S., Sato, T., et al.: Seventeen cases of coexistence of early gastric cancer and linear ulcer. Case 3: Early gastric cancer (type IIc+III) associated with linear ulcer of the anterior wall of the incisura region.(in Japanese) *I to Cho(Stomach and Intestine)*, 8:1035, 1973.

Nishi, M., Nakamura, M., Takagi, K., et al.: Multiple cancers of the stomach.(in Japanese) *Geka(Surgery)*, 31:1115, 1968.

Nishizawa, M., Nomoto, K., Mayama, S., et al.: Seventeen cases of coexistence of early gastric cancer and linear ulcer. Case 17: Early gastric cancer (type IIc+III) associated with linear ulcer along the lesser curvature.(in Japanese) *I to Cho(Stomach and Intestine)*, 8:1077, 1973.

Ogata, H.: A case of multiple intramucosal carcinomas of the stomach.(in Japanese) *Igaku no Ayumi(Progress of Medicine)*, 69:365, 1969.

Oguro, Y., Huang, Z., Fujita, K., et al.: Seventeen cases of coexistence of early gastric cancer and linear ulcer. Case 13: Early gastric cancer (type III) associated with linear ulcer.(in Japanese) *I to Cho(Stomach and Intestine)*, 8:1065, 1973.

Oohara, T., Tohma, H., Aono, G.: Relationship between multiple ulcers and linear ulcers of the stomach.(in Japanese with English abstract) *I to Cho(Stomach and Intestine)*, 12:1105, 1977.

Oshida, K., Nishida, K.: Seventeen cases of coexistence of early gastric cancer and linear ulcer. Case 1: Early gastric cancer (type IIc+III) associated with linear ulcer on the incisura.(in Japanese) *I to Cho(Stomach and Intestine)*, 1:1029, 1973.

Sakita, T.: Endoscopic comments about the cases of linear ulcer concomitant with early cancer.(in Japanese with English abstract) *I to Cho(Stomach and Intestine)*, 8:1025, 1973.

Sannohe, Y., Fukushima, K., Wakita, M.: Seventeen cases of coexistence of early gastric cancer and linear ulcer. Case 9: Early gastric cancer associated with linear ulcer resembling multiple ulcers.(in Japanese) *I to Cho (Stomach and Intestine)*, 8:1053, 1973.

Sato, K., Takeda, Y., Ozawa, Y., et al.: Seventeen cases of coexistence of early gastric cancer and linear ulcer. Case 16: Early gastric cancer (type IIc+III) associated with linear ulcer in the upper portion of the incisura.(in Japanese) *I to Cho(Stomach and Intestine)*, 8:1074, 1973.

Shinkai, M., Ueta, M., Kobayashi, Y., et al.: A small IIc+III type early gastric cancer on the anterior wall of the mid-body accompanying linear ulcer; Report of a case. (in Japanese with English abstract) *I to Cho(Stomach and Intestine)*, 8:1095, 1973.

Shirakabe, H.: Coexistence of early gastric cancer and linear ulcer; Roentgenologic comments.(in Japanese with English abstract) *I to Cho(Stomach and Intestine)*, 8:1019, 1973.

Sugiyama, N., Kumakura, K., Maruyama, M., et al.: Seventeen cases of coexistence of early gastric cancer and linear ulcer. Case 7: Early gastric cancer (type IIc+III) associated with linear ulcer of the incisura.(in Japanese) *I to Cho(Stomach and Intestine)*, 8:1047, 1973.

Toriya, S., Kawai, K., Kohli, Y.: Seventeen cases of coexistence of early gastric cancer and linear ulcer. Case 5: Advanced cancer resembling IIc+III early cancer associated with linear ulcer in the incisura.(in Japanese) *I to Cho(Stomach and Intestine)*, 8:1041, 1973.

Uchida, Y., Miura, T., Matsuo, M., et al.: Seventeen cases of coexistence of early gastric cancer and linear ulcer. Case 2: Early cancer (IIc) coexisting with linear ulcer on the incisura.(in Japanese) *I to Cho(Stomach and Intestine)*, 8:1032, 1973.

Yamazaki, S., Tsuda, S., Matsumoto, Y.: A case of multiple depressed early gastric cancer.(in Japanese) *I to Cho (Stomach and Intestine)*, 6:897, 1971.

Chapter 14 Radiographic Diagnosis of Cancer Smaller Than 10mm

References

Hirota, T., Itabashi, M., Suzuki, K., et al.: Clinico-pathological study on 63 cases of micro- and small early gastric cancer; Histogenesis of gastric cancer.(in Japanese with English abstract) *I to Cho(Stomach and Intestine)*, 14:1027, 1979.

Ikeda, S., Ibayashi, J., Mikuni, T., et al.: Minute IIb type early cancer of the stomach clinically diagnosed as such; A case report.(in Japanese) *I to Cho(Stomach and Intestine)*, 9:581, 1974.

Ito, M., Sukie, H., Yokochi, K.: A case of minute IIc type early cancer of the stomach associated with kissing ulcers.(in Japanese with English abstract) *I to Cho (Stomach and Intestine)*, 10:783, 1975.

Kumakura, K., Maruyama, M.: Retrospective study on X-ray findings of gastric minute cancer. 28th Annual Meeting of Nippon Societas Radiologica, Yonago, 1969.

Kawamura, S., Minute carcinoma of the stomach detected by biopsy.(in Japanese) *I to Cho(Stomach and Intestine)*, 9:56, 1974.

Maruyama, M.: Retrospective study on radiographic findings of microcarcinoma of the stomach.(in Japanese) *Nippon Igaku Hoshasen Gakkai Zasshi(Nippon Acta Radiologica)*, 29:149, 1969.

Maruyama, M., Kumakura, K., Takagi, K., et al.: Micro-carcinoma of the stomach.(in Japanese with English abstract) *I to Cho(Stomach and Intestine)*, 5:988, 1970.

Maruyama, M.: Diagnostic limits for early gastric cancer by radiography, *in* Marukami, T. (ed): *Early Gastric Cancer, GANN Monograph on Cancer Research*, vol. 11. Tokyo, University of Tokyo Press, 1971/Baltimore, University Park Press, 1972, pp 119—130.

Maruyama, M.: Early gastric cancer *in* Laufer, I. (ed): *Double Contrast Gastrointestinal Radiology with Endoscopic Correlation*. Philadelphia, W.B. Saunders Company, 1979, pp 241—288.

Murohisa, Y., Waki, S., Muto, Y., et al.: Two cases with minute early gastric cancer detected by lavage cytology. (in Japanese) *Nippon Rinsho Saibo Gakkai Zasshi(Journal of Japanese Society of Clinical Cytology)*, 17:244, 1978.

Nakamura, K., Sugano, H., Takagi, K., et al.: Histogenesis of gastric carcinoma: Microscopical, electron microscopical and statistical study on primary microcarcinoma.(in Japanese) *Gan no Rinsho(Japanese Journal of Cancer Clinics)*, 15:627, 1969.

Nakamura, K.: *Pathology of Gastric Cancer: Microcarcinoma and Its Histogenesis.*(in Japanese) Kyoto, Kimpo-do, 1972.

Ogata, H.: A case of multiple intramucosal carcinomas of the stomach.(in Japanese) *Igaku no Ayumi(Progress of Medicine)*, 69:365, 1969.

Oi, I., Iwazuka, M., Ichioka, S., et al.: A case of small IIb type early gastric cancer diagnosed by aiming biopsy.(in Japanese) *I to Cho(Stomach and Intestine)*, 5:469, 1970.

Oohara, T.: Clinico-pathology of Microcarcinoma; Gastric cancer less than 5 mm in the greatest diameter.(in Japanese with English abstract) *I to Cho(Stomach and Intestine)*, 14:1037, 1979.

Sakuma, Y., Kuwahara, N.: Multiple microcarcinomas of the stomach.(in Japanese) *Nippon Rinsho(Japanese Journal of Clinical Medicine)*, 35:3448, 1977.

Takekoshi, T., Sugiyama, N., Baba, Y.: The diagnostic progress and limitation of gastric carcinoma: Endoscopic study of microcarcinoma of stomach (smaller than 5 mm in diameter).(in Japanese) *Progr. Digest. Endoscopy*, 10:56, 1977.

Takekoshi, T.: Progress and future of diagnosis of early gastric cancer.(in Japanese) *Medicina*, 14:175, 1977.

Takekoshi, T., Takagi, K., Maruyama, M.: Endoscopic diagnosis of minute stomach cancer. IVth World Congress of Digestive Endoscopy, Madrid, 1978.

Tsukasa, S., Chuma, Y., Nakahara, N., et al.: A case of IIc type early gastric cancer (minute carcinoma).(in Japanese) *I to Cho(Stomach and Intestine)*, 8:655, 1973.

Tsukasa, S., Nakahara, N.: The status of the diagnosis of early IIb type gastric carcinoma.(in Japanese) *Gastroent. Endoscopy*, 16:675, 1974.

Yarita, T., Shirakabe, H., Nagahama, A., et al.: A case of multiple minute IIb–IIc early gastric cancer diagnosed before operation.(in Japanese with English abstract) *I to Cho(Stomach and Intestine)*, 13:1081, 1978.

Yarita, T., Shirakabe, H., Okada, F., et al.: X-Ray diagnosis of minute gastric cancer.(in Japanese with English abstract) *I to Cho(Stomach and Intestine)*, 14:1045, 1979.

Bibliography

Fukumoto, S.: A case of microcarcinoma of the stomach.(in Japanese with English abstract) *I to Cho(Stomach and Intestine)*, 5:986, 1970.

Fukutomi, H., Takezawa, H.: Endoscopic diagnosis of gastric carcinoma less than 1 cm in diameter.(in Japanese with English abstract) *I to Cho(Stomach and Intestine)*, 5:961, 1970.

Furusawa, M., Yoshinaga, H., Nakahara, K., et al.: A minute IIc type gastric carcinoma which was documented preoperatively.(in Japanese with English abstract) *I to Cho(Stomach and Intestine)*, 14:1071, 1979.

Hidano, H., Nakazawa, S.: A case of minute cancer of the stomach detected by X-ray.(in Japanese with English abstract) *I to Cho(Stomach and Intestine)*, 14:1065, 1979.

Hirabayashi, H., Nomura, M., Kiyama, T.: A case of microcarcinoma of the stomach.(in Japanese with English abstract) *I to Cho(Stomach and Intestine)*, 5:983, 1970.

Ichikawa, T., Ukawa, S.: A case of early gastric carcinoma of type IIc with diameter of 5 mm.(in Japanese) *Kosankinbyo Kenkyu Zasshi(Journal of Research Institute for Tuberculosis and Cancer)*, 30:120, 1978.

Kasugai, T., Kato, H., Tsubouchi, M., et al.: Gastric biopsy of minute carcinoma.(in Japanese with English abstract) *I to Cho(Stomach and Intestine)*, 5:817, 1970.

Kasugai, T.: Diagnosis of minute lesions; Endoscopy, cytology, biopsy.(in Japanese) *I to Cho(Stomach and Intestine)*, 5:1015, 1970.

Kojima, T., Kurauchi, Y., Siroeda, S., et al.: A minute carcinoma of the stomach; A case report.(in Japanese with English abstract) *I to Cho(Stomach and Intestine)*, 9:1201, 1974.

Maruyama, M., Kumakura, K., Fujii, A., et al.: Radiological diagnosis of minute gastric carcinoma (less than 10 mm).(in Japanese) *Gastroent. Endoscopy*, 12:50, 1970.

Miyoshi, M., Koyama, H., Hino, R., et al.: A case report of a minute gastric cancer diagnosed before operation.(in Japanese with English abstract) *I to Cho(Stomach and Intestine)*, 14:1081, 1979.

Murakami, H., Suzuki, S., Maruyama, M., et al.: A case of double minute gastric cancer diagnosed before operation.(in Japanese with English abstract) *I to Cho (Stomach and Intestine)*, 14:1077, 1979.

Nakamura, K., Sugano, H., Takagi, K.: Carcinoma of the stomach in incipient phase; Its histogenesis and histological appearances. *GANN(Japanese Journal of Cancer Research)*, 59:251, 1968.

Nishiyama, K., Inuo, T., Ito, S., et al.: Two cases of microcarcinoma of the stomach.(in Japanese) *Nippon Shokaki Byo Gakkai Zasshi(Japanese Journal of Gastroenterology)*, 73:739, 1976.

Nishizawa, M., Ito, I., Nomoto, K., et al.: The X-ray demonstrability of microcarcinoma.(in Japanese with English abstract) *I to Cho(Stomach and Intestine)*, 5:951, 1970.

Nomoto, K.: A case of microcarcinoma of the stomach.(in Japanese with English abstract) *I to Cho(Stomach and Intestine)*, 5:992, 1970.

Okazaki, Y., Fujita, K., Kawahara, K., et al.: Present status of endoscopic diagnosis of minute gastric cancer and its future.(in Japanese with English abstract) *I to Cho (Stomach and Intestine)*, 14:1059, 1979.

Okuda, S.: Diagnosis of microcarcinoma; Comparison of single and multiple cases.(in Japanese) *Gastroent. Endoscopy*, 12:26, 1970.

Saito, T.: The diagnostic progress and limitation of gastric carcinoma: Minute gastric carcinoma, type IIb early gastric carcinoma and gastric scirrhous.(in Japanese) *Progr. Dig. Endoscopy*, 10:50, 1977.

Sasahara, M., Kakizaki, G., Ishidate, T., et al.: A case with minute IIb type early gastric cancer.(in Japanese with

English abstract) *I to Cho(Stomach and Intestine)*, 11:1129, 1976.

Shida, S., Yasui, A.: Microcarcinoma of the stomach.(in Japanese) *Gastroent. Endoscopy*, 15:511, 1973.

Shirakabe, H., Kidokoro, T., Takagi, K.: Statistical figures of very small gastric carcinoma under 1 cm in diameter preoperatively diagnosed; based on the results of questionnaire to 24 institutions in Japan.(in Japanese) *I to Cho(Stomach and Intestine)*, 5:995, 1970.

Suzuki, H., Nagayo, T.: A method for pathological study of gastric microcarcinoma; alcian blue-hematoxylin method.(in Japanese with English abstract) *I to Cho (Stomach and Intestine)*, 14:1117, 1979.

Suzuki, S., Ichioka, S., Ide, H., et al.: Biopsy under direct vision for early gastric cancer small than 1 cm in diameter.(in Japanese with English abstract) *I to Cho (Stomach and Intestine)*, 5:971, 1970.

Takagi, K.: Macroscopic diagnosis of minute gastric cancer. (in Japanese with English abstract) *I to Cho(Stomach and Intestine)*, 5:939, 1970.

Takekoshi, T., Yamase, Y., Ochiai, H.: Multiple IIc type early microcarcinoma of the stomach; A case report.(in Japanese) *I to Cho(Stomach and Intestine)*, 7:1525, 1972.

Ujiie, T.: A case of microcarcinoma of the stomach.(in Japanese with English abstract) *I to Cho(Stomach and Intestine)*, 5:980, 1970.

Yagi, M., Kasugai, T.: A case of microcarcinoma of the stomach.(in Japanese with English abstract) *I to Cho (Stomach and Intestine)*, 5:977, 1970.

Yamada, T.: Point, minute and small cancers of the stomach at the early development stage detected by improved chymotrypsin lavage method for diagnostic cytology. *Acta Cytologica*, 22:460, 1978.

Yasui, A., Sang, S., Nakayama, A., et al.: Microcarcinoma of the stomach.(in Japanese) *I to Cho(Stomach and Intestine)*, 1:267, 1966.

Chapter 15   Miscellaneous Tumors of the Stomach

References

Christodoulopoulos, J.B., Klots, A.P.: Carcinoid syndrome with primary carcinoid tumor of the stomach. *Gastroenterology*, 40:429, 1961.

Crummy, A.B., Jr., Juhl, J.H.: Calcified gastric leiomyoma. *Amer. J. Roentgenol.*, 87:727, 1962.

Helwig, E.B., Ranier, A.: Inflammatory fibroid polyps of the stomach. *Surg. Gynecol. Obstet.*, 96:355, 1953.

Peskin, G.W., Orloff, M.J.: Carcinoids, the malignant carcinoid syndrome and 5-hydroxytryptamine (Serotonin). *Amer. J. Med. Sci.*, 237:224, 1959.

Vanek, J.: Gastric submucosal granuloma with eosinophilic infiltration. *Amer. J. Pathol.*, 25:397, 1949.

Bibliography

Bartlet, J.P., Adams, W.E.: Generalized giant hypertrophic gastritis simulating neoplasm; Differential diagnosis and report of case. *Arch. Surg.*, 60:543, 1950.

Berne, C.J., Gibson, W.R.: Giant hypertrophic gastritis. *West J. Surg.*, 57:388, 1949.

Bücker, J.: Die hyperplastiche Gastritis im Röntgenbild. *Fortschr. Röntgenstr.*, 71:246, 1949.

Bücker, J., Stössel, H.G.: Über gutartige Magentumoren. *Fortschr. Röntgenstr.*, 94:159, 1961.

Bücker, J.: Die Antrumgastritis. *Radiologe*, 6:264, 1966.

Butz, W.C.: Giant hypertrophic gastritis. *Gastroenterology*, 39:183, 1960.

Calenoff, L., Sparberb, M.: Gastric pseudolesions: Roentgenographic-gastrophotographic correlations. *Amer. J. Roentgenol.*, 173:139, 1971.

Davis, J.G., Adams, D.B.: The roentgen findings in gastric leiomyomas and leiomyosarcomas. *Radiology*, 67:67, 1956.

Debray, C., Martin, E.: Benign gastric tumors, *in* Bockus, H.L. (ed): *Gastroenterology*. Philadelphia, W.B. Saunders Company, 1974, pp 1018–1040.

Doi, H., Tobayashi, K., Yamada, T., et al.: Radiographic diagnosis of submucosal tumors of the stomach.(in Japanese) *I to Cho(Stomach and Intestine)*, 1:919, 1966.

Elliott, G.V., Wilson, H.M.: Mesenchymal tumors of stomach. *AMA Arch. Int. Med.*, 89:358, 1952.

Feldman, M., Weinberg, T.: Aberrant pancreas; A cause of duodenal syndrome. *JAMA*, 148:893, 1952.

Forrester-Wood, W.R.: Giant hypertrophic gastritis. *Brit. J. Surg.*, 37:278, 1950.

Goldberg, H.I., Margulis, A.R.: Adenomyoma of the stomach; Report of a case. *Amer. J. Roentgenol.*, 96:382, 1966.

Goldberg, H.I., O'Keiffe, D.O., Jenis, H., et al.: Diffuse esoinophilic gastroenteritis. *Amer. J. Roentgenol.*, 119:342, 1973.

Masuda, H., Inoue, S., Arakawa, H.: Radiographic diagnosis of submucosal tumors of the stomach.(in Japanese) *I to Cho(Stomach and Intestine)*, 1:931, 1966.

Nelson, R.S.: Malignant tumors of the stomach other than carcinoma, *in* Bockus, H.L. (ed): *Gastroenterology*. Philadelphia, W.B. Saunders Company, 1974, pp 998–1017.

Palmer, E.D.: Benign intramural tumors of the stomach; A review with special reference to gross pathology. *Medicine*, 30:81, 1951.

Phillips, J.C., Lindsay, J.W., Kendall, J.A.: Gastric leiomyosarcoma; Roentgenologic and clinical findings. *Amer. J. Dig. Dis.*, 15:239, 1970.

Seaman, W.B.: Non-neoplastic diseases of the stomach, *in* Margulis, A.R., Burhenne, H.J. (eds): *Alimentary Tract Roentgenology*, vol 1. St. Louis, The C.V. Mosby Company, 1973, p 607.

Siegelman, S.S., Gold, J.A., Simon, M., et al.: Ulceration of intramural gastric neoplasms. *Amer. J. Dig. Dis.*, 14:127, 1969.

Wolf, W.: Benign Magen Tumoren. *Dtsch. Med. Wschr.*, 81:1081, 1956.

Yao, T., Watanabe, H., Okada, Y., et al.: A case of carcinoid of· the stomach.(in Japanese with English abstract) *I to Cho(Stomach and Intestine)*, 5:1247, 1970.

Index

Author Index

Subject Index